HANDBOOK OF PSYCHOTHERAPY
CASE FORMULATION

HANDBOOK OF PSYCHOTHERAPY CASE FORMULATION

Second Edition

Edited by
TRACY D. EELLS

THE GUILFORD PRESS
New York   London

© 2007 The Guilford Press
A Division of Guilford Publications, Inc.
72 Spring Street, New York, NY 10012
www.guilford.com

Printed in the United States of America

This book is printed on acid-free paper.

Last digit is print number: 9   8   7   6   5   4   3   2

Library of Congress Cataloging-in-Publication Data

Handbook of psychotherapy case formulation / edited by Tracy D. Eells. 2nd ed.
    p. ; cm.
 Includes bibliographical references and index.
 ISBN 978-1-59385-351-8 (hardcover: alk. paper)
 ISBN 978-1-60623-942-1 (paperback: alk. paper)
 1. Psychiatry—Case formulation.   2. Psychiatry—Differential therapeutics.
 3. Psychotherapy—Methodology.   I. Eells, Tracy D.
 [DNLM: 1. Psychotherapy—methods. WM 420 H23232 2006]
 RC473.C37H46 2006
 616.89'14—dc22

                                           2006010632

To my parents

And to Bernadette, Elias, Aidan, and Lillian

About the Editor

Tracy D. Eells, PhD, received his doctorate in clinical psychology at the University of North Carolina, Chapel Hill, and completed a postdoctorate fellowship at the John D. and Catherine T. MacArthur Foundation Program on Conscious and Unconscious Mental Processes at the University of California, San Francisco. He is currently Associate Professor of Psychiatry and Behavioral Sciences and Associate Dean for Faculty Affairs at the University of Louisville School of Medicine. He has a busy individual and group psychotherapy practice and teaches psychotherapy to psychiatry residents and clinical psychology graduate students. Dr. Eells has published several papers on psychotherapy case formulation and has conducted workshops on the topic for professionals. He is on the editorial board of multiple psychotherapy journals and currently serves as Executive Officer of the Society for Psychotherapy Research.

Contributors

Marna S. Barrett, PhD, Department of Psychiatry, University of Pennsylvania School of Medicine, Philadelphia, Pennsylvania

Franz Caspar, PhD, Psychologie Clinique, Université de Genève, Geneva, Switzerland

Travis A. Cos, MS, Department of Psychology, Drexel University, Philadelphia, Pennsylvania

John T. Curtis, PhD, Department of Psychiatry, University of California, San Francisco School of Medicine, San Francisco, California

Tracy D. Eells, PhD, Department of Psychiatry and Behavioral Sciences, University of Louisville, Louisville, Kentucky

Rhonda Goldman, PhD, Argosy University, Schaumburg, and Illinois School of Professional Psychology, Schaumburg, Illinois

Leslie S. Greenberg, PhD, Department of Psychology, York University, Toronto, Ontario, Canada

Mardi J. Horowitz, MD, Department of Psychiatry, University of California, San Francisco School of Medicine, San Francisco, California

Shannon M. Kelly, MS, Department of Counseling and Educational Psychology, Indiana University, Bloomington, Indiana

Kelly Koerner, PhD, Evidence Based Practice Collaborative, Seattle, Washington

Hanna Levenson, PhD, Wright Institute, Berkeley, California; Brief Psychotherapy Program, Psychiatry Department, California Pacific Medical Center, and Levenson Institute for Training (LIFT), San Francisco, California

Lester Luborsky, PhD, Center for Psychotherapy Research, Department of Psychiatry, University of Pennsylvania School of Medicine, Philadelphia, Pennsylvania

John C. Markowitz, MD, Department of Psychiatry, New York State Psychiatric Institute, New York, New York

Stanley B. Messer, PhD, Graduate School of Applied and Professional Psychology, Rutgers University, Piscataway, New Jersey

Arthur M. Nezu, PhD, Department of Psychology, Drexel University, Philadelphia, Pennsylvania

Christine Maguth Nezu, PhD, Department of Psychology, Drexel University, Philadelphia, Pennsylvania

Jacqueline B. Persons, PhD, San Francisco Bay Area Center for Cognitive Therapy and Psychology, University of California, Berkeley, Berkeley, California

Charles R. Ridley, PhD, Department of Counseling and Educational Psychology, Indiana University, Bloomington, Indiana

George Silberschatz, PhD, Department of Psychiatry, University of California, San Francisco School of Medicine, San Francisco, California

Hans H. Strupp, PhD, Psychology Department, Vanderbilt University, Nashville, Tennessee

Holly A. Swartz, MD, University of Pittsburgh School of Medicine, Pittsburgh, Pennsylvania

Michael A. Tompkins, PhD, San Francisco Bay Area Center for Cognitive Therapy and Psychology Department, University of California, Berkeley, Berkeley, California

David L. Wolitzky, PhD, Department of Psychology, New York University, New York, New York

Preface

The primary goal envisioned for the first edition of *Handbook of Psychotherapy Case Formulation* was to address the gap between the almost universally recognized importance of case formulation as a core psychotherapy skill and the reported lack of adequate training in this skill. The *Handbook* also aimed to bring several research-based and statistically reliable methods of case formulation to a wider clinical audience. Since the first edition, case formulation has received more attention, as evidenced by the publication of several texts (e.g., Bruch & Bond, 1998; Hersen & Porzelius, 2002; Horowitz, 2005; Meier, 2003; Needleman, 1999; Nezu, Nezu, & Lombardo, 2004) and articles (e.g., Bieling & Kuyken, 2003; Caspar, Berger, & Hautle, 2004; Eells & Lombart, 2003; Eells, Lombart, Kendjelic, Turner, & Lucas, 2005; Tarrier & Calam, 2002; Westmeyer, 2003) on the topic. Therefore, a revision is needed to incorporate developments in psychotherapy training, and recent research and thinking about case formulation. All chapters on topics covered in the original edition have been updated to include developments in the method, revisions, new research, and improvements in training individuals to use the method. The case formulation methods included represent currently existing and practiced approaches.

Additional goals of this second edition have been to increase the clinical utility of the book by asking each contributor to include an example of a completed formulation as it would be developed in practice; to better integrate the chapters and the book as a whole by adding a concluding chapter comparing and contrasting each of the formulation methods presented earlier; and to add material on multicultural competence training in case formulation. The latter goal was addressed in two ways. A chapter was added discussing the rationale for considering cultural factors, and presenting a multiculturally focused method of case formulation. In addition, each chapter presenting a case formulation method includes a section discussing multicultural considerations and how they would affect the case formulation process and product.

A hallmark of the first edition was that each chapter describing a method of case formulation followed the same organizational format. With minor changes, the second edition retains this format. The reasons for the standard format are to facilitate comparisons among the methods, to ensure that similar categories of information are provided for each method, and to increase the book's ease of use. All contributors were asked to organize their chapters according to the following headings: historical background of their approach, conceptual framework, multicultural and inclusion/exclusion criteria, steps in case formulation construction, application to psychotherapy technique, case example, training, and research support for the approach. The following sections describe what was asked of each author.

• *Historical Background of the Approach.* In this section, authors describe the historical and theoretical origins of their case formulation approach.

• *Conceptual Framework.* The goal of this section is to present *what* is formulated and *why.* Authors were asked to consider the following questions: What assumptions about psychopathology and healthy psychological functioning underlie the approach? What assumptions about personality structure, development, self concept, affect regulation, and conflict (if any) are made? What are the components of the case formulation and what is the rationale for including each component? How are treatment goals incorporated into the model? Does the formulation predict the course and outcome of therapy, including obstacles to success? If so, how?

• *Multicultural and Inclusion/Exclusion Criteria.* How suitable is the approach for patients of diverse ethnic and cultural backgrounds? How are these varying sociocultural contexts accounted for within the formulation? More generally, which patients are appropriate and inappropriate for formulation with the method? What type and range of problems is the method suitable for?

• *Steps in Case Formulation Construction.* The goal of this section is to provide a detailed, step-by-step description of *how* to construct a case formulation with the method under discussion. After reading this section, readers should be able to make an attempt at constructing a case formulation using method. Questions authors were asked to address included the following: How much time is required to formulate the case? What materials are used (e.g., interviews, questionnaires, progress notes)? Does the patient participate in constructing the formulation? Are structured interview techniques or other special procedures required to make the formulation? What provisions are made for evaluating, amending, or correcting the formulation? What form does the final product take?

• *Application to Psychotherapy Technique.* This section addresses how the therapist might use the formulation in therapy. For example, is the formulation shared directly with the patient, and if so, in what form?

• *Case Example.* A concrete case example is presented to illustrate how the method is applied in the treatment of a specific individual. Authors were encouraged to present actual materials used in case formulation, for example, interview transcripts, questionnaires, or diagrams.

• *Training.* This section addresses how individuals are best trained to use the case formulation method. The reason for including this section was to provide interested readers with concrete steps to take in order to learn the method described.

• *Research.* This section summarizes scientific evidence for the reliability and validity of the method. The decision to include this section was based on the assumption that a case formulation method can be treated as a psychometric instrument, and therefore, is subject to similar empirical scrutiny.

It is my hope that this revised text, including the standard format, the focused questions, the expanded focus on multiculturalism, the greater integration of material, and the grounding in evidence, provides readers with multiple and varied tools to draw upon in therapy. As a mentor of mine once said, "It is always helpful to add another string to your bow."

REFERENCES

Bieling, P. J., & Kuyken, W. (2003). Is cognitive case formulation science or science fiction? *Clinical Psychology: Science and Practice, 10,* 52–69.

Bruch, M., & Bond, F. W. (Eds.). (1998). *Beyond diagnosis: Case formulation approaches in CBT.* New York: Wiley.

Caspar, F., Berger, T., & Hautle, I. (2004). The right view of your patient: A computer-assisted, individualized module for psychotherapy training. *Psychotherapy: Theory, Research, Practice, Training, 41*(2), 125–135.

Eells, T. D., & Lombart, K. G. (2003). Case formulation and treatment concepts among novice, experienced, and expert cognitive-behavioral and psychodynamic therapists. *Psychotherapy Research, 13*(2), 187–2004.

Eells, T. D., Lombart, K. G., Kendjelic, E. M., Turner, L. C., & Lucas, C. (2005). The quality of psychotherapy case formulations: A comparison of expert, experienced, and novice cognitive-behavioral and psychodynamic therapists. *Journal of Consulting and Clinical Psychology, 73,* 579–589.

Hersen, M., & Porzelius, L. K. (Eds.). (2002). *Diagnosis, conceptualization, and treatment planning for adults: A step-by-step guide.* Mahwah, NJ: Lawrence Erlbaum.

Horowitz, M. (2005). *Understanding psychotherapy change: A practical guide to configurational analysis.* Washington, DC: American Psychological Association.

Meier, S. T. (2003). *Bridging case conceptualization, assessment, and intervention.* Thousand Oaks, CA: Sage.

Needleman, L. D. (1999). *Cognitive case conceptualization: A guidebook for practitioners.* Mahwah, NJ: Lawrence Erlbaum.

Nezu, A. M., Nezu, C. M., & Lombardo, E. R. (2004). *Cognitive-behavioral case formulation and treatment design: A problem-solving approach.* New York: Springer.

Tarrier, N., & Calam, R. (2002). New developments in cognitive-behavioural case formulation. Epidemiological, systemic and social context: An integrative approach. *Behavioural and Cognitive Psychotherapy, 30*(3), 311–328.

Westmeyer, H. (2003). On the structure of case formulations. *European Journal of Psychological Assessment, 19*(3), 210–216.

Contents

Contents

PART I

INTRODUCTION

Chapter 1

History and Current Status
of Psychotherapy Case Formulation

Tracy D. Eells

Recognition of the central role that case formulation plays in psychotherapy planning and intervention has increased since the first edition of this handbook. Evidence for this claim includes the publication of several books that focus exclusively or primarily on case formulation, including those by Bruch and Bond (1998), Horowitz (1997, 2005), Hersen and Porzelius (2002), Meier (2003), Needleman (1999), and Nezu, Nezu, and Lombardo (2004), as well as the publication of several books on methods of psychotherapy that include chapters on formulation as a key step in the method (e.g., Benjamin, 2003; Binder, 2004; Silberschatz, 2005). In addition, significant research and methodological/theoretical articles on the topic of case formulation have been published (Bieling & Kuyken, 2003; Eells, Lombart, Kendjelic, Turner, & Lucas, 2005; Caspar, Berger, & Hautle, 2004; Eells & Lombart, 2003; Tarrier & Calam, 2002; Westmeyer, 2003), and two peer-reviewed journals focusing on case presentations and review have started (Fishman, 2000; Hersen, 2002). Both involve the presentation of cases in a standard format that includes a section on case formulation.

With these developments in mind, my task in this chapter is to trace the history of the concept of formulation in psychotherapy. My primary goal is to provide a context in which to better understand the chapters on specific case formulation methods that follow. I begin with a working definition and then review major historical and contemporary influences on the form and content of a psychotherapy case formulation. Next, I propose five tensions that influence the psychotherapy case formulation process. Finally,

I discuss the psychotherapy case formulation as an object of and a tool for scientific study. A guiding theme throughout the chapter is that case formulation is a core psychotherapy skill that lies at an intersection of diagnosis and treatment, theory and practice, science and art, and etiology and description.

A WORKING DEFINITION

A psychotherapy case formulation is a hypothesis about the causes, precipitants, and maintaining influences of a person's psychological, interpersonal, and behavioral problems. A case formulation helps organize information about a person, particularly when that information contains contradictions or inconsistencies in behavior, emotion, and thought content. Ideally, it contains structures that permit the therapist to understand these contradictions and to categorize important classes of information within a sufficiently encompassing view of the patient. A case formulation also serves as a blueprint guiding treatment and as a marker for change. It should help the therapist experience greater empathy for the patient and anticipate possible ruptures in the therapy alliance (Safran, Muran, Samstag, & Stevens, 2002; Samstag, Muran, & Safran, 2004).

As a hypothesis, a case formulation may include inferences about predisposing or antecedent vulnerabilities based on early childhood traumas, a pathogenic learning history, biological or genetic influences, sociocultural influences, currently operating contingencies of reinforcement, or maladaptive schemas and beliefs about the self or others. The nature of this hypothesis can vary widely depending on which theory of psychotherapy and psychopathology the clinician uses. Psychodynamic approaches focus primarily on unconscious mental processes and conflicts (Messer & Wolitzky, Chapter 3, this volume; Perry, Cooper, & Michels, 1987; Summers, 2003); a cognitive therapy formulation might focus on maladaptive thoughts and beliefs about the self, others, the world, or the future (e.g., Beck, 1995; Freeman, 1992; Persons & Tompkins, Chapter 10, this volume); in contrast, a behavioral formulation traditionally does not emphasize intrapsychic events but, rather, focuses on the individual's learning history and a functional analysis related to environmental contingencies of reinforcement and inferences about stimulus–response pairings (Haynes & O'Brien, 1990; Wolpe & Turkat, 1985). Contemporary behavioral formulations increasingly incorporate cognition and affect as components in the functional analysis (Nezu, Nezu, & Cos, Chapter 12, this volume; Persons & Tompkins, Chapter 10, this volume). Biological explanations might also be interwoven into a case formulation. Some experts advocate pursuing rigorous causal connections between a psychopathological condition and its determinants (Haynes, Spain, & Oliveira, 1993), whereas others stress achieving an explanatory narrative that may not have a factual basis in "historical truth," but is nevertheless therapeutic in that it provides a conceptual account of the patient's condition and a procedure for improving it (Frank & Frank, 1991; Spence, 1982). As a hypothesis, a case formulation is also subject to revision as new information emerges, as tests of the working hypothesis indicate, and as a clinician views the patient through the lens of an alternate theoretical framework.

Case formulation involves both content and process aspects. Content aspects comprise several components that together paint a holistic picture of the individual and his or her problems. They may also include a prescriptive component that flows directly from the earlier descriptions and hypotheses and proposes a plan for treatment (Sperry, Gudeman, Blackwell, & Faulkner, 1992). The treatment plan may include details such as the type of therapy or interventions recommended, the frequency and duration of meetings, therapy goals, obstacles toward achieving these goals, a prognosis, and a referral for adjunctive interventions such as pharmacotherapy, group therapy, substance abuse treatment, or a medical evaluation. Alternatively, interventions other than psychotherapy, or no interventions at all, might be recommended.

The process aspects of case formulation refer to the clinician's activities aimed at eliciting the information required to develop the formulation content; typically, this process primarily involves conducting a clinical interview. Two general categories of information should be kept in mind during a formulation-eliciting interview. The first is *descriptive* information, which includes demographics; the presenting problems; coping steps taken by the patient; any history of previous mental health problems or care; medical history; and developmental, social, educational, and work history. Although the selection of descriptive information can never be free of the influence of theory or perception, there is usually no attempt to interpret or infer meaning in this section; instead, the emphasis is on providing a reliable information base. The second category is *personal meaning* information, which refers to how the patient experienced and interprets the events described. To elicit this information, the therapist asks and observes how descriptive events affected the patient's thoughts, feelings, and behavior. The therapist can also infer personal meaning information from narratives the patient tells.

HISTORICAL AND CONTEMPORARY INFLUENCES

In this section I review five influences on the psychotherapy case formulation. These are the medical examination and case history, models of psychopathology and its classification, models of psychotherapy, psychometric assessment, and case formulation research.

The Medical Examination and Case History

The major influences on the form and logic of the psychotherapy case formulation are the medical examination and case study, which have their
roots in Hippocratic and Galenic medicine.[1] The rise of Hippocratic medicine in the 5th century B.C. marked a repudiation of polytheism and my-
thology as sources of illness or cure. It also signaled an embrace of reason,
logic, and observation in understanding illness, and the conviction that
only natural forces are at play in disease. The Hippocratic physicians believed that diagnosis must rest on a firm footing of observation and employed prognostication as a means of corroborating their diagnoses. They
took a holistic view of disease, viewing the patient as an active participant
in his or her cure. Foreshadowing contemporary physicians who propound
"wellness" and psychotherapists advocating a focus on patients' "problems
in living" (Sullivan, 1954), the Hippocratics viewed disease as an event occurring in the full context of the patient's life. Their treatment efforts were
aimed at restoring a balance of natural forces in the patient.

Working within erroneous theoretical assumptions involving humoral
interaction, vitalism, and "innate heat," the basic task of the Hippocratic
physician was to determine the nature of a patient's humor imbalance. Toward this end, a highly sophisticated physical examination developed in
which the physician, using his five senses, sought objective evidence to determine the underlying cause of the observed symptoms. According to
Nuland (1988), Hippocratic case reports included descriptions of changes
in body temperature, color, facial expression, breathing pattern, body position, skin, hair, nails, and abdominal contour. In addition, Hippocratic physicians tasted blood and urine; they examined skin secretions, ear wax,
nasal mucus, tears, sputum, and pus; they smelled stool; and observed
stickiness of the sweat. Once the physician had gathered and integrated this
information, he used it to infer the source of humoral imbalance and how
far the disease had progressed. Only then was an intervention prescribed.
The main point to be appreciated is the empirical quality of this examination. Symptoms were not taken at face value, nor were they assumed to be
the product of divine intervention; instead, objective evidence of the body's
ailment was sought.

The focus on observation and empiricism by Hippocrates and his students laid the foundation for physical examinations performed today. It
also serves as a worthwhile credo for the modern psychotherapy case
formulation. Importantly, the Hippocratics also provide modern psychotherapy case formulators with the caveat that even concerted efforts at objectivity and empiricism can fall prey to an overbelief in a theoretical framework into which observations are organized.

Before it could be described as modern, the Hippocratic ethos required
two additional ingredients: a focus on anatomical (and subanatomical)

structure and function as the foundation of disease, and the establishment of planned experimentation as a means of understanding anatomy and disease. These ingredients were supplied more than 500 years after Hippocrates by another Greek physician, Galen of Pergamon. Before Galen, a detailed knowledge of the body's anatomy and how disease disrupts it was considered ancillary information in medical training, at best. Galen's emphasis on anatomy and structure can be seen as a physiological precursor to current psychological theories that posit central roles for mental structures. These include psychodynamic concepts of id, ego, and superego, as well as self-representations, or schemas, which both cognitive and some psychodynamic theorists and researchers emphasize (Segal & Blatt, 1993).

Galen was the first to prize experimentation as a method for understanding anatomy. In a series of simple and elegant experiments, he proved that arteries contain blood, and that arterial pulsations originate in the heart. Consistent with this Galenian spirit, experimentation to test formulations about the "psychological anatomy" of individual psychotherapy patients has been proposed by several psychotherapy researchers and methodologists (e.g., Barlow & Hersen, 1984; Carey, Flasher, Maisto, & Turkat, 1984; Edelson, 1988; Edwards, Dattillio, & Bromley, 2004; Fishman, 2002; Morgan & Morgan, 2001; Stiles, 2003). Note also that many of the authors of chapters in this volume explicitly link their case formulation methods to empirically supported psychotherapies and to a tradition of empiricism.

Another significant advance in medical science with regard to diagnosis occurred many centuries after Galen. This was the publication, in 1769, of Giovanni Morgagni's *De Sedibus et Causis Morborum per Anatomen* (*The Seats and Causes of Disease Investigated by Anatomy*). Morgagni's work is a compilation of over 700 well-indexed clinical case histories, each linking a patient's symptom presentation to a report of pathology found at autopsy and any relevant experiments that had been conducted. *De Sedibus* was a remarkable achievement in that it firmly established Galen's "anatomical concept of disease." Although we now understand that illness is not only the product of diseased organs but also of pathological processes occurring in tissues and cellular and subcellular structures, the reductionist concept of disease still predominates. An 18th century physician using *De Sedibus* to treat a patient could use the index to look up his patient's symptoms, which could be cross-referenced to a list of pathological processes that may be involved. Morgagni's credo, that symptoms are the "cry of suffering organs," parallels the guiding assumption of some psychotherapy case formulation approaches that symptoms represent the "cry" of underlying psychopathological structures and processes.

A second accomplishment of Morgagni's is his foundation of the clinicopathological method of medical research, in which correspondences are examined between a patient's symptoms and underlying pathology re-

vealed at autopsy. Although there is no psychological equivalent of the conclusive autopsy, the advent of the clinicopathological method foreshadowed an emphasis on obtaining independent, corroborating evidence to
substantiate hypothesized relationships in psychology. Morgagni's *De Sedibus*
also demonstrated how advances in medical science can occur on a case-by-
case basis, and how the integration and organization of existing information can advance a science. The creation of online case study journals, such
as *Pragmatic Case Studies in Psychotherapy* (Fishman, 2000), provides a
database of psychotherapy cases with standard, researchable categories of
information included. Such efforts may mark the beginning of a psychological *De Sedibus*.

By extending the reach of our five senses, the tools and technologies of
medicine have also added immensely to diagnostic precision; in doing so,
medicine has provided a model for psychotherapy case formulations. Examples of developments in medicine that aided diagnosis include Laennec's
invention of the stethoscope in the early 19th century, Roentgen's discovery
of x-rays, and recent developments in brain imaging techniques. If parallels
exist in psychology, one might cite Freud's free association, Skinner's demonstration of the power of stimulus control over behavior, the technology
of behavior genetics, and the advent of psychometrics. Each of these "technologies" has added to our understanding of individual psychological and
psychopathological functioning. Later in this chapter, I discuss the potential
for structured case formulation methods to serve as research tools.

As this review of the medical examination and case study has shown,
the structure and logic of a traditional psychotherapy case formulation are
modeled closely after medicine. Specific aspects borrowed include an emphasis on observation; the assumption that symptoms reflect underlying
disease processes; experimentation as a means of discovery; an ideal of
postmortem (or posttreatment) confirmation of the formulation; and an increasing reliance upon technology to aid in diagnosis.

Models of Psychopathology and Its Classification

A clinician's assumptions about what constitutes psychopathology and how
psychopathological states develop, are maintained, and are organized, will
frame how that clinician formulates cases. These assumptions impose a set
of axiological constraints about what the clinician views as "wrong" with a
person, what needs to change, how possible change is, and how change
might be effected. Although an extended discussion of the nature and classification of psychopathology is beyond the scope of this chapter, three
themes that underlie ongoing debates on this topic are relevant to case formulation. (For an expanded discussion, see Blashfield, 1984; Kendell,
1975; or Millon, 1996.)

Etiology Versus Description

Throughout its history, psychiatry has oscillated between descriptive and etiological models of psychopathology (Mack, Forman, Brown, & Frances, 1994). The tension between these approaches to nosology reflects both dissatisfaction with descriptive models and the scientific inadequacy of past etiological models. During the 20th century, this trend is seen as Kraepelin's descriptive psychiatry gave way to a psychosocial focus inspired by Adolf Meyer and Karl Menninger, as well as a Freudian emphasis on unconscious determinants of behavior. A focus on description to the virtual exclusion of etiology was revived in 1980 with the publication of DSM-III. With etiological considerations relegated to the background at present, a conceptual vacuum has been created that case formulation attempts to fill, perhaps as an interim measure until a more empirically sound etiological nosology is established.

Categorical versus Dimensional Models

Just as psychopathologists have oscillated between etiological and descriptive nosologies, so have they debated the merits of categorical versus dimensional models of psychopathology. The categorical or "syndromal" view is that mental disorders are qualitatively distinct from each other and from "normal" psychological functioning. The categorical approach expresses the "medical model" of psychopathology, which, in addition to viewing disease as discrete pathological entities, also adheres to the following precepts: (1) diseases have predictable causes, courses, and outcomes; (2) symptoms are expressions of underlying pathogenic structures and processes; (3) the primary but not exclusive province of medicine is disease, not health; and (4) disease is fundamentally an individual phenomenon, not social or cultural. The categorical approach to psychopathology is traceable in recent history to Kraepelin's "disease concept" and is embodied in DSM-III and its successors. In recent years it has exerted a pervasive influence on psychopathology and psychotherapy research and clinical practice (Wilson, 1993).

Those advocating a dimensional approach claim that psychopathology is better viewed as a set of continua from normal to abnormal. Widiger and Frances (1994) argue that dimensional approaches help resolve classification dilemmas, especially regarding "poorly fitting" cases; that they retain more information than categorical models about "subclinical" functioning; and that they are more flexible in that cutoff scores can be used to create categories when clinical or research goals require them.

With regard to case formulation, what difference does it make whether a nosology is dimensional or categorical? Three factors can be identified:

potential for stigmatization, goodness-of-fit to one's view of personality organization, and ease of use.

Compared to dimensional models, categorical approaches may be more prone to stigmatize patients due to a greater tendency to reify what is actually a theoretical construct. For example, being told that one "has" a personality disorder can produce or exacerbate feelings of being defective, especially when proffered as an "explanation" of one's condition. This "formulation" can also have an unnecessarily demoralizing effect on the therapist. Dimensional approaches may be less prone toward stigmatization because dimensions are assumed to vary from normal to abnormal ranges and are not assumed to represent discrete psychological conditions.

When expressed in experience-near, functional, and context-specific terms, a case formulation can serve as a therapeutic adjunct to a categorical system, thus reducing the potential for stigmatization. For example, instead of labeling a person as having a personality disorder, the therapist might offer formulation-based interventions such as, "Could it be that when threatened by abandonment, you hurt yourself in an attempt to bring others close; but instead, you only drive them away?"; or "I wonder if you are letting others decide how you feel, instead of deciding for yourself."

The dimensional–categorical debate also has implications for the case formulator's frame of reference in understanding personality. If one views personality in an intraindividual context (Valsiner, 1986, 1987), that is, as an internally organized system of interconnecting parts, then the categorical approach is a closer fit. This view of personality is consistent with those offered by Allport (1961) and Millon (1996), among others. The categorical approach assumes that signs, symptoms, and traits cluster together, forming a whole that constitutes an organization greater than the sum of its parts. Thus, from the intraindividual standpoint, if a patient exhibits grandiosity in an interview, suggesting narcissistic personality disorder, the case formulator might examine more closely for interpersonal exploitativeness or entitlement, which are other features of this disorder. Reaching beyond DSM-IV-TR to other accounts of narcissism, the interviewer might also prepare for sudden fluctuations in the individual's self-esteem or for depressive episodes that come and go quickly, or he or she might examine for evidence of using others as "selfobjects" (Kohut, 1971, 1977, 1984).

On the other hand, the dimensional approach is the better fit if one views individual personality in an interindividual frame of reference (Valsiner, 1986, 1987); that is, as an array of traits that do not necessarily interrelate and which are best understood according to how they compare with their expression in other individuals. Dimensional approaches such as the five-factor model (Costa & Widiger, 1994) are built on the assumption that the dimensions are not correlated. Thus, an individual's score on the trait "agreeableness" would not help one predict his degree of "conscientiousness." A clinician working from an interindividual frame might propose a set of cardinal traits as comprising the core of a case formulation.

Ease of use is another consideration relevant to case formulation, as a case formulation must often be done quickly. As Widiger and Frances (1994) note, the categorical approach is better adapted to clinical decision making, which usually involves discrete decisions, such as to treat or not, to make intervention A or intervention B, and so on. Because the case formulation process involves a similar style of decision making, it may be more compatible with a categorical system. Categories may also have greater ease of use in helping a therapist and patient identify and label experiences. For example, a patient's salient "states of mind" might be incorporated into the case formulation and introduced into the therapy at an appropriate time (Horowitz & Eells, Chapter 5, this volume).

Normality versus Abnormality

Related to the issue of dimensional versus categorical models of psychopathology are decisions as to what is and what is not normal behavior and experience. These decisions are central to the task of psychotherapy case formulation. They not only guide the structure and content of the formulation, and the process by which the case formulation is identified, but also the clinician's intervention strategies and goals for treatment. First, it is important to recognize that all conceptions of psychopathology are social constructions, at least to some extent (Millon, 1996). They reflect culturally derived and consensually held views as to what is to be considered abnormal and what is not.

Several criteria can help in making decisions about what is normal or not. These include the following: statistical deviation from normative behavior, personal distress, causing distress in others, violation of social norms, deviation from an ideal of mental health, personality inflexibility, poor adaptation to stress, and irrationality (e.g., Millon, 1996; Widiger & Trull, 1991). These criteria provide a baseline and a context against which the patient's behavior and experiences can be compared. They enable the case formulator to better understand patients by comparing their stress responses to normative stress responses and to assess the separate contributions of dispositional versus situational, cultural, social, and economic factors to a patient's clinical presentation. The case formulator does not act as judge of the patient's experiences but uses knowledge about consensual views of normality and abnormality to help the patient adapt.

In sum, the content and structure of a psychotherapy case formulation is inextricably linked to the therapist's implicit or explicit views regarding the etiology of emotional problems, the dimensional versus categorical debate about mental disorders, and assumptions about what is normal and abnormal in one's psychological functioning.

Models of Psychotherapy

The therapist's approach to psychotherapy will, of course, greatly influence the case formulation process and end product. In this section, I review four major models of psychotherapy with a focus on their contributions to case formulation. These approaches are psychoanalytic, humanistic, behavior, and cognitive therapies.

Psychoanalysis

Psychoanalysis has had at least three major influences on the psychotherapy case formulation process. The principal contribution is that Freud and his successors developed models of personality and psychopathology that have significantly shaped our understanding of normal and abnormal human experience and behavior. Among the most significant psychoanalytic concepts are psychic determinism and the notion of a dynamic unconscious; the overdetermination, idiogenesis, and symbolic meaning of symptoms; symptom production as a compromise formation; ego defense mechanisms as maintainers of psychic equilibrium; and the tripartite structural model of the mind. Beginning with the early formulation that "hysterics suffer mainly from reminiscences" (Breuer & Freud, 1893/1955, p. 7), psychoanalysis has provided therapists with a general framework for understanding experiences that patients report in psychotherapy. More recent formulations by object relations theorists (e.g., Kernberg, 1975, 1984) and self psychologists (Kohut, 1971, 1977, 1984) have added to our understanding of individuals with personality disorders.

A second contribution of psychoanalysis to case formulation relates to an expanded view of the psychotherapy interview. Before Freud, the psychiatric interview was viewed similarly to an interview in a medical examination. It was highly structured and focused on obtaining a history and mental status review, reaching a diagnosis, and planning treatment (Gill, Newman, & Redlich, 1954). Since Freud, therapists recognize that patients often enact their psychological problems, and especially interpersonal problems, in the course of describing them to the therapist. The interview process itself became an important *source* of information for the formulation. That is, the manner in which patients organize their self-presentations and thoughts, approach or avoid certain topics, and behave nonverbally has become part of what the therapist formulates.

A third contribution of psychoanalysis to formulation is its emphasis on the case study. Although the value of the case history continues to be debated (e.g., Morgan & Morgan, 2001; Runyan, 1982; Stiles, 2003), there is little question that Freud elevated the method's scientific profile. The case study was the principal vehicle through which Freud presented and supported psychoanalytic precepts.

Interestingly, psychoanalysis has not traditionally incorporated the concept of a medical diagnosis into a formulation (Gill et al., 1954). Freud's own disinterest in diagnosis is revealed in the index of the *Standard Edition* of his complete works, which shows no entries for "diagnosis" or "formulation," although a few under "anamnesis." Pasnau (1987) and Wilson (1993) argue that psychoanalysts' lack of emphasis on diagnosis contributed to the "demedicalization" of psychiatry earlier this century. These writers argue that the "disease concept" was not seen as compatible or relevant to psychoanalysts' focus on unconscious psychological determinants of symptoms as opposed to organic determinants, nor to an emphasis on motivational states, early life history, or interpersonal relationship patterns.

Along with its contributions to case formulation, psychoanalysts have also been criticized for applying general formulations to patients when they do not fit. One prominent example may be Freud's case study of Dora (see Lakoff, 1990). Psychoanalytic formulations have also been criticized for being overly speculative (Masson, 1984), for exhibiting a male bias (Horney, 1967), and for lack of scientific rigor (Grunbaum, 1984).

Humanistic Therapy

Proponents of humanistically oriented psychotherapies have traditionally taken the view that case formulation, or at least "psychological diagnosis" is unnecessary and even harmful. According to Carl Rogers (1951), "psychological diagnosis . . . is unnecessary for [client-centered] psychotherapy, and may actually be detrimental to the therapeutic process" (p. 220). Rogers was concerned that formulation places the therapist in a "one up" position in relation to the client and may introduce an unhealthy dependency into the therapy relationship, thus impeding a client's efforts to assume responsibility for solving his or her own problems. In Rogers's (1951) words, "There is a degree of loss of personhood as the individual acquires the belief that only the expert can accurately evaluate him, and that therefore the measure of his personal worth lies in the hands of another" (p. 224). Rogers (1951) also expressed the social philosophical objection that diagnosis may in the long run place "social control of the many [in the hands of] the few" (p. 224). While Rogers's criticisms serve as a caveat, they also seem based on the assumption that the practice of "psychological diagnosis" necessarily places the therapist and patient in a noncollaborative relationship in which the formulation is imposed in a peremptory fashion rather than reached jointly and modified as necessary. It is also noteworthy that contemporary exponents of phenomenological therapies are less rejecting of formulation than was Rogers but tend to emphasize formulation of the moment-to-moment experiences of the client rather than proposing global patterns that describe a client (Greenberg & Goldman, Chapter 13, this volume).

Contributions of humanistic psychology to case formulation include its emphasis on the client as a person instead of a "disorder" that is "treated," its focus on the here-and-now aspect of a human encounter rather than an intellectualized "formulation," and its view of the therapist and client as equals in their relationship. Humanistic psychology also takes a holistic rather than a reductionist view of humankind. Methodologically, humanistic approaches have also contributed techniques that facilitate insight and a deepening of experience and, therefore, contribute to a case formulation. These include role playing and the "empty chair" technique. Taken as a whole, these influences have tempered what some have viewed as the potential dehumanizing effects of case formulation.

Behavior Therapy

Behavior therapists have historically tended to neglect assessment (Goldfried & Pomeranz, 1968) and criticize the concept of diagnosis for similar reasons. These include an emphasis on unobservable mental entities or forces, a focus on classification per se, and concerns about lack of utility in helping individuals (Hayes & Follette, 1992). These therapists prefer to focus on a "functional analysis" of behavior, which involves identifying relevant characteristics of the individual in question, his or her behavior, and environmental contingencies or reinforcement, then applying behavioral principles to make alterations. Some behaviorists have acknowledged limitations in the functional analysis approach to case formulation, primarily due to difficulties in replicability and resulting problems in studying patients scientifically (Hayes & Follette, 1992). More recently, behavior therapists have broadened the notion of functional analysis and focused it into a case formulation format (Haynes & Williams, 2003; Nezu, Nezu, & Cos, Chapter 12, this volume).

Notwithstanding the criticisms just cited, behaviorists have made at least three major contributions to the case formulation process. First is an emphasis on symptoms. Behaviorists have strived to understand the "topography" of symptomatology, including relevant stimulus–response associations and contingencies of reinforcement. In contrast to dynamic thinkers who view symptoms as *symbolic* of a more fundamental problem, behaviorists focus on symptoms *as* the problem and aim directly at symptom relief. Second, more than other practitioners, behaviorists have emphasized environmental sources of distress. As a consequence, greater attention has been placed on changing the environment rather than the individual. A formulation that is more balanced in attributing maladaptive behavior to the individual and his or her environment is less stigmatizing. Third, behaviorists have emphasized empirical demonstrations to support the effectiveness of their approaches. This includes measuring symptomatology, isolating potential causal variables, and systematically varying them and examining the effects on behavior. This tradition dates back to Watson's demonstration with Little Albert that specific phobias can be produced and extinguished according to principles of classical conditioning.

Cognitive Therapy

In a series of influential volumes, Beck and his colleagues have set forth general formulations about the causes, precipitants, and maintaining influences in depression (Beck, Freeman, Davis, & Associates, 2004), anxiety disorders (Beck, Emery, & Greenberg, 1985), personality disorders (Beck, Rush, Shaw, & Emery, 1979, and substance abuse (Beck, Wright, Newman, & Liese, 1993). Within the cognitive framework, specific mechanisms have been theorized for specific disorders such as panic disorder (Clark, 1986) and social phobia (Clark & Wells, 1995). These formulations emphasize a set of cognitive patterns, schemas, and faulty information processes, each specific to the type of disorder. Depressed individuals, for example, tend to view themselves as defective and inadequate, the world as excessively demanding and as presenting insuperable obstacles to reaching goals, and the future as hopeless. The thought processes of depressed individuals are described as revealing characteristic errors, including making arbitrary inferences, selectively abstracting from the specific to the general, overgeneralizing, and dichotomizing. In contrast, formulations of anxious individuals tend to center around the theme of vulnerability, and those of substance-abusing individuals may focus on automatic thoughts regarding the anticipation of gratification and increased efficacy when using drugs or symptom relief that will follow drug intake. Until recently, cognitive psychologists tended to focus on general formulations for these disorders rather than in dividualistic variations constructed for a specific patient (Persons & Tompkins, Chapter 10, this volume). Since Persons (1989) published her book on case formulation from the cognitive-behavioral perspective, there is increased interest on individualized formulations (e.g., Tarrier & Calam, 2002). As Persons and Tompkins (Chapter 10, this volume) note, the jury is still out on whether individualized formulations have a differential impact on the outcome of cognitive-behavioral therapy than when generalized formulations are used.

Psychometric Assessment

Among clinical psychology's contributions to understanding psychopathology are the development of reliable and valid personality tests, standards for constructing and administering these tests, and the application of probability theory to assessment. The influence of these developments on psychotherapy case formulation has been indirect, however, and not what it potentially might be. One reason may be a tendency among many clinical psychologists to see psychotherapy and psychometric assessment as separate, and perhaps incompatible, enterprises. Second, questions have regularly arisen about the practical value of psychological assessment for psychotherapy (e.g., Bersoff, 1973; Hayes, Nelson, & Jarrett, 1987; Korchin & Schuldberg, 1981; Meehl, 1958). In fact, very little research has examined the incremental benefit of psychological assessment on treatment planning, implementation, and outcome, despite the availability of research strategies for addressing this issue (Hayes et al., 1987).

What are the potential contributions of psychometrics and psychometric thinking to psychotherapy case formulation? First is the use of validated personality and symptom measures themselves in the case formulation process. As the reader of this volume will see, several authors routinely use symptom measures as part of their case formulation method. Other authors have discussed psychotherapy applications of frequently used measures, including the Minnesota Multiphasic Personality Inventory—Second Edition (Butcher, 1993), Rorschach (Aronow, Rezinikoff, & Moreland, 1994), and Thematic Apperception Test (Bellak, 1993). In addition, Widiger and Sanderson (1995) advocate the use of semistructured interviews to assess the presence of personality disorders more reliably. Quantitative approaches to evaluating psychopathology and life history events might also provide a powerful means of understanding a patient's dynamics, as suggested by Meehl (1958) and developed by Bruhn (1995) with regard to early memories and by Shedler and Westen with regard to personality disorders (Shedler & Westen, 1998; Westen & Shedler, 1999a, 1999b).

A second potential contribution to case formulation relates to the way of thinking that is associated with psychometric assessment. An awareness of concepts such as reliability, validity, and standardization of administration of a measure may increase the fit of a case formulation to the individual in question. For example, just as standardized administration of psychological tests is important for a reliable and valid interpretation of the results, so might it be important for the therapist to adopt a standard approach in an assessment interview to understand the client more accurately and empathically. In accomplishing this goal, the therapist should not be rigid or wooden in an attempt to adopt a standardized approach but, instead, should strive to be close enough to the patient's thoughts and feelings while also sufficiently distant as to remain a reliable instrument for assessing the patient's problems, including the possible expression of those problems in the therapy relationship. Maintaining such a stance is particularly important during the psychotherapy interview because it is the most frequently used tool for assessing psychotherapy patients and is also highly subject to problems with reliability (Beutler, 1995).

Case Formulation Research

The value of a case formulation is relative to its reliability and validity. Reliability here refers to how well clinicians can independently construct similar formulations based on the same clinical material; it can also refer to the extent to which they agree as to how well an already-constructed formulation or its components fit a particular set of clinical material. Predictive validity refers to how well the formulation predicts psychotherapy process events or outcome.

In 1966, a Chicago psychoanalyst, Philip Seitz (1966), published an article detailing the efforts of a small research group to study what he termed "the consensus problem in psychoanalytic research" (p. 209). For 3 years, the group of six psychoanalysts independently reviewed either detailed interview notes from a single case of psychotherapy or dreams taken from several psychotherapy cases. Each formulator wrote an essay-style narrative addressing the precipitating situation, focal conflict, and defense mechanisms at play in the clinical material. The participants also reported their interpretive reasoning and evidence both supporting and opposing their formulation. After the formulations were written, they were distributed to each member of the group who then had the opportunity to revise his formulation in light of clues provided in the formulations of others. The group met weekly to review its findings. Despite the group's initial enthusiasm, the results were disappointing, even if predictable. Seitz reported that satisfactory consensus was achieved on very few of the formulations.

The primary value of Seitz's paper is that it alerted the community of psychotherapy researchers and practitioners to the "consensus problem." If psychotherapy research aspired to be a scientific enterprise, progress had to be made in the consistency with which clinicians describe a patient's problems and way of managing them. Seitz's (1966) paper is also valuable for its presentation of why the clinicians had difficulty obtaining agreement. A general reason was the "inadequacy of our interpretive methods" (p. 214). One of these inadequacies was the tendency of group members to make inferences at an overly deep level, for example making references to "phallic–Oedipal rivalry" and "castration fears." Seitz (1966) also recognized that the group placed "excessive reliance upon intuitive impressions and insufficient attention to the systematic and critical checking of our interpretations" (p. 216). These remarks foreshadowed those of current researchers who have identified limitations and biases in human information-processing capacities (Kahneman, Slovic, & Tversky, 1982; Turk & Salovey, 1988).

In the years following the publication of Seitz's paper, multiple researchers focused on improving the reliability and validity of psychotherapy case formulations. The first to successfully achieve this was Lester Luborsky (1977; Luborsky & Barrett, Chapter 4, this volume) with his core conflictual relationship theme (CCRT) method. Over 15 structured case formulations methods have been proposed in the literature (Luborsky et al., 1993). Although most of these methods were developed within a psychodynamic framework, methods from behavioral, cognitive-behavioral, cognitive-analytic, and eclectic/integrative schools have also been proposed. The reliability and validity of several have been tested (Barber & Crits-Christoph, 1993). A sampling of these methods includes the CCRT (Luborsky & Crits-Christoph, 1990), the plan formulation method (Curtis, Silberschatz, Sampson, Weiss, & Rosenberg, 1988), the role relationship model configuration method (Horowitz, 1989, 1991), the cyclic maladaptive pattern (Johnson, Popp, Schacht, Mellon, & Strupp, 1989; Schacht & Henry, 1994), the idiographic conflict formulation method (Perry, 1994; Perry, Augusto, & Cooper, 1989), the consensual response formulation method (Horowitz, Rosenberg, Ureño, Kalehzan, & O'Halloran, 1989), cognitive-behavioral case formulation (Persons, 1989, 1995), and Plan Analysis (Caspar, 1995). Several of these methods are described in detail in this volume and their commonalities are discussed in the last chapter.

A surprising amount of research has been conducted on the topic of case formulation, in addition to that on reliability and validity of formulations. This work may be categorized broadly as focusing either on outcomes or processes (Westmeyer, 2003). The former category is by far the greater of the two, and investigates a formulation as a completed product, which, essentially, is a putative hypothesis about an individual's psychological functioning. From this standpoint, investigators have assessed the psychometric properties of case formulation methods, specifically their reliability and validity, as discussed earlier (Barber & Crits-Christoph, 1993; Luborsky & Crits-Christoph, 1998; Persons & Bertagnolli, 1999); the contribution of case formulations to psychotherapy processes (Messer, Tishby, & Spillman, 1992; Silberschatz, Curtis, & Nathans, 1989; Silberschatz, Fretter, & Curtis, 1986) and outcomes (Chadwick, Williams, & Mackenzie, 2003; Tarrier & Calam, 2002); and the value of case formulations as explanatory models of specific psychological processes, for example, symptom formation (L. Luborsky, 1996), grief (Fridhandler, Eells, & Horowitz, 1999; Horowitz et al., 1993), and role reversal (Eells, 1995).

Case formulation from the process standpoint focuses on questions such as "How do therapists actually construct formulations?" (Eells, Kendjelic, & Lucas, 1998), "Are more experienced or expert therapists better at case formulation than novices?" (Eells, Lombart, Kendjelic, Turner, & Lucas, 2005; Mayfield, Kardash, & Kivlighan, 1999), and "How can one best train therapists in case formulation?" (Caspar, Berger, & Hautle, 2004; Lauterbach & Newman, 1999).

Further evidence that the scientific aspects of case formulation are being given greater attention recently is the development of a new online journal, *Pragmatic Case Studies in Psychotherapy*, that provides innovative, quantitative, and qualitative knowledge about psychotherapy processes and outcomes, based on a case formulation methodology (Fishman, 2000). An exciting aspect of this effort is the creation of a large database of therapy case studies, each of which will be organized under common headings, including one addressing the therapist's formulation of the client. This database may provide opportunities for research and insights into psychotherapy processes and outcomes that other methodologies have not. In addition, some psychotherapy researchers are calling for more systematic study of case formulations (e.g., Bieling & Kuyken, 2003; Tarrier & Calam, 2002). Theoretical rationales for programs of single-subject, case formulation research have been offered by Kuyken (in press), Westmeyer (2003), and Eells (1991).

In this section, I have traced historical and contemporary influences that have shaped the process and content of the psychotherapy case formulation to what it is today. As reviewed, its form and structure originated in Hellenic days and are deeply embedded in medicine but have also been altered in significant ways by psychoanalytic, humanistic, behavioral, and cognitive psychology. Psychotherapy case formulation has also been influenced by how psychopathology is understood, by the development of psychometric assessment, and by recent research in which the reliability and validity of a case formulation have been examined.

TENSIONS INHERENT IN THE CASE FORMULATION PROCESS

I now examine five tensions that must be handled in developing a comprehensive case formulation. Each tension represents competing and incompatible goals faced by the clinician in attempting to understand a patient. The clinician must reconcile each of these tensions if the case formulation is to serve as an effective tool for psychotherapy.

Immediacy versus Comprehensiveness

The task of case formulation is foremost a pragmatic one. From the first hour of therapy, the clinician needs to develop an idea of the patient's symptoms, core problems, goals, obstacles, coping or defense mechanisms, interpersonal style, maladaptive behavior patterns, life situation, and so on. For this reason, a case formulation is needed relatively early in treatment. At the same time, the more comprehensive a case formulation is, without loss of clarity or focus, the better it will serve the clinician and patient. The priority given to practicality necessarily exacts a cost in comprehensiveness.

Some writers have advised that a case formulation should be completed in a single hour session with a patient (Kaplan & Sadock, 1998;

Morrison, 1993). It may be unrealistic, however, to produce a sufficiently comprehensive case formulation on the basis of a single hour. Nevertheless, it is worth noting that experienced physicians begin to entertain and rule out diagnostic possibilities from the earliest minutes of medical interviewing (Elstein et al., 1978). The same may be the case for experienced psychotherapists.

Another aspect of the tension between immediacy versus comprehensiveness is that the clinician observes a restricted behavior sample in a relatively controlled interview context. This may promote a selection bias and obscure a patient's capabilities and limitations that would be apparent in other contexts.

In sum, as the therapist seeks to balance the goals of immediacy and comprehensiveness, he or she must efficiently identify what is needed to help the patient and avoid areas that may be intriguing or interesting but have little to do directly with helping the patient get better.

Complexity versus Simplicity

One can construe the case formulation task in relatively simple or complex terms. If an overly simple construction is offered, important dimensions of the person's problems may go unrecognized or misunderstood. If overly complex, the formulation may be unwieldy, too time-consuming, and impractical. In addition, the more complex a case formulation method, the more difficult it may be to demonstrate its reliability and validity. Thus, a balance between complexity and simplicity is an important aim in case formulation construction.

Of course, even the most complex of formulations falls far short of the complexity of the actual person one interviews. As the writer Robertson Davies (1994) asks, then answers: "How many interviewers, I wonder, have any conception of the complexity of the creature they are interrogating? Do they really believe that what they can evoke from their subject is the whole of their 'story'? Not the best interviewers, surely" (p. 20).

Clinician Bias versus Objectivity

A third tension in the case formulation process is between a therapist's efforts at accurate understanding of a patient and inherent human flaws in every therapist's ability to do so. There is a long tradition of research demonstrating the limits of clinical judgment, inference, and reasoning (Garb, 1998; Kahneman et al., 1982; Kleinmuntz, 1968; Meehl, 1954; Turk & Salovey, 1988). These errors include heuristic biases, illusory correlation, neglecting base rates, and "halo" and recency effects. Meehl (1973) identifies multiple examples of logical and statistical errors that can undermine clinical judgment. These include either overpathologizing patients on the basis of their "differentness" from the clinician or underpathologizing them on the basis of their "sameness"; presuming merely on the basis of the co-existence of symptoms and intrapsychic conflict that the latter are causing the former; conflating "softheartedness" with "softheadedness"; and treating all clinical evidence as equally good.

Psychoanalysts have also long been aware of how distortions in a therapist's understanding of a patient can affect the therapy. This awareness is reflected in terms such as "countertransference," "projection," and "suggestion" (see also Meehl, 1983).

Observation versus Inference

Fourth, all case formulations are built on both observation and inference about psychological processes that organize and maintain an individual's symptoms and problematic behavioral patterns. If a clinician relies too heavily on observable behavior, he or she may overlook meaningful patterns organizing a patient's symptoms and problems in living. If the clinician weights the formulation excessively on inference, the risk of losing its empirical basis increases. Thus, a clinician must achieve a balance between observation and inference. The clinician should be able to provide an empirical link between psychological processes that are inferred and patient phenomena that are observed. It may aid the clinician to label inferences according to how close or distant to observable phenomena they lie.

Individual versus General Formulations

A case formulation is fundamentally a statement about an individual and is thus tailored to that specific individual's life circumstances, needs, wishes, goals, blind spots, fears, thought patterns, and so on. Nevertheless, in arriving at a conceptualization of a patient, the therapist must rely on his or her general knowledge about psychology and knowledge of the psychotherapy and psychopathology research literature, as well as past experiences working with other individuals, especially those who seem similar to the person in question. The goodness-of-fit from the general or theoretical to the specific or individual is never perfect.

When attempting to balance the individual and the general in constructing case formulations, two kinds of errors are possible. First is the error of attempting to make a patient fit a generalized formulation that really does not fit. As mentioned earlier, Freud's analysis of Dora has been criticized on this point. Examples are not restricted to psychoanalysis. In the cognitive-behavioral realm, for example, attributing a patient's panic symptoms entirely to catastrophic interpretations of bodily sensations may neglect significant life history events or relationship patterns that also contribute to the onset and maintenance of the symptoms, as well as to the meaning they have for the patient. Overgeneralizing can also result from stereotyping patients on the basis of ethnicity, age, gender, appearance, socioeconomic background, or education.

A second kind of error is to overindividualize a formulation, neglecting one's knowledge of psychology, psychopathology, and past work with psychotherapy patients. If each patient is taken as a complete *tabula rasa* with experiences that are so unique that the therapist must throw away all previous knowledge, then the therapist is doing the patient a disservice.

Thus, a balance must be reached between an individual and general formulation. Humility is an asset in this respect. The match between any model and any individual is inherently imperfect, and the formulation is never more than an approximation of the individual in distress.

CASE FORMULATION AS A SCIENTIFIC TOOL

Earlier, I discussed how psychotherapy case formulations have become *objects* of scientific scrutiny through studies of their reliability and validity. As objects of study, one can also investigate study case formulation from the interindividual framework—for example, by comparing differences between expert and novice case formulators regarding the process of case formulation (Eells & Lombart, 2003; Eells et al., 2005) or by evaluating methods of training case formulators (e.g., Caspar, Berger, & Hautle, 2004; Kendjelic & Eells, 2006).

With demonstrations of the reliability and validity of case formulation methods, one can also use a case formulation as a research *tool*, that is, as a means through which knowledge about individual psychological functioning might be advanced. Although case study research in psychology has traditionally been viewed as within the discovery rather than the confirmation context of science, other scientific disciplines and even some within psychology have benefited from the aggregation of individual case studies within the confirmation context. Notable examples include medicine (Nuland, 1988), ethnography (Rosenblatt, 1981), and neuropsychology (Shallice, 1989). Single-participant research has a long history in experimental psychology; in fact, the entire operant conditioning research tradition is built on it (Morgan & Morgan, 2001).

Within psychotherapy and psychopathology research, a number of epistemological questions arise as one considers the possibility that a case formulation might serve as a tool in both the discovery *and* the confirmation phases of science. One of these questions is, How might the use of case formulations as research tools affect the nature of the scientific knowledge that subsequently accumulates? A complete answer to this question depends on many factors, not the least of which is the ingenuity, structure, design, comprehensiveness, reliability, and validity of the specific case formulation method in question. Nevertheless, there may be two classes of psychological knowledge for which a structured case formulation method would be particularly well suited.

One of these is knowledge about intraindividual psychological functioning. As noted earlier, the intraindividual frame of reference focuses on the individual as an internally organized system of interconnecting parts. Because a case formulation focuses on one person and how the internal organization of that person has gone awry to produce distress, research designs based on case formulations may permit the study of individuals while preserving the systemic nature of those individuals. Such an approach would diverge from the dominant research strategies in psychology, which Valsiner (1986) describes as based on an interindividual frame of reference. According to Valsiner (1986), the interindividual frame involves "comparison of an individual subject (or samples of subjects) with other individuals (samples) in order to determine the standing of these subjects relative to one another" (p. 396). Statements such as "The experimental group scored higher on variable X than the control group" or "John obtained a WAIS-R IQ of 112, which is at the 79th percentile" reflect an interindividual frame of reference. These conclusions provide comparative information, but do not address intraindividual issues such as how variable X interacts with variables Y or Z within any individual; nor do they address John's preferred problem-solving strategies, or how well his intelligence, affective style, or motivations are integrated. In sum, although useful for answering questions about differences *between* systems, the interindividual frame does not address variation *within* the systems that are compared, except as error variance.

The distinction between the intraindividual and interindividual frames of reference is particularly important in light of a significant body of literature addressing epistemological problems that arise when one conflates these two frames (Eells, 1991; Hilliard, 1993; Kim & Rosenberg, 1980; Kraemer, 1978; Lewin, 1931; Morgan & Morgan, 2001; Sidman, 1952; Thorngate, 1986; Tukey & Borgida, 1983). In clinical psychology, this conflation typically takes the form of a mismatch between the research questions and the means used to answer them. In an informal review, Eells (1991) found that most articles in a prestigious psychology journal framed research questions in terms of intraindividual psychological functioning, analyzed these questions from the interindividual frame, then returned to the intraindividual frame of reference when interpreting the results. At first glance, this incongruity between hypothesis, method, and interpretation may appear innocuous, as interindividual methodologies such as analysis of variance and correlational analysis dominate the research training of most psychologists, and hence, we are in the habit of "thinking interindividually" even about intraindividual problems. However, a variety of studies suggests harmful consequences of such mismatches (e.g., Kim & Rosenberg, 1980;

Kraemer, 1978; Tukey & Borgida, 1983). Each of these studies explored a research question from within the interindividual frame and then explored the same question from the intraindividual frame using the same sample of individuals. In each study, the results from each frame led to widely divergent conclusions. The logical basis for this divergence has been discussed by Sidman (1952), Thorngate (1986), Valsiner (1986), and others.

Although a psychotherapy case formulation can facilitate the construction of hypotheses at the intraindividual level of analysis and can provide a framework for the interpretation of results, there is also a need to apply methodologies that are appropriate for analyzing data at the level of the individual. Several such methods have been developed, proposed, or demonstrated (e.g., Bakeman & Gottman, 1986; Barlow & Hersen, 1984; Eells, 1995; Eells, Fridhandler, & Horowitz, 1995; Fonagy & Moran, 1993; Gottman 1980; Jones, Cumming, & Pulos, 1993; Rosenberg, 1977: Rudy & Merluzzi, 1984).

The second class of psychological knowledge for which the use of case formulations as research tools might be well suited is that growing from an "individual–socioecological" frame of reference (Valsiner, 1986). According to Valsiner, this frame emphasizes individuals in transactions with others, focusing on how assistance from one individual influences problem solving that emerges when two individuals interact. Problems are viewed as both created and constrained by the structure of the interpersonal environment and by the goals of the individual in question. "In this reference frame, an individual's actions and thinking to solve a problem that has emerged in the person–environment transaction is not a solitary, but a social event" (Valsiner, 1986, p. 400). One example of research from the individual–socioecological frame is Vygotsky's "zone of proximal development" (Van der Veer & Valsiner, 1991; Wertsch, 1985.)

The development of a case-formulation-based program of research from the individual–socioecological frame may be particularly helpful in improving our understanding of the therapeutic alliance, which is one of the most powerful predictors of outcome (Horvath & Greenberg, 1994). Such a program could also help us better understand individual changes processes in psychotherapy and how processes such as imitation, introjection, identification, and role reversal may create conditions for both psychopathology as well as psychological health.

CONCLUSIONS

At the outset of this chapter, I described psychotherapy case formulation as lying at an intersection of diagnosis and treatment, theory and practice, science and art, and etiology and description. To conclude the chapter, I return to this point. With respect to diagnosis and treatment, a case formulation provides a pragmatic tool to supplement and apply a diagnosis to the specifics of an individual's life. It also serves as a vehicle for converting a diagnosis into a plan for treatment, in terms of both general treatment strategies as well as "tactics" with respect to one's choice of specific interventions. A psychotherapy case formulation provides a link between theories of psychotherapy and psychopathology, on the one hand, and the application of these theories to a specific individual, on the other. The case formulation reflects a transposition of theory into practice. As both science and art, a case formulation should embody scientific principles and findings but also an appreciation of the singularity and humanity of the person in question. In sum, a psychotherapy case formulation is an integrative tool. In the hands of a psychotherapist who knows how to construct and use it, a case formulation is indispensable.

NOTE

1. Much of the material in this section is based on Nuland (1988).

REFERENCES

Allport, G. W. (1961). *Pattern and growth in personality.* New York: Holt, Rinehart & Winston.

Aronow, E., Rezinikoff, M., & Moreland, K. L. (1994). *The Rorschach technique: Perceptual basics and content analysis.* Needham Heights, MA: Allyn & Bacon.

Bakeman, R., & Gottman, J. M. (1986). *Observing interaction: An introduction to sequential analysis.* Cambridge, UK: Cambridge University Press.

Barber, J. P., & Crits-Christoph, P. (1993). Advances in measures of psychodynamic formulations. *Journal of Consulting and Clinical Psychology, 61,* 574–585.

Barlow, D. H., & Hersen, M. (1984). *Single case experimental designs: Strategies for studying behavior.* New York: Pergamon Press.

Beck, A. T., Emery, G., & Greenberg, R. (1985). *Anxiety disorders and phobias: A cognitive perspective.* New York: Basic Books.

Beck, A. T., Freeman, A., Davis, D. D., & Associates. (2004). *Cognitive therapy of personality disorders* (2nd ed.). New York: Guilford Press.

Beck, A. T., Rush, A. J., Shaw, B. F., & Emery, G. (1979). *Cognitive therapy of depression.* New York: Guilford Press.

Beck, A. T., Wright, F. D., Newman, C. F., & Liese, B. (1993). *Cognitive therapy of substance abuse.* New York: Guilford Press.

Beck, J. S. (1995). *Cognitive therapy: Basics and beyond.* New York: Guilford Press.

Bellak, L. (1993). *The Thematic Apperception Test, the Children's Apperception Test and the Senior Apperception Test in clinical use* (5th ed.). Needham Heights, MA: Allyn & Bacon.

Benjamin, L. S. (2003). *Interpersonal reconstructive therapy: Promoting change in nonresponders.* New York: Guilford Press.

Bersoff, D. N. (1973). Silk purses into sow's ears: The decline of psychological testing and a suggestion for its redemption. *American Psychologist, 28,* 892–899.

Beutler, L. E. (1995). The clinical interview. In L. E. Beutler & M. R. Berren (Eds.) *Integrative assessment of adult personality* (pp. 94–120). New York: Guilford Press.

Bieling, P. J., & Kuyken, W. (2003). Is cognitive case formulation science or science fiction? *Clinical Psychology: Science and Practice, 10,* 52–69.

Binder, J. L. (2004). *Key competencies in brief dynamic psychotherapy: Clinical practice beyond the manual.* New York: Guilford Press.

Blashfield, R. K. (1984). *The classification of psychopathology: Neo-Kraepelinian and quantitative approaches.* New York: Plenum Press.

Breuer, J., & Freud, S. (1955). On the psychical mechanism of hysterical phenomena: Preliminary communication. In J. Strachey (Ed.), *The standard edition of the complete psychological works of Sigmund Freud* (Vol. 2, pp. 1–17). London: Hogarth Press. (Original work published 1893)

Bruch, M., & Bond, F. W. (Eds.). (1998). *Beyond diagnosis: Case formulation approaches in CBT.* New York: Wiley.

Bruhn, A. R. (1995). Early memories in personality assessment. In J. N. Butcher (Ed.), *Clinical personality assessment: Practical approaches* (pp. 278–301). New York: Oxford University Press.

Butcher, J. N. (1993). *Use of the MMPI-2 in treatment planning.* New York: Oxford University Press.

Carey, M. P., Flasher, L. V., Maisto, S. A., & Turkat, I. D. (1984). The a priori approach to psychological assessment. *Professional Psychology Research and Practice, 15,* 515–527.

Caspar, F. (1995). *Plan analysis: Toward optimizing psychotherapy.* Seattle: Hogrefe & Huber.

Caspar, F., Berger, T., & Hautle, I. (2004). The right view of your patient: A computer-assisted, individualized module for psychotherapy training. *Psychotherapy: Theory, Research, Practice, Training, 41*(2), 125–135.

Chadwick, P., Williams, C., & Mackenzie, J. (2003). Impact of case formulation in cognitive behaviour therapy for psychosis. *Behaviour Research and Therapy, 41*(6), 671–680.

Clark, D. M. (1986). A cognitive approach to panic disorder. *Behaviour Research and Therapy, 24,* 461–470.

Clark, D. M., & Wells, A. (1995). A cognitive model of social phobia. In R. G. Heimberg & M. R. Liebowitz (Eds.), *Social phobia: Diagnosis, assessment, and treatment* (pp. 69–93). New York: Guilford Press.

Costa, P. T., & Widiger, T. A. (Eds.). (1994). *Personality disorders and the five-factor model of personality.* Washington, DC: American Psychological Association.

Curtis, J. T., Silberschatz, G., Sampson, H., Weiss, J., & Rosenberg, S. E. (1988). Developing reliable psychodynamic case formulation: An illustration of the Plan Diagnosis method. *Psychotherapy, 25,* 256–265.

Davies, R. (1994). *The cunning man.* New York: Penguin Books.

Edelson, M. (1988). *Psychoanalysis: A theory in crisis.* Chicago: University of Chicago Press.

Edwards, D. J. A., Dattilio, F. M., & Bromley, D. B. (2004). Developing evidence-based practice: The role of case-based research. *Professional Psychology: Research and Practice, 35*(6), 589–597.

Eells, T. (1991, August). *Single subject research: An epistemological argument for its scientific value.* Paper presented at the meeting of the American Psychological Association, San Francisco, CA.

Eells, T. D. (1995). Role reversal: A convergence of clinical and quantitative evidence. *Psychotherapy Research, 5,* 297–312.

Eells, T. D., Fridhandler, B., & Horowitz, M. J. (1995). Self schemas and spousal bereavement: Comparing quantitative and clinical evidence. *Psychotherapy, 32,* 270–282.

Eells, T. D., Kendjelic, E. M., & Lucas, C. P. (1998). What's in a case formulation?: Development and use of a content coding manual. *Journal of Psychotherapy Practice and Research, 7*(2), 144–153.

Eells, T. D., & Lombart, K. G. (2003). Case formulation and treatment concepts among novice, experienced, and expert cognitive-behavioral and psychodynamic therapists. *Psychotherapy Research, 13*(2), 187–2004.

Eells, T. D., Lombart, K. G., Kendjelic, E. M., Turner, L. C., & Lucas, C. (2005). The quality of psychotherapy case formulations: A comparison of expert, experienced, and novice cognitive-behavioral and psychodynamic therapists. *Journal of Consulting and Clinical Psychology, 73,* 579–589.

Eells, T. D., Lombart, K. G., Kendjelic, E. M., Turner, L. C., & Lucas, C. (in press). The quality of psychotherapy case formulations: A comparison of expert, experienced, and novice cognitive-behavioral and psychodynamic therapists. *Journal of Consulting and Clinical Psychology.*

Fishman, D. B. (2000). Transcending the efficacy versus effectiveness research debate: Proposal for a new, electronic "Journal of Pragmatic Case Studies." *Prevention and Treatment, 3,* [online] Article 8. Available from http://journals.apa.org/prevention/.

Fishman, D. B. (2002). From single case to data base: A new method for enhancing psychotherapy, forensic, and other psychological practice. *Applied and Preventive Psychology, 10,* 275–304.

Fonagy, P., & Moran, G. (1993). Selecting single case research designs for clinicians. In N. E. Miller, L. Luborsky, J. P. Barber, & J. P. Docherty (Eds.), *Psychodynamic treatment research: A handbook for clinical practice* (pp. 62–95). New York: Basic Books.

Frank, J. D., & Frank, J. B. (1991). *Persuasion and healing: A comparative study of psychotherapy* (3rd ed.). Baltimore: Johns Hopkins University Press.

Freeman, A. (1992). Developing treatment conceptualizations in cognitive therapy. In A. Freeman & F. Dattilio (Eds.), *Casebook of cognitive-behavioral therapy* (pp. 13–23). New York: Plenum Press.

Fridhandler, B., Eells, T. D., & Horowitz, M. (1999). Psychoanalytic explanation of pathological grief: Scientific observation of a single case. *Psychoanalytic Psychology, 16*(1), 1–24.

Garb, H. N. (1998). *Studying the clinician: Judgment research and psychological assessment.* Washington, DC: American Psychological Association.

Gill, M., Newman, R., & Redlich, F. C. (1954). *The initial interview in psychiatric practice.* New York: International Universities Press.

Goldfried, M. R., & Pomeranz, D. M. (1968). Role of assessment in behavior modification. *Psychological Reports, 23,* 75–87.

Gottman, J. M. (1980). *Time-series analysis: A comprehensive introduction for social scientists.* Cambridge, UK: Cambridge University Press.

Grunbaum, A. (1984). *The foundations of psychoanalysis: A philosophical critique.* Berkeley: University of California Press.

Hayes, S. C., & Follette, W. C. (1992). Can functional analysis provide a substitute for syndromal classification? *Behavioral Assessment, 14,* 345–365.

Hayes, S. C., Nelson, R. O., & Jarrett, R. B. (1987). The treatment utility of assessment: A functional approach to evaluating assessment quality. *American Psychologist, 42,* 963–974.

Haynes, S. N., & O'Brien, W. H. (1990). Functional analysis in behavior therapy. *Clinical Psychology Review, 10,* 649–668.

Haynes, S. N., Spain, E. H., & Oliveira, J. (1993). Identifying causal relationships in clinical assessment. *Psychological Assessment, 5,* 281–291.

Haynes, S. N., & Williams, A. E. (2003). Case formulation and design of behavioral treatment programs: Matching treatment mechanisms to causal variables for behavior problems. *European Journal of Psychological Assessment, 19*(3), 164–174.

Hersen, M. (2002). Rationale for clinical case studies: An editorial. *Clinical Case Studies, 1*(1), 3–5.

Hersen, M., & Porzelius, L. K. (Eds.). (2002). *Diagnosis, conceptualization, and treatment planning for adults: A step-by-step guide.* Mahwah, NJ: Erlbaum.

Hilliard, R. B. (1993). Single-case methodology in psychotherapy process and outcome research. *Journal of Consulting and Clinical Psychology, 61,* 373–380.

Horney, K. (1967). *Feminine psychology.* New York: Norton.

Horowitz, L. M., Rosenberg, S. E., Ureño, G., Kalehzan, B. M., & O'Halloran, P. (1989). Psychodynamic formulation, consensual response method and interpersonal problems. *Journal of Consulting and Clinical Psychology, 57,* 599–606.

Horowitz, M. (1997). *Formulation as a basis for planning psychotherapy treatment.* Washington, DC: American Psychiatric Press.

Horowitz, M. (2005). *Understanding psychotherapy change: A practical guide to configurational analysis.* Washington, DC: American Psychological Association.

Horowitz, M., Stinson, C., Fridhandler, B., Milbrath, C., Redington, D., & Ewert, M. (1993). Pathological grief: An intensive case study. *Psychiatry: Interpersonal and Biological Processes, 56,* 356–374.

Horowitz, M. J. (1989). Relationship schema formulation: Role-relationship models and intrapsychic conflict. *Psychiatry, 52,* 260–274.

Horowitz, M. J. (Ed.). (1991). *Person schemas and maladaptive interpersonal patterns.* Chicago: University of Chicago Press.

Horvath, A. O., & Greenberg, L. S. (1994). *The working alliance: Theory, research, and practice.* New York: Wiley.

Johnson, M. E., Popp, C., Schacht, T. E., Mellon, J., & Strupp, H. H. (1989). Converging evidence for identification of recurrent relationship themes: Comparison of two methods. *Psychiatry, 52,* 275–288.

Jones, E. E., Cumming, J. D., & Pulos, S. M. (1993). Tracing clinical themes across phases of treatment by a Q-Set. In N. E. Miller, L. Luborsky, J. P. Barber, & J. P.

Docherty (Eds.), *Psychodynamic treatment research: A handbook for clinical practice* (pp. 14–36). New York: Basic Books.

Kahneman, D., Slovic, P., & Tversky, A. (1982). *Judgment under uncertainty: Heuristics and biases.* New York: Cambridge University Press.

Kaplan, H. I., & Sadock, B. J. (1998). *Kaplan and Sadock's synopsis of psychiatry: Behavioral sciences/clinical psychiatry* (8th ed.). Baltimore: Williams & Wilkins.

Kendell, R. (1975). *The role of diagnosis in psychiatry.* Oxford, UK: Blackwell Scientific.

Kendjelic, E. M., & Eells, T. D. (2006). *Generic psychotherapy case formulation training improves formulation quality.* Manuscript submitted for publication.

Kernberg, O. (1975). *Borderline conditions and pathological narcissism.* New York: Jason Aronson.

Kernberg, O. (1984). *Severe personality disorders.* New Haven, CT: Yale University Press.

Kim, M. P., & Rosenberg, S. (1980). Comparison of two structural models of implicit personality theories. *Journal of Personality and Social Psychology, 38,* 375–389.

Kleinmuntz, B. (1968). The processing of clinical information by man and machine. In B. Kleinmuntz (Ed.), *Formal representation of human judgment* (pp. 149–186). New York: Wiley.

Kohut, H. (1971). *Analysis of the self.* New York: International Universities Press.

Kohut, H. (1977). *Restoration of the self.* New York: International Universities Press.

Kohut, H. (1984). *How analysis cures.* New York: International Universities Press.

Korchin, S. J., & Schuldberg, D. (1981). The future of clinical assessment. *American Psychologist, 36,* 1147–1158.

Kraemer, H. C. (1978). Individual and ecological correlation in a general context. *Behavioral Science, 23,* 67–72.

Kuyken, W. (in press). Evidence-based case formulation: Is the emperor clothed? In N. Tarrier (Ed.), *Case formulation in cognitive behaviour therapy?: The treatment of challenging and complex cases.* New York: Routledge.

Lakoff, R. T. (1990). *Talking power: The politics of language.* New York: Basic Books.

Lauterbach, W., & Newman, C. F. (1999). Computerized intrapersonal conflict assessment in cognitive therapy. *Clinical Psychology and Psychotherapy, 6*(5), 357–374.

Lewin, K. (1931). The conflict between Aristotelian and Galileian modes of thought in contemporary psychology. *Journal of General Psychology, 5,* 141–177.

Luborsky, L. (1977). Measuring a pervasive psychic structure in psychotherapy: The core conflictual relationship theme. In N. Freedman & S. Grand (Eds.), *Communicative structures and psychic structures* (pp. 367–395). New York: Plenum Press.

Luborsky, L. (1996). *The symptom-context method: Symptoms as opportunities in psychotherapy.* Washington, DC: American Psychological Association.

Luborsky, L., Barber, J. P., Binder, J., Curtis, J., Dahl, H., Horowitz, L., et al. (1993). Transference-based measures: A new class based on psychotherapy sessions. In N. E. Miller, L. Luborsky, J. P. Barber, & J. P. Docherty (Eds.), *Psychodynamic treatment research: A handbook for clinical practice* (pp. 326–341). New York: Basic Books.

Luborsky, L., & Crits-Christoph, P. (1990). *Understanding transference: The CCRT method*. New York: Basic Books.

Luborsky, L., & Crits-Christoph, P. (1998). *Understanding transference: The Core Conflictual Relationship Theme method* (2nd ed.). Washington, DC: American Psychological Association.

Mack, A. H., Forman, L., Brown, R., & Frances, A. (1994). A brief history of psychiatric classification: From the ancients to DSM-IV. *Psychiatric Clinics of North America, 17,* 515–523.

Masson, J. M. (1984). *The assault on truth: Freud's suppression of the seduction theory.* New York: Farrar, Strauss and Giroux.

Mayfield, W. A., Kardash, C. M., & Kivlighan, D. M. (1999). Differences in experienced and novice counselors' knowledge structures about clients: Implications for case conceptualization. *Journal of Counseling Psychology, 46*(4), 504–514.

Meehl, P. E. (1954). *Clinical versus statistical prediction.* Minneapolis: University of Minnesota Press.

Meehl, P. E. (1958). Some ruminations on the validation of clinical procedures. *Canadian Journal of Psychology, 13,* 102–128.

Meehl, P. E. (1973). Why I do not attend case conferences. In *Psychodiagnosis: Selected papers* (pp. 225–302). New York: Norton.

Meehl, P. E. (1983). Subjectivity in psychoanalytic inference: The nagging persistence of Wilhelm Fliess's Achensee question. In J. Earman (Ed.), *Minnesota studies in the philosophy of science: Vol. 10. Testing scientific theories* (pp. 349–411). Minneapolis: University of Minnesota Press.

Meier, S. T. (2003). *Bridging case conceptualization, assessment, and intervention.* Thousand Oaks, CA: Sage.

Messer, S. B., Tishby, O., & Spillman, A. (1992). Taking context seriously in psychotherapy: Relating therapist interventions to patient progress in brief psychodynamic therapy. *Journal of Consulting and Clinical Psychology, 60,* 678–688.

Millon, T. (1996). *Disorders of personality: DSM-IV and beyond.* New York: Wiley.

Morgan, D. L., & Morgan, R. K. (2001). Single-participant research design: Bringing science to managed care. *American Psychologist, 56*(2), 119–127.

Morrison, J. (1993). *The first interview.* New York: Guilford Press.

Needleman, L. D. (1999). *Cognitive case conceptualization: A guidebook for practitioners.* Mahwah, NJ: Erlbaum.

Nezu, A. M., Nezu, C. M., & Lombardo, E. R. (2004). *Cognitive-behavioral case formulation and treatment design: A problem-solving approach.* New York: Springer.

Nuland, S. B. (1988). *Doctors: The biography of medicine.* New York: Vintage Books.

Pasnau, R. O. (1987). The remedicalization of psychiatry. *Hospital and Community Psychiatry, 38,* 145–151.

Perry, J. C. (1994). Assessing psychodynamic patterns using the idiographic conflict formulation method. *Psychotherapy Research, 4,* 239–252.

Perry, J. C., Augusto, F., & Cooper, S. H. (1989). Assessing psychodynamic conflicts: I. Reliability of the ideographic conflict formulation method. *Psychiatry, 52,* 289–301.

Perry, S., Cooper, A. M., & Michels, R. (1987). The psychodynamic formulation: Its purpose, structure and clinical application. *American Journal of Psychiatry, 144,* 543–550.

Persons, J. B. (1989). *Cognitive therapy in practice: A case formulation approach.* New York: Norton.

Persons, J. B. (1995). Interrater reliability of cognitive-behavioral case formulations. *Cognitive Therapy and Research, 19,* 21–34.

Rogers, C. R. (1951). *Client-centered therapy: Its current practice, implications, and theory.* Boston: Houghton Mifflin.

Rosenberg, S. (1977). New approaches to the analysis of personal constructs in person perception. In A. W. Landfield (Ed.), *Nebraska Symposium on Motivation, 1976. Personal construct psychology* (pp. 179–242). Lincoln: University of Nebraska Press.

Rosenblatt, P. C. (1981). Ethnographic case studies. In M. B. Brewer & B. E. Collins (Eds.), *Scientific inquiry and the social sciences: A volume in honor of Donald T. Campbell* (pp. 194–225). San Francisco: Jossey-Bass.

Rudy, T. E., & Merluzzi, T. V. (1984). Recovering social–cognitive schemata: Descriptions and applications of multidimensional scaling for clinical research. In P. C. Kendall (Ed.), *Advances in cognitive-behavioral research and therapy* (Vol. 3, pp. 61–102). New York: Guilford Press.

Runyan, W. B. (1982). In defense of the case study method. *American Journal of Orthopsychiatry, 52,* 440–446.

Safran, J. D., Muran, J. C., Samstag, L. W., & Stevens, C. (2002). Repairing alliance ruptures. In J. C. Norcross (Ed.), *Psychotherapy relationships that work: Therapist contributions and responsiveness to patients.* (pp. 235–254). London: Oxford University Press.

Samstag, L. W., Muran, J. C., & Safran, J. D. (2004). Defining and identifying alliance ruptures. In D. P. Charman (Ed.), *Core processes in brief psychodynamic psychotherapy: Advancing effective practice* (pp. 187–214). Mahwah, NJ: Erlbaum.

Schacht, T. E., & Henry, W. P. (1994). Modeling recurrent patterns of interpersonal relationship with the Structural Analysis of Social Behavior: The SASB-CMP. *Psychotherapy Research, 4,* 208–221.

Segal, Z. F., & Blatt, S. J. (Eds.). (1993). *The self in emotional distress: Cognitive and psychodynamic perspectives.* New York: Guilford Press.

Seitz, P. F. (1966). The consensus problem in psychoanalytic research. In L. Gottschalk & L. Auerbach (Eds.), *Methods of research and psychotherapy* (pp. 209–225). New York: Appleton-Century-Crofts.

Shallice, T. (1989). *From neuropsychology to cognitive neuroscience.* Hillsdale, NJ: Erlbaum.

Shedler, J., & Westen, D. (1998). Refining the measurement of Axis II: A Q-sort procedure for assessing personality pathology. *Assessment, 5*(4), 333–353.

Sidman, M. (1952). A note on functional relations obtained from group data. *Psychological Bulletin, 49,* 263–269.

Silberschatz, G. (2005). *Transformative relationships: The control–mastery theory of psychotherapy.* New York: Routledge.

Spence, D. P. (1982). *Historical truth and narrative truth.* New York: Norton.

Sperry, L., Gudeman, J. E., Blackwell, B., & Faulkner, L. R. (1992). *Psychiatric case formulations.* Washington, DC: American Psychiatric Press.

Stiles, W. B. (2003). When is a case study psychotherapy research? *Psychotherapy Bulletin, 38,* 6–11.

Sullivan, H. S. (1954). *The psychiatric interview.* New York: Norton.

Summers, R. F. (2003). The psychodynamic formulation updated. *American Journal of Psychotherapy, 57*(1), 39–51.

Tarrier, N., & Calam, R. (2002). New developments in cognitive-behavioural case formulation. Epidemiological, systemic and social context: An integrative approach. *Behavioural and Cognitive Psychotherapy, 30*(3), 311–328.

Thorngate, W. (1986). The production, detection, and explanation of behavioral patterns. In J. Valsiner (Ed.), *The individual subject and scientific psychology* (pp. 71–93). New York: Plenum Press.

Tukey, D. D., & Borgida, E. (1983). An intrasubject approach to causal attribution. *Journal of Personality, 51,* 137–151.

Turk, D. C., & Salovey, P. (Eds.). (1988). *Reasoning, inference, and judgment in clinical psychology.* New York: Free Press.

Valsiner, J. (Ed.). (1986). *The individual subject and scientific psychology.* New York: Plenum Press.

Valsiner, J. (1987). *Culture and the development of children's action.* New York: Wiley.

Van der Veer, R., & Valsiner, J. (1991). *Understanding Vygotsky: A quest for synthesis.* Cambridge, UK: Blackwell.

Wertsch, J. V. (1985). *Vygotsky and the social formation of mind.* Cambridge, MA: Harvard University Press.

Westen, D., & Shedler, J. (1999a). Revising and assessing axis II, Part I: Developing a clinically and empirically valid assessment method. *American Journal of Psychiatry, 156*(2), 258–272.

Westen, D., & Shedler, J. (1999b). Revising and assessing axis II, Part II: Toward an empirically based and clinically useful classification of personality disorders. *American Journal of Psychiatry, 156*(2), 273–285.

Westmeyer, H. (2003). Clinical case formulation: Introduction to the special issue. *European Journal of Psychological Assessment, 19*(3), 161–163.

Widiger, T. A., & Frances, A. J. (1994). Toward a dimensional model for the personality disorders. In P. T. Costa & T. A. Widiger (Eds.), *Personality disorders and the five-factor model of personality* (pp. 19–39). Washington, DC: American Psychological Association.

Widiger, T. A., & Sanderson, C. J. (1995). In J. N. Butcher (Ed.), *Clinical personality assessment: Practical approaches* (pp. 380–394). New York: Oxford University Press.

Widiger, T. A., & Trull, T. A. (1991). Diagnosis and clinical assessment. *Annual Review of Psychology, 42,* 109–133.

Wilson, M. (1993). DSM-III and the transformation of American psychiatry: A history. *American Journal of Psychiatry, 150,* 399–410.

Wolpe, J., & Turkat, I. D. (1985). Behavioral formulation of clinical cases. In I. D. Turkat (Ed.), *Behavioral case formulation* (pp. 5–36). New York: Plenum Press.

Chapter 2

Multicultural Considerations in Case Formulation

CHARLES R. RIDLEY
SHANNON M. KELLY

The mental health field usually attracts people who have good intentions. Students training to be counselors, psychologists, psychiatrists, and social workers typically look forward to improving others' lives, and they resolutely commit to protecting their clients' welfare. Unfortunately, such good intentions are not good enough. Despite the heightened attention multicultural issues have received in research, training, and ethical codes over the past 30 years, unfair treatment and oppression continue to permeate most corners of the field (Heppner, Casas, Carter, & Stone, 2000; Ridley, 2005). Indeed, more than a half century of research highlights the pervasiveness of racism in the mental health system (Ridley, 2005).

Psychological assessment is not exempt from this trend. Practitioners often misinterpret minority clients' test scores because they overlook these clients' cultural backgrounds, motivations, and circumstances (Cuéllar, 1998; Ridley, 2005). At the same time, clinicians often fail to consider their own biases during the assessment process (Dana, 2005; Ridley, 2005). They also tend to equate assessment with standardized testing and diagnosis rather than with the array of techniques necessary for developing a comprehensive picture of clients (Dana, 2005; Ridley, 2005). Furthermore, one of the most commonly used assessment tools, the *Diagnostic and Statistical Manual of Mental Disorders* (DSM; American Psychiatric Association, 2000), has been widely criticized for emphasizing individual origins of mental disorders and harboring Eurocentric conceptions of normality.

33

Thus, practitioners easily can neglect the influences of acculturation, racial identity, and immigration on the human experience, not to mention social problems such as racism, sexism, and homophobia (Kress, Eriksen, Rayle, & Ford, 2005; Velásquez, Johnson, & Brown-Cheatham, 1993). Given these factors, psychological assessment is vulnerable to the same stereotyping, prejudice, and systematic bias that pervades both the broader mental health system and society at large.

Conducting multiculturally competent assessments can seem daunting, however. As Malgady (1996) observed, "Limited empirical data and even sparser theoretical preconceptions hinder researchers, professional practitioners, and policy makers in deciding whether or not—and if so, how—a culturally informed mental health assessment ought to take place" (p. 73). Trainees might find multicultural assessment particularly intimidating. After all, training curricula usually teach cultural considerations separately from general theories and skills, often relegating them to special multicultural classes (Ridley, Kelly, Mollen, & Kleiner, 2005). Given training programs' difficulty integrating culture and practice, it is no wonder that students feel lost as they attempt to incorporate cultural considerations into assessment.

The purpose of this chapter is twofold: (1) to explain why practitioners must consider culture when developing case formulations, and (2) to offer a procedure for incorporating cultural factors into clinical decision making. To achieve our objectives, we organize the chapter into eight major sections. First, we present a definition of culture. Next, we discuss the importance of considering culture in case formulation and highlight some critical issues in multicultural assessment. We then describe the conceptual framework underlying the multicultural assessment procedure (MAP), which we outline in detail in the fifth section. In the sixth section, we explore how the MAP applies to a variety of case formulation techniques. We then show this procedure in action by presenting a case example. Next, we suggest steps trainees can take to learn the MAP. Finally, we discuss the empirical support underlying this approach to assessment and case formulation.

DEFINITION OF CULTURE

This chapter addresses cultural considerations in assessment and case formulation, but what exactly is culture, anyway? This question might seem simple, but a widely accepted answer has eluded psychologists. Whereas some scholars equate culture with concepts such as race and ethnicity, for example, others only vaguely define the relationship between these constructs. In this chapter, we accept Marsella and Kameoka's (1989) definition of culture:

Culture is shared learned behavior that is transmitted from one generation to another for purposes of human adjustment, adaptation, and growth. Culture has both internal and external referents. External referents include artifacts, roles, and institutions. Internal referents include attitudes, values, beliefs, expectations, epistemologies, and consciousness. (p. 233)

This definition highlights two key features of culture. First, culture permeates all realms of human experience; practitioners therefore must uncover and integrate a broad range of data throughout the helping process. Second, culture has external and internal dimensions. Consider an Arab client who presents with depressive symptoms after losing his job, for example. His external cultural referent is the traditional expectation that Arab men must provide for their families. His internal cultural referent is his shame about not satisfying this role. Often, the external aspects of clients' psychological presentation are more obvious than the internal aspects (Ridley, Li, & Hill, 1998).

Individuals vary in their adherence to external and internal cultural referents, however. Indeed, although the aforementioned Arab client believes strongly in his culture's traditional male provider role, another Arab man might not. Thus, a third feature of culture comprises within-group differences among people of similar backgrounds. Given these variations, clinicians should expect to encounter clients who embrace values, attitudes, beliefs, and behaviors that deviate from their native cultural norms. These idiosyncrasies comprise a fourth feature of culture. A fifth and final aspect of culture is its inclusive nature. Because "culture" applies to any group with a shared learned behavior for the purpose of adjustment, adaptation, and growth, cultures include groups defined by race, ethnicity, age, socioeconomic status, sexual orientation, religion, and a variety of other characteristics (Ridley et al., 1998).

THE IMPORTANCE OF CONSIDERING CULTURE IN CASE FORMULATION

As described earlier, culture touches all corners of human experience. Therapy is no exception. Indeed, culture is an invisible and silent participant in every clinician–client interaction, including psychological assessment (Draguns, 1989; Good & Good, 1986). The therapeutic relationship occurs against the cultural backdrop of towns, cities, regions, and countries, and both clinicians and clients are products of their respective cultures (Rollock & Terrell, 1996). Culture therefore influences therapy via three channels: the client, the clinician, and the setting in which their relationship develops.

The interaction among these cultural factors can be difficult to manage. In fact, many clinicians who claim to consider culture in case formulation cannot articulate how they do so, and they often feel incompetent assessing clients' assimilation and acculturation (Lopez & Hernandez, 1987; Ramirez, 1994; Ramirez, Wassef, Paniagua, & Linskey, 1996). When practitioners fail to account for cultural influences in counseling, however, miscommunication, misunderstanding, and mistreatment often occur. Indeed, clinicians who ignore or minimize culture overlook the realities of their clients' lives, their own lives, and the counseling context. These oversights virtually guarantee inaccurate perceptions of clients' circumstances, poor case formulations, and misdiagnoses (Ridley et al., 1998; Rogler, 1992, 1993a, 1993b).

Edwards (1982) described two types of diagnostic errors that can occur when practitioners fail to consider culture in assessment. Type I error involves concluding that clients' functioning is pathological when it actually is normal given their cultural context and circumstances. Illustrating this error, Thompson, Blueye, Smith, and Walker (1983) described a Native American client whom hospital staff considered violent and impulsive until a resident realized this behavior reflected unfulfilled basic needs. In contrast, Type II error involves failing to identify pathology when it truly exists. Lewis, Balla, and Shanok (1979) uncovered this error when practitioners considered hallucinations, paranoia, and grandiosity to be normal and adaptive for a sample of low-income, urban African American adolescents, even though the adolescents actually suffered from psychiatric disorders. Both Type I and Type II errors often lead to inappropriate interventions and poor treatment outcomes (Rollock & Terrell, 1996). Cultural sensitivity, on the other hand, maximizes opportunities for therapeutic gain and improves the diagnostic process (Ridley, Mendoza, Kanitz, Angermeier, & Zenk, 1994; Ridley et al., 1998; Rogler, 1992, 1993a, 1993b).

CRITICAL ISSUES IN MULTICULTURAL ASSESSMENT

Clearly, accounting for clients' culture is essential for sound case formulation and fair, effective service. But how does this happen? Given culture's omnipresence in therapeutic relationships, clinicians might wonder how they possibly could integrate this complex construct into practice. Later, we offer the MAP to guide trainees and practitioners as they tackle this challenging but necessary task. Like any counseling technique, however, clinicians cannot employ the MAP in a vacuum. Indeed, to understand and harness the concepts embedded in our model, practitioners must view the procedure in context by considering the therapeutic relationship, relevant research, professional trends, and societal patterns. Before describing the MAP, we therefore discuss nine critical issues in multicultural assessment.

Equitable Service Delivery

More than 175 separate studies and commentaries have uncovered racism in the mental health system (Ridley, 2005). These publications have revealed that minority clients are more likely than white clients to be dissatisfied with their treatment, to be misdiagnosed, and to be assigned to junior staff (Ridley, 2005). Several professional organizations have decried these discrepancies and called for equitable service delivery. One of these outlets, the American Psychological Association, Office of Ethnic Minority Affairs (1993), offered "Guidelines for Providers of Psychological Services to Ethnic, Linguistic, and Culturally Diverse Populations," including Guideline 8d, which is especially pertinent to multicultural case formulation: "Psychologists are cognizant of the sociopolitical contexts in conducting evaluations and providing interventions; they develop sensitivity to issues of oppression, sexism, elitism, and racism" (p. 47).

Most clinicians do not realize that, even with the best intentions, they could be deviating from such guidelines (Ridley, 2005). To increase the likelihood of equitable service delivery, practitioners need reliable methods for multicultural assessment and case formulation. The MAP answers this call: It is highly intentional, is clearly outlined, and aims to enhance judgmental accuracy while diminishing bias.

Science–Practice Integrity

The scientist–practitioner model underlies many counselor training programs (Spengler, Strohmer, Dixon, & Shivy, 1995). We not only encourage trainees to conduct and consume research related to this realm but also urge them to approach assessment and case formulation from a scientific perspective. Indeed, to reduce the risk of racism and biased judgments and to enhance the soundness of clinical decisions and treatment, practitioners should formulate and test hypotheses regarding their clients, operationalize their decision-making strategies, self-observe, self-correct, and evaluate their assessment outcomes (Spengler et al., 1995). The fusion of science and practice is integral to the MAP and to sound assessment and case formulation.

The Problem of Pseudoetic Criteria

In the United States, psychological theory and practice are based on predominantly Western cultural values (Fernández & Kleinman, 1994). For example, professional conceptualizations of personality and psychopathology tend to favor individualism over interdependence, even though Asian, Latin American, and African cultures often prize social relationships (Bond & Smith, 1996; Markus & Kitayama, 1991). Unfortunately, American practitioners often draw from Western-based mental health constructs regardless of their clients' cultural backgrounds, which usually results in misdiagnosis (Ridley et al., 1998). The term "pseudoetic" refers to this trend (Triandis, Malpass, & Davidson, 1973); clinicians using a pseudoetic approach apply culturally specific (emic) criteria to clients of other cultures as if these criteria were culturally universal (etic). The MAP can help mental health professionals avoid this pitfall by grounding assessment and case formulation in the scientist–practitioner model.

The Clinician–Client Relationship

As mentioned earlier, the clinician–client relationship is culturally complex. Although this complexity can enhance therapy, it also can impede accurate assessment and case formulation. Good (1993) proposed two reasons behind this hurdle. First, clients must self-disclose in the therapeutic relationship, but cultures vary in the level of intimacy required for such self-disclosure. Second, the transference and countertransference that stem from cultural differences in the clinician–client relationship can complicate eliciting and interpreting clinical data.

The MAP honors the importance of the complex relationship between clinicians and clients. It urges cultural sensitivity during the clinical interview, and it reminds practitioners to nurture the therapeutic relationship by monitoring their attitudes and feelings toward clients, attending to their clients' attitudes and feelings toward them, and addressing the interaction of both.

The Clinician's Cognitive and Behavioral Flexibility

When we speak of clinicians' cognitive complexity, we refer to the intricacy of their information processing and decision making. Cognitive complexity is essential to developing expertise across occupations, including those in the mental health field (Ridley et al., 2005). Highlighting this point, Goodyear (1997) proposed that cognitive complexity distinguishes novice from expert counselors; indeed, how practitioners conceptualize cases, determine their approach with clients, and maintain motivation is more important than their in-session behaviors. Along these lines, Ronnestad and Skovholt (2003) noted that regardless of their experience level, practitioners must continuously self-reflect to avoid stagnation and to ensure sustained professional development.

Once clinicians develop complex thinking skills, they are primed to behave with greater flexibility. Cognitively complex practitioners tend to seek out and integrate more clinical information than do those with lower cognitive complexity, for example, and they tend to diagnose more accurately (Holloway & Wolleat, 1980; Spengler & Strohmer, 1994; Watson,

1976). Furthermore, given that integrating science and practice requires complex thinking skills, cognitive complexity increases clinicians' chances of approaching case formulation scientifically (Ridley et al., 1998). As described earlier, this scientific perspective is essential to reducing bias and error in the assessment process. Our MAP therefore incorporates specific examples of cognitive complexity and behavioral flexibility, as well as ample opportunity to execute and evaluate these skills.

Linguistic Competency

The assessment process is primarily verbal (Ridley et al., 1998). Given this central role of language, multicultural assessment is ripe for miscommunication between clinicians and clients. The language spoken during the assessment process can affect emotional expression, for example, and it can influence diagnostic outcomes (Altarriba & Santiago-Rivera, 1994; Guttfreund, 1990).

When practitioners are linguistically competent, however, language can be a clinical asset. As Santiago-Rivera (1994) explained, linguistically competent clinicians realize clients' language is "the method by which knowledge, beliefs, and traditions are transmitted and is closely related to an individual's history and culture" (p. 74). Luckily, linguistic competency does not require learning every possible native language of one's clientele. Instead, practitioners can become linguistically competent through methods such as assessing clients' language dominance and preference, mastering key idioms and expressions from clients' native languages, and using interpreters effectively (Marcos, Alpert, Urcuyo, & Kesselman, 1973; Santiago-Rivera, 1995).

Linguistic competency is essential to executing our MAP, which holds verbal exchanges between clinicians and clients at its core. This competency is especially important when determining which data-gathering methods are necessary for comprehensive case formulation. Indeed, linguistically competent clinicians are open to using a variety of communication methods (e.g., storytelling) to uncover cultural data that language barriers might otherwise bury.

Ethics

Most training curricula for mental health professionals include at least one course on ethics. Ethical codes provide guidelines to ensure clinicians establish appropriate professional relationships and execute proper clinical procedures, and they require competence in practice (e.g., American Psychological Association, 2002). Although this competence encompasses a variety of clinical realms, it entails a general respect for human rights and dignity, as well as the ability to assess clients cross-culturally. Unfortunately, few assessment measures are valid for use with culturally diverse populations, and many clinicians lack a coherent framework for developing solid multicultural case formulations (Ridley et al., 1998). Nevertheless, practitioners are ethically mandated to assess clients fairly and accurately, regardless of cultural background. To help clinicians meet these ethical obligations, our MAP offers guidelines for psychological testing, shows how to integrate test data with other clinical data, and encourages practitioners to respect and to critically examine clients' cultural values.

The Press of Managed Care

Managed care refers to "any health care delivery system in which various strategies are employed to optimize the value of provided services by controlling their cost and utilization, promoting their quality, and measuring performance to ensure cost-effectiveness" (Corcoran & Vandiver, 1996, p. 309). Managed care affects multicultural assessment in several ways (Ridley et al., 1998). First, managed care corporations usually make short-term demands for diagnosis and treatment, which pressures clinicians to assess and diagnose clients extremely quickly (Miller, 1996a). Such rushed assessment can force practitioners to use cognitive shortcuts, which increases the risk of bias and deprives clients of thorough, accurate evaluations. Second, managed care companies often establish practice guidelines to maximize profits, a mentality that often leads to ineffective and inappropriate treatment (Miller, 1996b). Finally, on a more optimistic note, managed care generates standards for accountability (Richardson & Austad, 1991). Because managed care companies often want proof of clinical efficacy, practitioners need to choose the techniques best suited to individual clients and to execute these techniques appropriately. Both tasks will require multicultural competence, which encompasses the science-practice integrity, cognitive complexity, behavioral flexibility, and other qualities featured in the MAP.

Inadequacies of Current Approaches

Over the past three decades, mental health professionals' growing acknowledgement of multicultural considerations has yielded many suggestions for sound assessment. These guidelines vary widely, encouraging clinicians to use nonstandardized methods, employ culture-specific instruments, assess clients' psychocultural adjustment, conduct behavioral analyses, interpret culturally related defenses, validate clients' cultural belief system, and attempt myriad other tactics to promote multicultural competence (Ridley et al., 1998).

Although such suggestions have helped highlight culture's significance, their utility is limited because they often are outlined in a piecemeal fashion

(Ridley et al., 1998). The lack of a coherent framework for integrating such a variety of ideas makes it difficult not only to remember the long list of suggestions but also to orchestrate them smoothly and skillfully. Furthermore, most of the field's suggestions identify what needs to happen in multicultural assessment, but they offer no concrete guidance for satisfying those needs. Although descriptions of issues abound, direction and methodology are generally absent in discussions of multicultural assessment. Finally, many of the suggestions mentioned earlier lack a solid scientific basis and stem from multicultural assessment literature that is largely biased. Much of the literature cited in support of these suggestions focuses solely on white clinicians' assessment of minority clients, for example, which erroneously implies that (1) white practitioners lag behind non-white practitioners in multicultural competence and (2) minority clients require special considerations to be understood, whereas white clients do not. Our MAP addresses these deficiencies by outlining an empirically grounded conceptual framework that includes concrete clinical procedures to guide multicultural assessment.

CONCEPTUAL FRAMEWORK OF THE MAP

Before delving into a detailed discussion of the MAP, trainees must understand the philosophy behind our approach to multicultural assessment and case formulation. Too often the assumptions underlying therapeutic procedures and techniques go unspoken, which leads to confusion and hinders thorough scholarly critiques. We therefore have decided to make our philosophy of assessment and case conceptualization explicit. We consider psychological assessment to be the entire process of collecting, organizing, and interpreting psychological data about clients. Case conceptualizations, on the other hand, comprise decisions based on assessments. Ten principles underlie our assessment philosophy (Ridley et al., 1998).

- *First, a sound assessment is accurate and comprehensive.* Although most practitioners aspire toward this principle, assessment decisions often are inaccurate and incomplete. Many clinicians fail to consider medical roots of psychological conditions, for example, such as hyperthyroidism's tendency to produce depression-like symptoms. Incomplete assessments also might focus solely on clients' deficits rather than their strengths. Omitting such data can lead to inaccuracy, misdiagnosis, and unsound treatment.
- *Second, assessment is a larger concept than diagnostic classification.* Indeed, a diagnostic category is only one descriptor of an individual. Granted, diagnoses carry their own importance and are a valid feature of the assessment process. Assessments must move beyond labels, however, to

incorporate a broad range of information, including prognosis, severity, strengths, and social supports. Including these data promotes comprehensiveness and accuracy.

• *Third, psychological assessment is complex.* Clients' mental health status stems from interactions between psychological, biological, social, cultural, and organic factors. Sometimes, one of these aspects lies at the heart of a client's presenting issue. Other times, these issues are so inextricably intertwined that a problem's etiology cannot be traced to a sole cause. Given the intricacy inherent in clients' backgrounds, assessment is necessarily complicated and challenging.

• *Fourth, psychological assessment is a process of progressive decision making.* As mentioned earlier, the goal of psychological assessment is accurate, comprehensive case conceptualization. As a clinical picture gradually unfolds, practitioners must make a series of microdecisions; indeed, rushing into larger diagnostic decisions and skipping these microdecisions usually leads to inaccuracy and unsoundness. The MAP addresses the nine microdecisions shown in the decision tree in Figure 2.1:

1. After collecting salient data, will I make an assessment decision based solely on that information?
2. What methods should I use to collect nonsalient data?
3. How do I respond to all data (salient and nonsalient)?
4. Which data are cultural, and which are idiosyncratic?
5. How do base rates apply to cultural data?
6. Which stressors are dispositional, and which are environmental?
7. Which data are clinically significant, and which are insignificant?
8. What is my working hypothesis?
9. What is my conclusive assessment decision, including (a) What is the nature of psychopathology (if any)? and (b) How do non-pathological but clinically significant data fit into the assessment conclusion?

These microdecisions illuminate the process nature of assessment. Given the many decisions inherent in this endeavor, we propose that clinicians must be skillful, motivated, disciplined, and trained to carry out sound multicultural assessments and case formulations.

• *Fifth, as a decision-making process, assessment involves considerable subjectivity.* Although practitioners often base assessments on seemingly objective data, including test results, medical records, and behavioral observations, they also rely heavily on their personal perceptions. They decide what data to gather, and they determine how best to synthesize and interpret this data in psychological reports. Thus, subjectivity plays a crucial and valuable role in assessment and case formulation. Although clinicians must manage their subjectivity to minimize bias during the assessment pro-

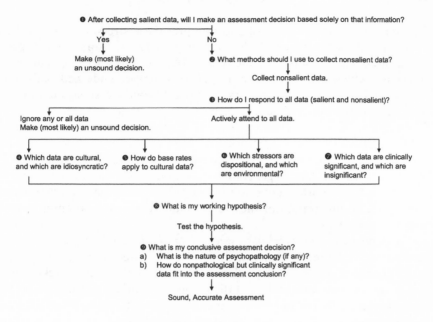

❶ After collecting salient data, will I make an assessment decision based solely on that information?

Yes → Make (most likely) an unsound decision.

No → **❷** What methods should I use to collect nonsalient data? → Collect nonsalient data.

❸ How do I respond to all data (salient and nonsalient)?

Ignore any or all data
Make (most likely) an unsound decision.

Actively attend to all data.

❹ Which data are cultural, and which are idiosyncratic?

❺ How do base rates apply to cultural data?

❻ Which stressors are dispositional, and which are environmental?

❼ Which data are clinically significant, and which are insignificant?

❽ What is my working hypothesis?

Test the hypothesis.

❾ What is my conclusive assessment decision?
a) What is the nature of psychopathology (if any)?
b) How do nonpathological but clinically significant data fit into the assessment conclusion?

Sound, Accurate Assessment

FIGURE 2.1. Assessment decision tree.

cess, they also should strive to balance it with objectivity and appreciate its ability to illuminate the intricacies of clients' experiences.

• *Sixth, a sound assessment has clinical utility.* Indeed, without sound assessments at their core, treatment plans would have little chance of being effective. To better understand this concept, consider the effects of an absent or unsound assessment. Clinicians who fail to conduct initial assessments of their clients have no way of measuring therapeutic change. Furthermore, if treatment plans stem from assessment data, inaccurate assessment data would yield misguided interventions. Accurate, complete assessments, on the other hand, form solid foundations for effective treatment plans.

• *Seventh, culture is always pertinent to psychological assessment.* Clinicians therefore should continuously ask themselves, "How is culture relevant to understanding this client?" rather than, "Is culture relevant to understanding this client?" This mind-set encourages practitioners to consider not only how minority and nonminority clients' backgrounds influence assessment but also how their own culture affects this process.

• *Eighth, assessment should include dispositional and environmental factors, either of which can impair normal functioning.* Stressors occur in a cultural context, and clients express them through unique cultural lenses, regardless of whether they stem from dispositional factors (e.g., personality), environmental factors (e.g., poverty), or a combination of both. Furthermore, practitioners observe and interpret these stressors through their own cultural lenses. Granted, disentangling social stressors from dispositional stressors often is difficult. Our MAP attempts to help clinicians determine where culture-specific normative behavior ends and pathology begins, and it guides practitioners to move beyond personal cultural assumptions while making clinical decisions.

• *Ninth, sound assessment requires a systematic methodology based on a conceptually coherent framework.* After all, given the complexity inherent in all clients' lives, clinicians must piece together a potentially overwhelming array of data to generate a case conceptualization. Some sort of conceptual framework is enormously helpful to guide the gathering, interpretation, and integration of these data. Our MAP is one attempt to provide this framework.

• *Tenth, psychological assessment is a challenging responsibility.* As we mentioned earlier, clinicians are ethically obligated to conduct accurate and complete assessments regardless of their clients' cultural background. We recognize that this task is difficult and potentially intimidating. We hope, however, that instead of shying away from this challenge, trainees and practitioners will consider our MAP and strive even harder to perform sound assessments.

THE MAP

Now that we have described our philosophy of assessment, outlined relevant critical issues, and established the necessity of considering culture in case formulation, the time has come to operationalize the MAP, which is depicted in Figure 2.2. The MAP features three distinguishing characteristics. First, it is pragmatic. As the figure indicates, it outlines concrete guidelines and microdecisions to promote sound multicultural assessment. Furthermore, the MAP is flexible. Although its guidelines are systematic and logical, it encourages complex cognition while discouraging simplistic, rigid thinking. Finally, the MAP is cyclical. When clinicians learn new information during the therapeutic process, they can recycle through the MAP to incorporate these data and, if necessary, modify their decisions. Indeed, we encourage practitioners to monitor their clinical thought processes and to maintain cultural self-awareness throughout assessment and case formulation. Such continuous self-reflection is critical to becoming an expert practitioner (Goodyear, 1997; Ridley et al., 2005; Ronnestad & Skovholt, 2003).

Aside from these general characteristics, the MAP encompasses three operational features. First, the MAP integrates decision points throughout the assessment process, allowing clinicians to address the microdecisions

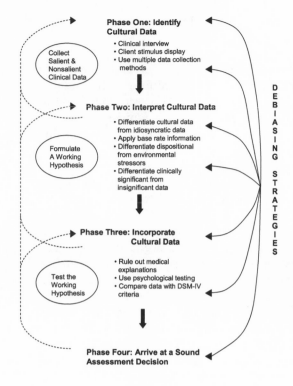

FIGURE 2.2. Multicultural assessment procedure.

outlined in Figure 2.1 and reminding them that each microdecision is vital
to sound assessment and case formulation. Second, the procedure comprises four progressive phases. The first phase, identify cultural data, involves gathering salient (overt) and nonsalient (covert) clinical data through
multiple data collection methods. The second phase, interpret cultural data,
asks practitioners to organize and interpret cultural information to arrive at
a working hypothesis. The third phase, incorporate cultural data, encompasses integrating cultural information with other relevant data so clinicians can test their working hypotheses. The fourth phase entails reaching a
sound assessment decision. We urge practitioners to recycle through the
procedure as necessary after this phase, as well as to examine their assessment decisions during the entire process. The MAP's final operational
feature comprises its debiasing strategies, which aim to minimize clinical
judgment errors. These strategies do not compose a separate phase of the
MAP; rather, clinicians can use them to improve accuracy throughout the
procedure. Before discussing these strategies, however, we describe the
MAP's fundamental phases in more detail.

Phase 1: Identify Cultural Data

Clinical Interview

Amidst the array of assessment methods available to practitioners, the clinical interview is the most popular tool for gathering data (Watkins, Campbell, Nieberding, & Hallmark, 1995). Although clinical interviews are susceptible to practitioners' flawed judgments (Meehl, 1966), they allow clinicians to acquire a wide variety of information during the assessment process. Indeed, according to Zimmerman (1994), asking about clients' medical, psychiatric, and social histories is essential to any clinical interview. Because culture always is relevant in assessment, exploring clients' cultural background also is crucial to a comprehensive clinical interview (Ridley et al., 1998).

Given that culture is a complex construct, trainees and practitioners might wonder where they should begin in identifying and gathering relevant cultural data. As a starting point, clinicians can ask their clients to describe and clarify their cultural background (Scott & Borodovsky, 1990). However, to avoid burdening clients with the responsibility of educating them, practitioners can use structured interviews, which will help maximize the thoroughness of their cultural data search. The Person-In-Culture Interview (Berg-Cross & Chinen, 1995), for example, comprises 24 open-ended questions to help clinicians gather cultural data and avoid stereotyping clients. Practitioners also can draw from Locke's (1992) list of 10 types of cultural information as they conduct clinical interviews: level of acculturation, economic issues, history of oppression, language, experience of racism and prejudice, sociopolitical issues, methods of childrearing, religious and spiritual practices, family composition, and cultural value.

Client Stimulus Display

When clients come to counseling, they bring with them a tremendous amount of information about their life and experiences. Clinicians usually do not know this information in advance, which is why they assess clients. Given the different types of data clients can harbor about themselves, assessment can pose quite a challenge. Granted, most clients present overt data that are easy to identify, including obvious mannerisms and self-disclosures. Many clinicians are tempted to end their assessments with this salient data (López & Hernandez, 1987), but doing so yields incomplete results, thereby increasing the likelihood of ineffective treatment. Thus, along with overt data, practitioners also must seek out and integrate covert data. Covert data are not automatically identifiable, and they can include issues such as unexpressed conflicts, implicit cultural values, and repressed memories.

As they conduct their assessments, practitioners can divide both overt and covert data into two subcategories: idiosyncratic and cultural data.

Cultural data encompass what would be expected of any person from the client's culture and usually reflect that client's cultural norms. Idiosyncratic data, on the other hand, are unique to the client and would not necessarily be expected of other clients from the culture in question.

As mentioned earlier, gathering overt data typically is not very labor intensive for clinicians because this information is largely obvious. Once they recognize these salient data, practitioners can work through the first decision point outlined in our assessment philosophy: After collecting salient data, will I make an assessment decision based solely on that information? At this point, some clinicians might feel ready to reach an assessment decision. They should remember, however, that initial interviews rarely yield enough data to inform a sound conclusion. Indeed, unless clients are especially open, cooperative, and insightful, practitioners will need to move beyond immediately obvious salient data and probe for more obscure nonsalient data. This situation brings practitioners to the second decision point: What methods should I use to collect nonsalient data?

Use Multiple Data Collection Methods

Although the clinical interview is the most common tool for gathering client data, other methods might be necessary to uncover the information needed for sound assessment. These alternative methods can be especially useful for ascertaining covert data, and they promote the cognitively complex approach to case formulation that we advocate. Dana (1993) recommended taking life histories, for example, which allow clients to tell their life stories without restriction from clinicians. He also suggested conducting behavioral observations to infer nonobservable personality traits from observable actions. Other data collection methods include assessing clients' development on psychological and cultural constructs, obtaining post-assessment narratives, and involving the family network in the assessment process (Ridley et al., 1998). After using multiple means of gathering overt and covert client information, practitioners can address the third decision point in our model: How do I respond to all data (salient and nonsalient)? This question brings us to our MAP's next phase.

Phase 2: Interpret Cultural Data

Differentiate Cultural from Idiosyncratic Data

After gathering overt and covert data through multiple methods, clinicians usually face a potentially overwhelming mountain of information. Granted, they could ignore some or all of these data, but this choice would signify incompetence: Even if the information proves to be unimportant, neglecting it can lead to Type II error, overlooking clinically significant information.

We therefore encourage practitioners to attend actively to all assessment data, at least to some degree.

Clinicians can begin actively attending to client information by asking themselves, Which data are cultural, and which are idiosyncratic? To answer this question, practitioners should ask their clients about their personal meanings and experiences and compare them with cultural norms. When these meanings and experiences overlap with established norms, it is safe to assume that cultural norms apply. For example, when clinicians ask their clients about their personal conception of gender roles, they can apply cultural gender norms if (and only if) their clients' notions coincide with those of their culture. Practitioners can arrive at four different conclusions when differentiating cultural from idiosyncratic data: They can correctly conclude data are cultural, incorrectly conclude data are cultural, correctly conclude data are idiosyncratic, and incorrectly conclude data are idiosyncratic. Arriving at a correct verdict requires counselors to consider another decision point: How do base rates apply to cultural data?

Apply Base Rate Information to Cultural Data

Some authors have argued that failing to use statistical norms, or base rates, in assessment is unethical (e.g., Norcross, 1991). Given the multitude of relevant research findings, however, many clinicians are uncertain about which base rate information to attend to. Base rates regarding psychological disorders, comorbid conditions, medical conditions that manifest psychological symptoms, and suicide rates in different populations probably are the most important for practitioners to learn (Ridley et al., 1998). Although no single, consolidated source exists as a base rate reference, PsycInfo and other database searches, as well as Internet searches, can direct practitioners to books, articles, and chapters devoted to topics of interest, which often will include base rate information. Once clinicians do locate pertinent base rates, they must be sure to apply them to cultural rather than idiosyncratic data. Indeed, interpreting idiosyncratic data, which is unique to the client, by using normative base rate information would be illogical. This caveat highlights the importance of the previous decision point: distinguishing cultural from idiosyncratic data.

Differentiate Dispositional Stressors from Environmental Stressors

To help organize the large mass of client information and to move toward a working hypothesis, clinicians should determine which symptoms stem from within-client origins (i.e., dispositional stressors) and which stem from outside-the-client circumstances (i.e., environmental stressors). Of course, separating dispositional from environmental stressors can be tricky: People rarely experience only one stressor at a time, and both types of stressors often occur simultaneously, usually becoming tightly intertwined (Ridley, 1984). Practitioners can ask themselves a series of questions to ease the categorization process, however, including: What is the typical amount of stress a person in similar circumstances with similar beliefs, values, and customs as my client would experience from particular types of stressors? What are culturally adaptive and culturally maladaptive reactions to such stressors in my client's culture? What type of reaction is my client exhibiting? How much control does my client have over stressors? What is the degree to which the stressors are desired and not desired? How many stressors must the client manage at one time? (Canino & Spurlock, 1994; Newhill, 1990; Sinacore-Guinn, 1995).

Differentiate Clinically Significant from Clinically Insignificant Data

Although we recommended earlier that clinicians attend to all clinical data, there comes a point where they must decide which information is significant and insignificant in generating a working hypothesis. Answers to the three previous decision points—distinguishing cultural from idiosyncratic data, applying base rates to cultural data, and differentiating dispositional from environmental stressors—usually provide insight into data's significance, so practitioners should reserve judgment in this realm until they have worked through the other steps of this phase. Once they have addressed these decision points, clinicians should obtain clients' perspectives on the assessment data. Five questions especially relevant to discussions about cultural data are:

1. What do you think has caused the symptom?
2. Why do you think it started when it did?
3. What do you think the symptom does to you?
4. How severe is the symptom? Will it last a long or short time?
5. What kind of treatment do you think will relieve the symptom (Kleinman, 1979; Ridley et al., 1998)?

Sometimes clients' answers will generate additional insight into their presenting issue. Other times, after reflecting on their knowledge and training, clinicians will determine that clients' interpretations are unsound. Nevertheless, collaborating with clients during this decision-making process will increase practitioners' likelihood of correctly categorizing data as significant or insignificant.

Formulate a Working Hypothesis

After working through the seven decision points involved in identifying and interpreting cultural data, clinicians are ready to construct a working hypothesis. We offer seven guidelines for tackling this task (Ridley et al., 1998). First, practitioners should determine the psychological consequences of a behavior for their client; is it self-defeating or self-enhancing? Second, they should determine whether clients' cultural values contribute to impairment in the context in which the client is living. Third, they should decide whether clients' cultural behaviors represent extremes, even for members of the client's native culture. Fourth, clinicians should reframe psychological deficits as possible assets and consider whether dynamics that initially seem to be strengths actually could be detrimental. Fifth, they should interpret clients' psychological functioning alongside environmental and sociocultural influences. Sixth, they should gather clients' interpretations of the presenting issue. Seventh, practitioners should avoid distorting clients' psychological presentation with their own cultural biases and assumptions.

Some of these guidelines will apply to every client (e.g., guideline 1), whereas others might not be relevant in certain cases (e.g., guideline 2). Still, if clinicians consider and work through each guideline, they can arrive at tentative conclusions regarding the normalcy and abnormality of assessment data. They key word here is "tentative," however: By nature, working hypotheses are subject to testing and revision. The next phase addresses three strategies for hypothesis testing.

Phase 3: Incorporate Cultural Data

Rule Out Medical Explanations

More than half of the diagnoses listed in DSM-IV-TR have potential organic causes (American Psychiatric Association, 2000). Clinicians therefore should try to determine if clients' psychological presentation might have biological roots. Although information gathered during the clinical interview can help practitioners rule out medical explanations to some degree, referring clients to physicians also might be appropriate for properly testing working hypotheses.

Use Psychological Testing

Rather than conducting "fishing expeditions" with batteries of tests to generate hypotheses, clinicians should use psychological testing to evaluate the working hypotheses from phase 2 (Spengler et al., 1995). Given the vast array of tests available, practitioners could not possibly be experts on all psychological measures. They therefore must recognize the limits of their competence and refer clients for testing when clients' needs fall outside these bounds. If clinicians lack supervised training in testing non-native English speakers, for example, they should refer these clients to someone who is competent in this area (American Psychological Association, 1985). Furthermore, when practitioners do administer tests themselves, they should recognize the bias and error inherent in many psychological measures (Helms, 1992; Hinkle, 1994; Prediger, 1994; Sedlacek, 1994).

Compare Data with DSM-IV Criteria

Because diagnoses can enhance communication among professionals and sometimes reflect clinical realities, they are an important part of the assessment process (Nelson-Gray, 1994). Nevertheless, many diagnoses are not valid across cultures (Castillo, 1997). Thus, although we encourage practitioners to compare client data with DSM-IV criteria, we view it as only one piece of the multicultural assessment puzzle and only one step in hypothesis testing. Indeed, only after clinicians have compared assessment information with DSM-IV criteria, employed psychological testing, and ruled out medical explanations should they proceed to the ninth decision point: What is my conclusive assessment decision? The steps outlined in phase 3 can help practitioners answer this question by clarifying the nature of any existing psychopathology, as well as the relevance of nonpathological but clinically significant data.

Phase 4: Arrive at a Sound Assessment Decision

By identifying, interpreting, and incorporating cultural data in the first three phases of the MAP, clinicians should generate sound, accurate, and complete multicultural assessment decisions. The work does not end at phase 4, however. Because the helping process is fluid, important client information can emerge at any time and must be incorporated into case formulations. The MAP's recyclable nature speaks to this fluidity and highlights the value of practitioners' flexibility and cognitive complexity.

Potential Pitfalls and Debiasing Strategies

Although subjectivity is a valuable aspect of multicultural assessment and case formulation, clinicians should work to minimize the effects of bias to reduce the likelihood of judgment errors. After all, the consequences of faulty assessment can be grave, including inappropriate and ineffective treatment that can prolong or worsen clients' conditions (Butcher, 1997; Hill & Spengler, 1997; Rollock & Terrell, 1996). We offer guidelines to promote practitioners' cognitive complexity and accuracy in assessment.

Judgmental Heuristics and Related Debiasing Strategies

Judgmental heuristics are quick decision rules that clinicians usually execute automatically, often short-circuiting the decision-making process and defeating the scientific, complex thinking essential to sound assessment (Ridley et al., 1998; Spengler et al., 1995). Three heuristics relate particularly closely to assessment: availability, anchoring, and representativeness. Availability heuristics involve making decisions based on the most salient, readily available clinical information (Kahneman, Slovic, & Tversky, 1982; Morrow & Deidan, 1992). A practitioner specializing in depression, for example, might focus on client information that conforms to depression criteria and make clinical judgments based solely on this information, even though equally important data might exist. Anchoring heuristics, on the other hand, entail focusing on the first information gathered in assessment and downplaying the data acquired later in the process (Friedlander & Stockman, 1983). For instance, a practitioner might base clinical decisions only on information collected during intakes and fail to incorporate subsequent data. Finally, representativeness heuristics involve depending on existing cognitive schemas, which can lead to assuming false relationships between client characteristics and diagnostic categories (Nisbett & Ross, 1980; Spengler et al., 1995). A clinician might assume that Asian clients are achievement oriented with few emotional problems, for example, without considering this population's high rate of psychosomatic issues (Ridley et al., 1998). Indeed, representativeness heuristics often entail stereotyping and ignoring base rates.

Luckily, there are several strategies for overcoming these heuristics. First, practitioners can search for alternative explanations of client behavior, including racism, nutritional deficiency, socioeconomic factors, and educational issues (Arkes, 1981; Ridley, 2005). Clinicians also can conceptualize alternative interpretations of behavior; reframing apparent weaknesses as strengths is one example of this strategy (Ridley et al., 1998). Finally, practitioners can delay decision making until they have devoted sufficient time to hypothesis testing (Spengler et al., 1995). The MAP incorporates this strategy by proposing four recyclable stages to work through before making final clinical conclusions.

Confirmatory Bias and Disconfirmatory Hypothesis Testing

When practitioners confirm their hypotheses without trying to disprove them, they show confirmatory bias (Dumont, 1993). This bias often leads to diagnosing pathology without sufficient evidence to support this conclusion (Rosenhan, 1973). To combat confirmatory bias, Morrow and Deidan (1992) suggest several strategies: Ask a combination of confirming and disconfirming questions about working hypotheses, remain open to data that contradict working hypotheses, and consider reasons why working hypotheses might be incorrect.

APPLICATION ACROSS CASE FORMULATION METHODS

Most of this book's remaining chapters describe various approaches to case formulation. These methods do share some similarities, but they are largely independent of each other. The MAP is different, however. Although the MAP is useful as a stand-alone process, it becomes especially powerful when combined with other approaches to assessment. Indeed, no matter what case formulation method or theoretical orientation clinicians adopt, they always must account for clients' culture. After all, as described earlier, culture permeates all aspects of human experience, and treatment always occurs within a cultural context. Given culture's central role in the helping process, ignoring or mishandling cultural considerations during case formulation likely will lead to misdiagnosis and mistreatment. On the other hand, basing case formulations on accurate, thorough, impartial assessment data can increase the probability of sound treatment. The MAP can guide clinicians in conducting the culturally sensitive assessments crucial to any case formulation procedure.

Because the MAP and the other methods outlined in this book share some features, blending these approaches should be relatively seamless. For example, the MAP rests on the scientist–practitioner model and its inherent hypothesis testing. This model permeates the plan formulation method (PFM), which views the plan formulation as a constantly evaluated working hypothesis. It also surfaces in cognitive-behavioral case formulations, which use working hypotheses as the basis of treatment plans. Furthermore, just as the MAP advocates recycling the assessment process throughout treatment, both the PFM and time-limited dynamic psychotherapy (TLDP) incorporate continual evaluation and refinement of working hypotheses.

The MAP also includes techniques that can supplement other approaches to case formulation. Clinicians can employ the MAP's debiasing strategies throughout the treatment process, for instance, regardless of their theoretical orientation. In addition, our MAP suggests a variety of assessment methods for identifying and attending to clients' cultural and idiosyncratic data. Some case formulation methods also encourage practitioners to gather a broad range of client information; configurational analysis, for example, advocates noting both verbal and nonverbal data. Other methods, including interpersonal psychotherapy of depression, rely mainly on clinical interviews and common standardized measures to assess clients. The data-gathering strategies and decision questions posed in the MAP can inform these methods and increase the likelihood of sound case formulation.

CASE EXAMPLE

To illustrate the application of the MAP, we provide the following case example from Ridley et al. (1998).

Maria is a 24-year-old single, Mexican American female. She went to her community mental health center because she "just hasn't felt herself lately." On the intake form, she indicated feeling "pretty down," "unhappy with herself," and "unable to do much lately." Maria was referred to a white male clinician with 2 years' experience.

Phase 1: Identify Cultural Data

The clinician began his work with Maria by conducting a clinical interview. In addition to the general clinical interview, he conducted the Person-In-Culture Interview (Berg-Cross & Chinen, 1995) to glean more personal meaning from Maria's cultural data. During this interview process, the clinician gathered overt clinical data. Maria's family had no history of psychological problems, but they did use social services after immigrating to the United States to ease their adjustment to a new culture. Maria was in first grade when her family left Mexico, and she took bilingual classes, which helped her adjust and succeed in school. She now lives in a predominately Hispanic community in a midwestern city. Maria described her current mood as depressed, and she said she has been isolating herself and sleeping more than usual. Although Maria was oriented to person, place, and time during the interview, she seemed disheveled and somewhat guarded.

After this initial session, the practitioner discussed Maria in supervision. The clinician and his supervisor first addressed Maria's guardedness and identified three possible interpretations of this behavior: Maria might have reacted to unintentional racism by the clinician; she might have shown cultural transference, guarding herself against the white clinician because of negative interactions with white people in the past; or the clinician might have exhibited cultural countertransference, guarding himself against the Mexican American client because of negative interactions with Mexican Americans in his life. The supervisor and practitioner decided they needed more information about Maria's guardedness, so they decided to monitor this issue instead of reaching a quick conclusion. Next, they addressed the first decision point in the MAP: After collecting salient data, will I make an assessment decision based solely on that information? Although the clinician had been assuming Maria was depressed, his supervisor cautioned that there was not enough evidence to make that conclusion. Recognizing his confirmatory bias, the clinician decided to delay his decision making and to search for additional data.

After supervision, the clinician considered the second decision point: What methods should I use to collect nonsalient data? He decided to conduct a behavioral analysis and asked Maria to track her interactions with others, which revealed Maria's avoidance behaviors when she faced interpersonal conflict. The clinician also used a postassessment narrative to clarify culture's role in Maria's clinical picture. This follow-up questioning illuminated the origin of Maria's avoidance: When Maria was in middle school, she was hit in the head with a rock when she became entangled in a confrontation between white and Hispanic students. She has avoided confrontation ever since. The postassessment narrative also revealed Maria's recent experience of racism in medical school, which led her to withdraw despite her full scholarship. The clinician then used other tools to uncover covert data, including the Acculturation Rating Scale for Mexican Americans (Cuéllar, Harris, & Jasso, 1980), which pointed toward Maria's healthy biculturalism and ethnic/racial identity. Also, with Maria's consent, the clinician interviewed her mother and sister, who said her depression likely stemmed from her withdrawal from medical school. The results of these assessments brought the clinician to the third decision point: How do I respond to all data (salient and nonsalient)?

Phase 2: Interpret Cultural Data

Although the clinician knew he must consider all cultural data to arrive at a sound working hypothesis, he doubted that everything he had learned about Maria was significant. He was tempted to discount Maria's family's interpretation of her feelings, but his supervisor identified this temptation as the anchoring heuristic: The clinician favored data consistent with depression presented earlier in the assessment process and hesitated to incorporate the information gathered later on. The clinician therefore decided to consider all data and began working through the next four decision points.

He first asked, Which data are cultural, and which are idiosyncratic? Among other issues, he considered Maria's avoidance tendencies and determined they were sometimes idiosyncratic and sometimes cultural. They were idiosyncratic when Maria avoided any type of interpersonal conflict, but they were cultural when she exhibited healthy cultural paranoia given her experiences with racism.

He next asked, How do base rates apply to cultural data? After consulting relevant research, he found that people at particularly great risk for high stress levels include first-generation Hispanic students (Billson & Terry, 1982) and those who experience interruptions while pursuing higher education (Luther & Dukes, 1982). Because this information applied to Maria, the clinician incorporated it into his assessment.

The clinician then asked, Which stressors are dispositional, and which are environmental? He determined that Maria's depressed mood, isolation, and hypersomnia were dispositional, whereas her experiences with racism was environmental.

Finally, the clinician considered, Which data are clinically significant, and which are insignificant? He decided that most of Maria's data were significant, but her need for bilingual classes early in her education was unrelated to her leaving medical school. In fact, her bilingualism actually reflected a strength the clinician could consider in his assessment.

After addressing these questions, the clinician began generating a working hypothesis. Although not every guideline for constructing working hypotheses applies to every multicultural assessment, the clinician drew from several of them, including:

• *Determine the psychological consequences of a behavior for the individual—that is, whether the dynamic is self-defeating or self-enhancing.* The clinician examined the psychological consequences of Maria's avoidance of interpersonal conflict and determined that this pattern both heightened her depressed mood and paralyzed her pursuit of her professional goals. The clinician therefore concluded this dynamic was self-defeating for Maria.

• *Determine whether a client's cultural behavior represents an extreme even for members of the client's culture.* The clinician recognized that one cultural value, *sympatía,* related to Maria's clinical picture. Sympatía is a "general tendency toward avoiding interpersonal conflict, emphasizing positive behavior in agreeable situations, and de-emphasizing negative behaviors in conflictual circumstances" (Triandis, Marín, Lisansky, & Betancourt, 1984). Although the clinician respected this value, he realized Maria exhibits an extreme version by avoiding interpersonal conflict at unhealthy costs.

• *Do not distort the psychological presentation with one's biases and assumptions.* The clinician considered his biases and assumptions about Maria when listening to audiotapes of his sessions during supervision. The tapes revealed the clinician using phrases such as "your people" and "I've seen other Hispanics who feel that way." The clinician and supervisor explored two issues: (1) cultural countertransference toward Maria given the clinician's previous emotionally challenging experiences with Hispanics and (2) Maria's low level of self-disclosure stemming from this countertransference. Reexamining Maria's guardedness, the clinician and supervisor concluded that countertransference sparked this behavior and that the guardedness therefore had a realistic cultural foundation.

After working through these guidelines, the clinician developed this working hypothesis: Maria is experiencing a mood disorder of the depressive type that is exacerbated by her past experiences with racism. In addition, she is experiencing avoidant personality disorder based on her avoidant behaviors, especially in the context of interpersonal conflict.

Phase 3: Incorporate Cultural Data

Adhering to the scientist–practitioner model, the clinician then tested his working hypothesis in three ways. First, he ruled out medical explanations by asking Maria to undergo a medical physical exam, as she had not seen her doctor in more than 2 years. The exam revealed hypothyroidism, which often yields depressive symptoms. The clinician therefore concluded Maria's depression might partly relate to this medical condition.

Next, the clinician used a battery of psychological tests to augment his assessment, including the Minnesota Multiphasic Personality Inventory, Second Edition (MMPI-2) (Hathaway & McKinley, 1991). He referred to

Velásquez et al. (1997) to ensure appropriate administration of the test; they recommended using the MMPI-2 with Mexican Americans; always administering the complete MMPI-2; considering Mexican American clients' test-taking history; and determining the most appropriate language for MMPI-2 testing. The MMPI-2 results indicated an open, nondefensive test-taking approach, moderately high elevation on depression with mild somatic complaints, and other clinical scales within normal limits. Other tests suggested that Maria was experiencing high occupational/economic stress and high family/cultural stress, as well as a strong concern with social affiliation. Given these results, the clinician concluded that Maria does not meet the criteria for full-blown avoidant personality disorder; instead, she exhibits avoidant personality features in specific situations.

Finally, the clinician compared Maria's clinical data with the diagnostic criteria of certain DSM disorders. To explore alternative interpretations of Maria's presentation, he considered major depressive disorder and dysthymic disorder given the client's depressed mood, hypersomnia, and social isolation. He ruled these out, however, because of Maria's thyroid condition, her lack of previous depressive or manic episodes, and her intact reality orientation. The clinician also reaffirmed ruling out avoidant personality disorder, as Maria's avoidance occurs only in interpersonally conflictual situations.

Phase 4: Arrive at a Sound Assessment Decision

In this phase, the clinician addressed the last decision point in the MAP: What is my conclusive assessment decision? He examined two subquestions: (1) What is the nature of psychopathology, if any? and (2) How do nonpathological but clinically significant data fit into the assessment conclusion? The clinician determined that Maria was experiencing a mood disorder with depressive symptoms that stem partly from hypothyroidism. Environmental stressors, including racism, exacerbated her dispositionally based depression. Furthermore, conflicting cultural expectations complicated her presenting problems. The value of sympatía reinforced Maria's tendency to avoid the interpersonal conflict she will encounter when facing the racism in medical school, but this avoidance has created distress for Maria, who always has been a dedicated student. In light of these data, the clinician assigned this five-axis diagnosis to Maria:

- Axis I: 293.93 Mood disorder due to hypothyroidism with depressive features
- Axis II: V71.09 Avoidant personality features
- Axis III: 244.9 Hypothyroidism
- Axis IV: Victim of racism, conflicting cultural expectations
- Axis V: Current GAF = 55, highest in the past year = 70

This clinical assessment provides direction for treatment planning. With the MAP to guide his assessment, the clinician could use debiasing strategies throughout the process and make culturally sensitive, comprehensive decisions. If he had relied solely on traditional assessment approaches, the clinician likely would have overlooked relevant cultural information, and the client's treatment plan might have been less sound.

IMPLICATIONS FOR TRAINING

We have tried to make the MAP as user-friendly as possible by describing clear, concrete phases and strategies in the multicultural assessment process. Nevertheless, students can take several steps to start learning and applying our model. For example, one key to sound assessment and case formulation is increasing one's cognitive complexity and practicing metacognition. These measures are central to developing expertise (Goodyear, 1997), and they relate to the MAP's emphasis on the scientist–practitioner model, reflection, and self-awareness. Students therefore should focus not only on helping skills but also on their cognition and affect throughout their training, including their motivation levels (Ericsson, Krampe, & Tesch-Romer, 1993). Through self-monitoring, self-evaluation, and supervision, trainees can start developing cultural self-awareness, identifying their biases, and learning their realm of competence (Paniagua, 1994; Solomon, 1992).

Students also can build their knowledge in several areas to enhance their ability to use the MAP. They should become familiar with the scientific method, for instance, which will increase their comfort with hypothesis formulation, testing, and revision. Trainees also should begin building a cultural knowledge base, including base rate information and cultural, social, political, and psychological issues likely to arise among the population with which they will work. In the classroom, considering how such cultural factors integrate into theory and practice will prepare students for incorporating culture into assessment (Constantine, 1998).

Trainees also can prepare to use the MAP by researching, learning, and practicing a variety of assessment methods. These methods should include behavioral observations, life histories, postassessment narratives, and involving the family network, and they collectively should yield a picture comprising both cultural and idiosyncratic data. When dealing with standardized tests, students should research the composition of standardization samples and search for any possible bias in the tests' construction, administration, and interpretation. Finally, when learning about diagnosis, trainees should consider the strengths and weaknesses of DSM diagnostic categories, especially in light of clients' cultural and individual backgrounds (Castillo, 1997).

RESEARCH SUPPORT FOR THE APPROACH

As of this writing, research examining the MAP has been limited. Although some theoretical explorations of the MAP have surfaced, including Levy and Plucker's (2003) discussion of the MAP's potential for assessing gifted and talented clients, the authors are unaware of any empirical studies examining the MAP as a whole. This lack of scientific investigation might stem from the MAP's relatively recent development; perhaps insufficient time has elapsed to allow for significant empirical study. Furthermore, given its multiple phases and strategies for culturally sensitive assessment and case formulation, the MAP is quite complex, so researching the entire process would be challenging. Nevertheless, all the MAP's phases and components are grounded in empirical research. Although page constraints prevent us from discussing this research in detail, readers can consult the citations listed throughout the chapter and Ridley et al. (1998) to learn more about the empirical support for our approach.

CONCLUSION

At the beginning of this chapter, we acknowledged the good intentions of trainees and practitioners in the mental health field. Most of these people want to generate comprehensive, accurate assessments and case formulations, regardless of their clients' cultural backgrounds. The problem is that many trainees and clinicians are unsure how to work toward this goal. The MAP was developed to provide them with much-needed direction. Granted, multicultural assessment and case formulation initially can seem overwhelming. However, we hope our model's concrete guidelines not only will prevent discouragement but also will inspire students and clinicians who genuinely want to follow their profession's ethical guidelines for multicultural competence.

REFERENCES

Altarriba, J., & Santiago-Rivera, A. L. (1994). Current perspectives on using linguistic and cultural factors in counseling the Hispanic client. *Professional Psychology: Research and Practice, 25*, 388–379.

American Psychiatric Association. (2000). *Diagnostic and statistical manual of mental disorders* (4th ed., text rev.). Washington, DC: Author.

American Psychological Association. (1985). *Standards for educational and psychological testing*. Washington, DC: Author.

American Psychological Association, Office of Ethnic Minority Affairs. (1993). Guidelines for providers of psychological services to ethnic, linguistic, and culturally diverse populations. *American Psychologist, 48*, 45–48.

American Psychological Association. (2002). Ethical principles and code of conduct. *American Psychologist, 57,* 1060–1073.

Arkes, H. R. (1981). Impediments to accurate clinical judgment and possible ways to minimize their impact. *Journal of Consulting and Clinical Psychology, 49,* 323–330.

Berg-Cross, L., & Chinen, R. T. (1995). Multicultural training models and the Person-In-Culture Interview. In J. G. Ponterotto, J. M. Casas, L. A. Suzuki, & C. M. Alexander (Eds.), *Handbook of multicultural counseling* (pp. 333–356). Thousand Oaks, CA: Sage.

Billson, J. M., & Terry, M. B. (1982). In search of the silken purse: Factors in attrition among first generation students. *College and University, 58,* 57–75.

Bond, M. H., & Smith, P. B. (1996). Cross-cultural, social, and organizational psychology. *Annual Review of Psychology, 47,* 205–235.

Butcher, J. N. (1997). Introduction to the special section on assessment in psychological treatment: A necessary step for effective intervention. *Psychological Assessment, 9,* 331–333.

Canino, I. A., & Spurlock, J. (1994). *Culturally diverse children and adolescents: Assessment, diagnosis, and treatment.* New York: Guilford Press.

Castillo, R. J. (1997). *Culture and mental illness: A client-centered approach.* Pacific Grove, CA: Brooks/Cole.

Constantine, M. G. (1998). Developing competence in multicultural assessment: Implications for counseling psychology training and practice. *The Counseling Psychologist, 26*(6), 922–929.

Corcoran, K., & Vandiver, V. (1996). *Maneuvering the maze of managed care.* New York: Free Press.

Cuéllar, I. (1998). Cross-cultural clinical psychological assessment of Hispanic Americans. *Journal of Personality Assessment, 70,* 71–86.

Cuéllar, I., Harris, L., & Jasso, R. (1980). An acculturation scale for Mexican American normal and clinical populations. *Hispanic Journal of Behavioral Science, 2,* 199–217.

Dana, R. H. (1993). *Multicultural assessment perspectives for professional psychology.* Boston: Allyn & Bacon.

Dana, R. H. (2005). *Multicultural assessment: Principles, applications, and examples.* Mahwah, NJ: Erlbaum.

Draguns, J. G. (1989). Dilemmas and choices in cross-cultural counseling: The universal versus the culturally distinctive. In P. B. Pedersen, J. G. Draguns, W. J. Lonner, & J. E. Trimble (Eds.), *Counseling across cultures* (3rd ed., pp. 21–33). Honolulu: University of Hawaii Press.

Dumont, F. (1993). Inferential heuristics in clinical problem formulation: Selective review of their strengths and weaknesses. *Professional Psychology: Research and Practice, 24,* 196–205.

Edwards, A. W. (1982). The consequences of error in selecting treatment for blacks. *Social Casework: The Journal of Contemporary Social Work, 63,* 429–433.

Ericsson, K. A., Krampe, R. T., & Tesch-Romer, C. (1993). The role of deliberate practice in the acquisition of expert performance. *Psychological Review, 100,* 363–406.

Fernandez, R. L., & Kleinman, A. (1994). Culture, personality, and psychopathology. *Journal of Abnormal Psychology, 103,* 67–71.

Friedlander, M. L., & Stockman, S. J. (1983). Anchoring and publicity effects in clinical judgment. *Journal of Consulting and Clinical Psychology, 39,* 637–643.

Good, B. (1993). Culture, diagnosis, and comorbidity. *Culture, Medicine, and Psychiatry, 16,* 427–446.

Good, B., & Good, B. (1986). The cultural context of diagnosis and therapy: A view from medical psychiatry. In M. Miranda & H. Kitano (Eds.), *Mental health research and practice in minority communities: Development of culturally sensitive training programs* (DHHS Publication No. ADM 86-1466, pp. 1–27). Washington, DC: National Institute of Mental Health.

Goodyear, R. K. (1997). Psychological expertise and the role of individual differences: An exploration of issues. *Educational Psychology Review, 9,* 251–265.

Guttfreund, D. G. (1990). Effects of language usage on the emotional experience of Spanish–English and English–Spanish bilinguals. *Journal of Consulting and Clinical Psychology, 58,* 604–607.

Hathaway, S. R., & McKinley, J. C. (1991). *Manual for administration and scoring MMPI-2.* Minneapolis: University of Minnesota Press.

Helms, J. E. (1992). Why is there no study of cultural equivalence in standardized cognitive ability testing? *American Psychologist, 47,* 1083–1101.

Heppner, P. P., Casas, J. M., Carter, J., & Stone, G. L. (2000). The maturation of counseling psychology: Multifaceted perspectives, 1978–1998. In S. D. Brown & R. W. Lent (Eds.), *Handbook of counseling psychology* (3rd ed., pp. 3–49). New York: Wiley.

Hill, C. L., & Spengler, P. S. (1997). Dementia and depression: A process model for differential diagnosis. *Journal of Mental Health Counseling, 19,* 23–29.

Hinkle, J. S. (1994). Practitioners and cross-cultural assessment: A practical guide to information and training. *Measurement and Evaluation in Counseling and Development, 27,* 103–115.

Holloway, E. L., & Wolleat, P. L. K. (1980). Relationship of clinician conceptual level to clinical hypothesis formulation. *Journal of Counseling Psychology, 27,* 539–545.

Kahneman, D., Slovic, P., & Tversky, A. (1982). *Judgment under uncertainty: Heuristics and biases.* London: Cambridge Press.

Kleinman, A. (1979). Sickness as cultural semantics: Issues for an anthropological medicine and psychiatry. In P. Ahmed & G. Coehlo (Eds.), *Toward a new definition of health: Psychosocial dimensions* (pp. 53–65). New York: Plenum Press.

Kress, V. E. W., Eriksen, K. P., Rayle, A. D., & Ford, S. J. W. (2005). The DSM-IV-TR and culture: Considerations for counselors. *Journal of Counseling and Development, 83,* 97–104.

Levy, J. J., & Plucker, J. A. (2003). Assessing the psychological presentation of gifted and talented clients: A multicultural perspective. *Counseling Psychology Quarterly, 16*(3), 229–247.

Lewis, D. O., Balla, D. A., & Shanok, S. S. (1979). Some evidence of race bias in the diagnosis and treatment of the juvenile offender. *American Journal of Orthopsychiatry, 49,* 53–61.

Locke, D. C. (1992). *Increasing multicultural understanding: A comprehensive model.* Newbury Park, CA: Sage.

Lopez, S., & Hernandez, P. (1987). When culture is considered in the evaluation and treatment of Hispanic patients. *Psychotherapy: Theory, Research, and Practice, 24,* 120–126.

Luther, G. H., & Dukes, F. (1982, May). *A study of selected factors associated with the prediction and prevention of minority attrition.* Paper presented at the meeting for the Association for Institutional Research, Denver, CO.

Malgady, R. G. (1996). The question of cultural bias in assessment of diagnosis in ethnic minority clients: Let's reject the null hypothesis. *Professional Psychology: Research and Practice, 27,* 73–77.

Marcos, L. R., Alpert, M., Urcuyo, L., & Kesselman, M. (1973). The effect of interview language on the evaluation of psychopathology in Spanish-American schizophrenic patients. *American Journal of Psychiatry, 130,* 549–553.

Markus, H. R., & Kitayama, S. (1991). Culture and self: Implications for cognition, emotion, and motivation. *Psychological Review, 98,* 224–253.

Marsella, A. J., & Kameoka, V. A. (1989). Ethnocultural issues in the assessment of psychopathology. In S. Wetzler (Ed.), *Measuring mental illness: Psychometric assessment for clinicians* (pp. 231–256). Washington, DC: American Psychiatric Press.

Meehl, P. E. (1966). *Clinical versus statistical prediction: A theoretical analysis and review of the evidence.* Minneapolis: University of Minnesota Press.

Miller, I. J. (1996a). Time-limited brief therapy has gone too far: The result is invisible rationing. *Professional Psychology: Research and Practice, 27,* 567–576.

Miller, I. J. (1996b). Some "short-term therapy values" are a formula for invisible rationing. *Professional Psychology: Research and Practice, 27,* 577–582.

Morrow, K. A., & Deidan, C. T. (1992). Bias in the counseling process: How to recognize and avoid it. *Journal of Counseling and Development, 70,* 571–577.

Nelson-Gray, R. O. (1994). The scientist–practitioner model revisited: Strategies for implementation. *Behavior Change, 11,* 61–75.

Newhill, C. E. (1990). The role of culture in the development of paranoid symptomatology. *American Journal of Orthopsychiatry, 60,* 176–185.

Nisbett, R., & Ross, L. (1980). *Human inference: Strategies and shortcomings of human judgment.* Englewood Cliffs, NJ: Prentice-Hall.

Norcross, J. C. (1991). Prescriptive matching in psychotherapy: An introduction. *Psychotherapy, 28,* 439–443.

Paniagua, F. A. (1994). *Assessing and treating culturally diverse clients: A practical guide.* Thousand Oaks, CA: Sage.

Pedersen, P. (1994). Series editor's introduction. In F. A. Paniagua (Ed.), *Assessing and treating culturally diverse clients: A practical guide* (pp. vii–ix). Thousand Oaks, CA: Sage.

Prediger, D. J. (1994). Multicultural assessment standards: A compilation for counselors. *Measurement and Evaluation in Counseling and Development, 27,* 68–73.

Ramirez, D. E. (1994). Toward a concept of the counselor as philosopher/practitioner: Commentary on Whitaker, Geller, and Webb. *Journal of College Student Psychotherapy, 9,* 63–74.

Ramirez, S. Z., Wassef, A., Paniagua, F. A., & Linskey, A. O. (1996). Mental health providers' perceptions of cultural variables in evaluating ethnically diverse clients. *Professional Psychology: Research and Practice, 27,* 284–288.

Richardson, L. M., & Austad, C. S. (1991). Realities of mental health practice in managed care settings. *Professional Psychology: Research and Practice, 22,* 52–59.

Ridley, C. R. (1984). Clinical treatment of the nondisclosing black client: A therapeutic paradox. *American Psychologist, 39,* 1234–1244.

Ridley, C. R. (2005). *Overcoming unintentional racism in counseling and psychotherapy: A practitioner's guide to intentional intervention* (2nd ed.). Thousand Oaks, CA: Sage.

Ridley, C. R., Kelly, S. M., Mollen, D. R., & Kleiner, A. (2005, August). Forging new ground: Addressing issues of complexity in counselor training. In C. R. Ridley (Chair), *Beyond microskills: Embracing the complexity of training and practice.* Symposium conducted at the annual meeting of the American Psychological Association, Washington, DC.

Ridley, C. R., Li, L. C., & Hill, C. L. (1998). Multicultural assessment: Reexamination, reconceptualization, and practical application. *The Counseling Psychologist, 26*(6), 827– 910.

Ridley, C. R., Mendoza, D. W., Kanitz, B. E., Angermeier, L., & Zenk, R. (1994). Cultural sensitivity in multicultural counseling: A perceptual schema model. *Journal of Counseling Psychology, 41*, 125–136.

Rogler, L. H. (1992). The role of culture in mental health diagnosis: The need for programmatic research. *Journal of Nervous and Mental Disease, 180*, 745–747.

Rogler, L. H. (1993a). Culturally sensitizing psychiatric diagnosis: A framework for research. *Journal of Nervous and Mental Disease, 181*, 401–408.

Rogler, L. H. (1993b). Culture in psychiatric diagnosis: An issue of scientific accuracy. *Psychiatry, 56*, 324–327.

Rollock, D., & Terrell, M. D. (1996). Multicultural issues in assessment: Toward an inclusive model. In J. L. DeLucia-Waack (Ed.), *Multicultural counseling competencies: Implications for training and practice* (pp. 113–153). Alexandria, VA: Association for Counselor Education and Supervision.

Ronnestad, M. H., & Skovholt, T. M. (2003). The journey of the counselor and therapist: Research findings and perspectives on professional development. *Journal of Career Development, 30*, 5–44.

Rosenhan, D. L. (1973). On being sane in insane places. *Science, 179*(4070), 250–258.

Santiago-Rivera, A. L. (1995). Developing a culturally sensitive treatment modality for bilingual Spanish-speaking clients: Incorporating language and culture in counseling. *Journal of Counseling and Development, 74*, 12–17.

Scott, N. E., & Borodovsky, L. (1990). Effective use of cultural role taking. *Professional Psychology: Research and Practice, 21*, 167–170.

Sedlacek, W. E. (1994). Issues in advancing diversity through assessment. *Journal of Counseling and Development, 72*, 549–553.

Sinacore-Guinn, A. L. (1995). The diagnostic window: Culture and gender sensitive diagnosis and training. *Clinician Education and Supervision, 35*, 18–31.

Solomon, A. (1992, June). Clinical diagnosis among diverse populations: A multicultural perspective. *Families in Society: The Journal of Contemporary Human Services, 73*, 371– 377.

Spengler, P. M., & Strohmer, D. C. (1994). Clinical judgment biases: The moderating roles of clinician complexity and clinician preferences. *Journal of Counseling Psychology, 41*, 1–10.

Spengler, P. M., Strohmer, D. C., Dixon, D. N., & Shivy, V. A. (1995). A scientist-practitioner model of psychological assessment: Implications for training, practice, and research. *The Counseling Psychologist, 23*, 506–534.

Thompson, J. W., Blueye, H. B., Smith, C. R., & Walker, R. R. (1983). Cross-cultural curriculum content in psychiatric residency training: An American Indian and Alaska Native perspective. In J. C. Chunn, II, P. J. Dunston, & F. Ross-Sherrif (Eds.), *Mental health and people of color: Curriculum development and change* (pp. 269–288). Washington, DC: Howard University Press.

Triandis, H. C., Malpass, R. S., & Davidson, A. R. (1973). Psychology and culture. In P. H. Mussen & M. R. Rosenziveig (Eds.), *Annual review of psychology* (Vol. 24, pp. 355–378). Palo Alto, CA: Annual Review.

Triandis, H. C., Marín, G., Lisansky, J., & Betancourt, H. C. (1984). Simpatía as a cultural script of Hispanics. *Journal of Personality and Social Psychology, 47,* 1363–1375.

Velásquez, R. J., Gonzales, M., Butcher, J. N., Castillo-Canez, I., Apodaca, J. X., & Chavira, D. (1997). Use of the MMPI-2 with Chicanos: Strategies for counselors. *Journal of Multicultural Counseling and Development, 25,* 107–120.

Velásquez, R. J., Johnson, R., & Brown-Cheatham, M. (1993). Teaching counselors to use the *DSM-III-R* with ethnic minority clients: A paradigm. *Counselor Education and Supervision, 32,* 323–331.

Watkins, C. E., Campbell, V. L., Nieberding, R., & Hallmark, R. (1995). Contemporary practice of psychological assessment by clinical psychologists. *Professional Psychology: Research and Practice, 26,* 54–60.

Watson, R. S. (1976). *Clinician complexity and the process of hypothesizing about a client: An exploratory study of clinicians' information processing.* Unpublished doctoral dissertation, University of California, Santa Barbara.

Zimmerman, M. (1994). *Interview guide for evaluating DSM-IV psychiatric disorders and the mental status exam.* Philadelphia: Psych Products Press.

PART II

STRUCTURED CASE FORMULATION METHODS

Chapter 3

The Psychoanalytic Approach to Case Formulation

STANLEY B. MESSER
DAVID L. WOLITZKY

In this chapter we present an account of psychoanalytic case formulation as it is used clinically in conjunction with psychoanalytic treatment. Because it was developed in a clinical context, it is less formal and systematic than other approaches in this volume which are research based. For example, the psychoanalytic clinician does not typically record sessions, prepare verbatim transcripts, or have a panel of judges formally rate such material. At the same time, the psychoanalytic case formulation implicitly includes many of the concepts reviewed in other chapters, such as the Core Conflictual Relationship Theme (CCRT) (see Luborsky & Barrett, Chapter 4, this volume) and cyclical maladaptive behavior (see Levenson & Strupp, Chapter 6, this volume).

For present purposes we may define the psychoanalytic case formulation as a hierarchically organized set of clinical inferences about the nature of a patient's psychopathology, and, more generally, about his or her personality structure, dynamics, and development. These inferences which are generated in the course of the psychoanalytically informed interview include the presumed reasons for the patient's experience and behavior such as symptoms, dreams, fantasies, and maladaptive patterns of interpersonal relationships. For example, the clinician might observe that whenever the patient begins a new emotional involvement with a woman, he experiences an upsurge in claustrophobic symptoms. The patient might express anxiety about being in a crowded elevator and its getting stuck between floors. The psychoanalytic explanation might be that these symptoms reveal an unconscious fear of being trapped in a relationship, which may lead to a loss of a sense of personal identity.

The inferences and the interpretations that follow in the course of therapy often include the therapist postulating a probable sequence of historical events and the meanings assigned to them by the patient, many of which have continued to be unavailable to the latter's awareness. The nature of the evidence and clinical reasoning that lead to such clinical inferences and the means of attempting to validate interpretations based on them are addressed below.

HISTORICAL BACKGROUND OF THE APPROACH

The clinical case history method originated with Freud, and his early case studies continue to be taught as models of psychoanalytic thinking. Although other theorists such as Morton Prince (1905) also used the case study method, it was Freud's extensive reliance on this method and the insights it yielded that leads us to emphasize his key role in the development of the case formulation approach. It is interesting to note Freud's own, rare statement about the case history approach. In his discussion of Elisabeth von R., Freud (1900/1953) wrote:

> It still strikes me as strange that the case histories I write read like short stories and that, as one might say, they lack the serious stamp of science. I must console myself with the reflection that the nature of the subject is evidently responsible for this, rather than any preference of my own. . . . [A] detailed description of mental processes such as we are accustomed to find in the works of imaginative writers enables me, with the use of a few psychological formulas, to obtain at least some kind of insight into the course of that affliction [i.e., hysteria].

And, Freud continued, the case histories provide "an intimate connection between the story of the patient's suffering and the symptoms of his illness" (p. 160).

The history of efforts at psychodynamic case formulation began with Freud's search for treatment methods more effective than rest, hydrotherapy, and faradic stimulation (the application of low-voltage electrical stimulation to afflicted areas of the body). Freud began experimenting with hypnosis and eventually came to prefer the method of free association in which he directed the patient to say everything that came to mind. As we now know, this method became central to the evolution of psychoanalysis.

Freud was searching for the most efficacious way to facilitate the recall of so-called pathogenic memories. The theory he was developing was that the onset of symptoms coincided with a disagreeable experience that the patient forgot, that the quota of affect associated with this experience was "converted" to symptoms, and that the recovery of this experience and its associated affects was essential to the alleviation of the symptom (Breuer & Freud, 1893–1895/1955). The experience was both wished for and simultaneously dreaded in that it violated the person's moral code. As is well-known by now, Freud came to the idea that hysterics suffer from reminiscences connected to unacceptable sexual wishes.

From the start Freud tried to present plausible accounts of why and how the patient's symptoms developed and were ameliorated. Faced with a stream of seemingly disconnected, often bizarre sequences of verbal associations, Freud wanted to construct a meaningful explanation of the patient's often irrational behavior. He was particularly struck by gaps in the patient's memory, by the patient's tendency to avoid certain material, and by the inexplicable nature of the patient's symptoms. The assumptions of psychic determinism and unconscious motivation were central to his attempts at a rational explanation of the patient's difficulties. The subsequent development of psychoanalytic theory showed an increasingly complex and subtle understanding of human experience, particularly from the perspective of unconscious, intrapsychic conflict, a core notion of Freudian theory. The major tenets of the theory can be found in Brenner (1973).

Rapaport and Gill (1959), two important later figures who contributed to the structure of psychoanalytic case formulation, argued that a comprehensive case formulation would have to include the following multiple perspectives: dynamic, structural, genetic, adaptive, topographic, and economic. That is, corresponding to the order of the preceding terms, the formulation would have to address the patient's major conflicts (dynamic: e. g., wishes, and defenses against those wishes), those aspects of the patient's personality involved in the conflicts (structural: e.g., id vs. superego), the historical and developmental etiology of the conflicts (genetic), the adaptive and maladaptive compromise formations involved in the patient's defensive and coping strategies (adaptive), the conscious versus unconscious status of the conflicts (topographic), and the "economic" consequences of the preceding factors, not in the original sense of the distribution of "mobile" and "bound" cathexes but in the more descriptive sense of how constricted and brittle the patient's adjustment is by virtue of the excessive "energy" invested in his or her defensive maneuvers. Although contemporary case formulations generally contain less metapsychological language than in the past, with the exception of the economic viewpoint, they do attempt to cover the perspectives just outlined.

CONCEPTUAL FRAMEWORK

There are three major conceptual models in contemporary, mainstream psychoanalysis in North America—traditional Freudian, object relations, and self psychology.[1] Each model makes different assumptions about human beings and their core motivational dynamics. Some clinicians elect to adopt a multimodel approach in which they bring to bear each theoretical perspective with every patient (e.g., Silverman, 1986). Others use whichever model seems to fit a given case best, while some therapists stick to one of the models for most cases. Pine (1990) argues that each of the models refers to an important domain of human experience and each has a place in a comprehensive, multifaceted understanding of the patient. Unfortunately, we do not have a body of empirical evidence concerning the relative clinical utility of the different formulations offered by the several models. Nor do we know whether using any particular model or some combination of models is better than using no model at all beyond a commonsense, implicit personality theory. Clearly, these are issues for empirical study, as we note in the research section at the end of the chapter.

Following are the core propositions of the different models, focusing on what is formulated and why. (For a more detailed account of each model, see Greenberg & Mitchell, 1983.) According to the *Freudian drive/ structural model*, human behavior is determined by sexual and aggressive drives, which have four attributes: a source, an aim, an impetus, and an object. The *source* of the drives is somatic processes that make a demand on the mind. The *aim* of the drive is gratification through discharge, and the *impetus* is the drive's intensity. The *object* of the drive is the most variable aspect; gratification could be sought through an inanimate object, another person, or a part of one's body. The system operates according to the pleasure principle (i.e., people's goals are to reduce tension to an optimal level, maximize drive gratification, and minimize unpleasure). The person's major motivational thrust is to seek satisfaction of the wishes which are the psychological derivatives of the instinctual drives. Wishes are attempts to reinstate "perceptual identity" with the memories of past gratifications (Freud, 1900/1953). Obstacles to the immediate or long-term gratification of wishes are inevitable, creating intrapsychic conflicts. That is, the person seeks to gratify the wish but simultaneously avoids seeking gratification when wishes threaten to give rise to anxiety, guilt, or fear of external punishment. In brief, Freudian theory conceptualizes human behavior from the perspective of intrapsychic conflict.

In the tripartite, structural model of id/ego/superego, the id is the repository of the drives, the superego represents the internalized standards and prohibitions of the parents and the culture, and the ego modulates drive discharge by automatically instituting defenses. Defenses are activated by "signal anxiety" based on the ego's appraisal that the awareness or expression of certain wishes is apt to lead to traumatic anxiety. The principal anxieties, or danger situations of childhood, are loss of the object, loss of the object's love, castration anxiety, and superego anxiety (Brenner, 1982). These anxieties correspond to the psychosexual stages of oral, anal, phallic, and genital development. These key Freudian concepts are part of the larger, complex structure of interlocking concepts that constitute the framework for organizing the clinical material. A formulation based on these concepts that takes account of the aforementioned metapsychological points of view will focus principally on the patient's repetitive reenactments of core unconscious conflicts and fantasies; their defensive, adaptive, and developmental aspects; and their influence on character styles and object relationships (Perry, Cooper, & Michels, 1987).

A key feature of a Freudian formulation is an emphasis on unconscious fantasy, the conflicts expressed in such fantasy, and the influence of such conflicts and fantasies on the patient's behavior both within and outside the consulting room. A corollary assumption is that the current, unconscious fantasies are based on core conflicts originating in childhood. Current maladaptive behavior is seen to be largely motivated by unconscious fantasies, even if patients experience their behavior as lacking a sense of personal agency or as attributable primarily to external circumstance. Indeed, a significant aspect of the interpretive work in the course of treatment is to help patients realize the nature and extent of their intentional, though not conscious, disavowal of motives and affects that clash with their conscious values and attitudes.

In general terms, Freudian analysts emphasize the importance of unresolved Oedipal conflicts whereas adherents of object relations theories and of self psychology stress the significance of pre-Oedipal issues. Stated briefly, pre-Oedipal issues refer to anxieties arising in the first 2–3 years of life in relation to concerns about loss of the "object" (i.e., the principal caretakers) and the loss of the object's love, anxieties which correspond, respectively, to the oral and anal Freudian psychosexual stages of development. These anxieties are potentially present throughout life and the fear of their full-blown eruption is what triggers defensive reactions. The principal anxiety of the next psychosexual stage, the phallic stage, is castration anxiety which is said to arise in relation to the boy's Oedipal complex (i.e., his wish to destroy the rival for his mother's love and affection, namely, his father). For the models presented below it is issues of trust, safety, self-esteem, cohesion and preservation of self, and conflicted ties to parental figures who have also been significant sources of psychic pain that are seen as relatively more important than Oedipal conflicts in the development and maintenance of psychopathology.

From an *object relations perspective* (and for present purposes we combine the different theorists who represent this approach) the emphasis is on the internalized mental representations of self and other and their interactions, particularly the affective coloring of these interactions. This approach emphasizes the tendency to split self and other representations into "good" versus "bad" and the difficulty of integrating these representations. Concepts of introjective and projective identification figure prominently in these formulations. Many clinicians find these concepts especially useful in describing the difficulties people diagnosed with borderline personality disorder have in internalizing a stable, soothing introject and in establishing a differentiated, integrated sense of self. In contrast to traditional Freudians, object relations theorists stress human relatedness rather than drive discharge as human beings' central motivational aim. Correspondingly, their developmental formulations place relatively more weight on pre-Oedipal experience (e.g., the absence of "good enough" mothering and other environmental failures).

Case formulations based on this perspective will of course draw on concepts central to one or another version of object relations theories, principally those proposed by Klein (1948), Fairbairn (1952), Winnicott (1965), or Guntrip (1971), to mention only the more popular proponents of this point of view. Because this perspective stresses the patient's difficulty integrating "good" and "bad" mental representations of self and other, case formulations can be expected to focus on the patient's splitting off and disavowal of rage against parental figures in order not to threaten one's tie to the object on whom one also depends. As part of this defensive effort the patient may present a facade of "good" behavior (e.g., appear to conform to the parents' values and standards) along with a tendency to project onto others aspects of one's "bad self." The fully developed case formulation in this or any theoretical perspective emerges in the course of acquiring an in-depth knowledge of the patient in an intensive, exploratory psychotherapy.

There is general psychoanalytic consensus, particularly among object relations theorists that in their adult relationships patients reenact internalized object relations established in childhood. This is especially true for conflicted and unresolved relationships. Among the important clues to the nature of these internalized object relations are the patient's recall of what have been referred to as "model scenes" (Lachmann & Lichtenberg, 1992) or "schemas" (Slap & Slap-Shelton, 1991). These kinds of memories are organizing experiences or prototypes of the person's key issues and may be reenacted in the relationship with the interviewer or therapist. In monitoring ongoing interaction with patients, clinicians should be alert to the interpersonal implications of patients' communications as much as their content. The relationship episodes that patients relate often are allusions to wishes and fears of what might occur in the course of therapy.

The *self psychology model,* developed originally by Kohut (1971, 1977, 1984), centers on the development and maintenance of a cohesive self and the factors that promote healthy versus pathological narcissism. Kohut's self psychology focuses on the failure of parents to provide the experiences necessary for the child to form a cohesive sense of self and to actualize joyfully its ambitions and ideals. A key notion for Kohut is the parents' failure in empathic responsiveness, a failure that does not allow the child to use the parents as idealized selfobjects or as mirroring selfobjects. Observations of transference patterns are crucial to formulating the patient's narcissistic problems and the manner in which the patient has attempted to compensate for his or her self-defects. Although Kohut's theory is closer in some respects to Carl Rogers's views than to Freud's, his work has remained in the mainstream of American psychoanalysis.

The concept of selfobject refers to a generally unconscious, mental representation in which one person regards another as an extension of the self to be used to regulate aspects of his or her own sense of self (e.g., sense of cohesion or self-esteem). The two major classes of selfobjects are mirroring selfobjects and idealized selfobjects (Kohut, 1971, 1977). Both enhance the self by the self leaning on the perceived qualities contained in the mental representation of others, especially their perceived power, strength, and reliability. In the case of a mirroring selfobject, the person can have an experience such as "You admire me, and therefore I feel affirmed as a person of worth." In the case of an idealized selfobject, the schematic equivalent would be, "I admire you, therefore my sense of self and self-worth are enhanced by my vicarious participation in your strength and power." An everyday example of a mirroring selfobject experience is the young child's observation of the attentive, joyful gleam in its mother's eye, as might occur when the child masters a new skill. A common example of an experience of an idealized selfobject is the vicarious sense of power the young child feels when sitting on the shoulders of a parent.

For Kohut these kinds of experiences are reflections of parental empathy regarding the child's needs and constitute crucial building blocks in the development of a firm, cohesive sense of self, or what he would call the development of healthy narcissism. It is only the excessive reliance on selfobject needs that is associated with pathology of the self. An essential emphasis in the Kohutian approach to treatment is to provide patients with the missing selfobject experiences on the assumption that this will help repair the self-defects which are said to originate from the parents' failure to serve as phase-appropriate selfobjects. For therapists operating from this vantage point, the emergence of the mirror and idealizing transferences will provide vital data for an eventual case formulation specific to a particular patient.

Clinicians who prefer one or another of the aforementioned theories will make different psychodynamic formulations both at the outset of treatment and as the treatment progresses. For example, sexual difficulties are apt to be seen by the Kohutian in terms of disturbances in a cohesive sense of self, while in Freudian theory the notion of a fragmented self is more likely to be formulated as a derivative expression of castration anxiety.

What the Kohutian takes at face value is, for the Freudian, merely manifest content suggestive of a "deeper" meaning, and vice versa for the followers of Kohut.

Perry et al. (1987) state that a psychodynamic formulation, like a clinical diagnosis, has as its "primary function . . . to provide a succinct conceptualization of the case and thereby guide a treatment plan" (p. 543; but see McWilliams, 1998, for a contrast of DSM and psychoanalytic diagnoses). Such a formulation, *based on whatever theoretical perspectives one prefers*, "concisely and incisively clarifies the central issues and conflicts, differentiating what the therapist sees as essential from what is secondary" (p. 543). They urge that following any initial evaluation clinicians should write out at least a brief (i.e., 500–750 words) dynamic formulation as a working guide to understand and treat the case. The formulation, as they conceive of it, should focus on patients' current problems in light of their individual histories and current situations; sketch the dynamic and other factors that seem to explain the clinical picture; offer surmises about patients' individual backgrounds; and predict the likely impact of the foregoing factors on the process and outcome of therapy. We follow such a plan in the example given below.

THE NATURE OF PSYCHOANALYTIC INFERENCE

Before turning to a discussion of how the psychoanalytic clinician goes about formulating an actual case, it is useful to consider the process of clinical inference that undergirds case formulations. In line with the recognition that we can no longer speak of *the* theory of psychoanalysis, we have the increasingly accepted notion that, when formulating a case, the clinician creates a narrative structure.[2] This structure is an attempt to provide a coherent, comprehensive, plausible, and we hope accurate account of the individual's personality development and current functioning that is based on the life history of a particular patient as that history is told, lived, and retold by the patient in the course of the psychoanalytic encounter. However, there is no single, definitive, unchanging narrative to be told (Schafer, 1992). Implicit in this view is that there is no such thing as a psychoanalytic fact when we are talking about the reading of intentionality and meaning in patients' behavior and experience. There are observations of overt behavior from which inferences are drawn concerning the multiple psychological meanings of what is observed. Furthermore, what is observed (i.e., what is attended to selectively), stored, and retrieved from memory to arrive at a case formulation at a given point in time is influenced by the nature of the patient–therapist interaction and the evolving narrative structure into which it is placed. In other words, observation as well as inference is theory-saturated (Messer, Sass, & Woolfolk, 1988). It is no wonder that

Freudian patients are found to have Freudian dreams, and Jungian patients Jungian dreams.

The higher the level of inference in case formulation, the stronger the influence of the particular narrative structures through which the material is being conceptualized. Theoretical concepts can be thought of as a series of lenses through which the data of observation are filtered. For example, if a patient's first response to Card I of the Rorschach is "a mask," clinicians would probably agree that the response connotes "concealment." However, once we go beyond the inference of "concealment" to hypothesize what it is that is being concealed and why, we are increasingly guided by our preferred theory. As suggested earlier, traditional Freudian theory posits that adaptation to the environment requires that the id be socialized, renounce its unrealizable aims, and instead secure for the individual as much instinctual gratification with as little pain as possible. This developmental narrative of "the beast within that needs to be tamed" is consonant with the idea that the pleasure principle has to accommodate to the reality principle if the organism is to survive and adapt adequately. As Schafer (1992) points out, Freud's other major narrative structure was that of the organism as machine in which behavior is strictly determined through shifts in the quantity of psychic energies.

Freudian analysts will formulate case material from these (and related) Freudian perspectives at various degrees of distance from the clinical data. That is, one can speak in experience-distant terms of transformations of psychic energies and/or on a more experience-near level in terms of wishes, fears, and conflicts. Thus, for the Freudian, the inference of "concealment" is likely to generate hypotheses about defense against sexual and/or aggressive wishes. For an object relations theorist influenced by Winnicott (1965), the same inference will likely lead to formulations in terms of the "true self" and the "false self." As another example, whether we create a narrative in which idealization is seen primarily as a defense against hostility (i.e., a reaction formation), or whether it is regarded as stemming mainly from the search for an idealized selfobject to shore up one's sense of personal cohesiveness and strength, would partly depend on whether we prefer Freud's or Kohut's theory. Those adopting a multimodel approach (e.g., Silverman, 1986) would more freely entertain both inferences.

The clinician brings to the analytic situation not only one or more psychoanalytic frameworks within which to order and organize the clinical data but other cognitive frameworks that interact with the psychoanalytic lenses through which the clinical material is viewed. It is useful, following Peterfreund (1976), to think of a *series* of "working models" that are brought to bear on the material. First, we have our *commonsense working model* of psychological functioning, or what might be called our implicit theories of personality. Included here are such everyday notions as the following: if mother favors one sibling over another, the less favored sibling is apt to feel hurt, unlovable, and angry; reality is often more disappointing than the wishful fantasy would suggest; and past experiences have a psychological impact on future behavior.

Second, we have a *working model of ourselves* based on both the commonsense model noted earlier and on one or more *psychoanalytic models* through which we have come to understand ourselves. The *commonsense* and *psychoanalytic models* influence the *model of ourselves*, and these three models interact to influence our beginning understanding of the patient. A fourth model that influences our understanding of a particular patient is based on *the aggregate of one's experiences with previous patients*. Thus, the multiple, overlapping working models we employ include a commonsense mode, a preferred theoretical model, a model of ourselves based on these, and a model based on experience with previous patients.

In general, one could say that the telling and retelling of narratives is a means of situating the protagonist in relation to his or her mental life. In terms of Schafer's (1976, 1992) action language conception, this would mean attempting to develop a coherent, plausible narrative in which the patient comes to an "appropriate" appreciation of his or her role as the author of and actor in the script which is being enacted. From this perspective, behaviors that are initially understood as merely "happenings" are retold as intentional actions. Alternate theoretical models with their different etiological emphases would yield different story lines, even though they all share a recognition of the adverse impact of childhood trauma. For example, in the Freudian story line, one would tend to emphasize the operation of defense as a kind of disclaimed action and, in general, see the patient as responsible for his or her emotional dilemmas. By contrast, Kohutian story lines probably tend to cast the patient in the role of victim. At the extremes, Freudians could be seen as "blaming" the victim while Kohutians could be seen as "blaming" the parents. In turn, these perspectives could result in subtle differences in one's sense of personal responsibility for who one has become and for one's future.

Aside from what we may call the preferred story line, analysts share certain assumptions about how the mind works. These assumptions guide clinical listening and the evolving psychodynamic formulation. To explicate them all would require at least a chapter-length treatment. Therefore, we confine ourselves to the major assumptions, which include psychic determinism, unconscious motivation, the ideas of displacement, and symbolic equivalence.

Psychic determinism refers to the assumption of lawful regularity in mental life. That is, significant psychological events do not occur on a chance basis. Thus, if the patient switches the topic in the course of the session, a working hypothesis that guides the psychodynamic formulation is that the shift is not random but is likely to be dynamically linked to the earlier topics. This assumption operates at the clinical level in terms of the principle of contiguity. For example, suppose the patient says, in the first session, that she is afraid that if she starts to speak freely she will not be able to contain herself and will lose emotional control. She pauses momentarily, then asks where the women's bathroom is located. The clinician assumes that these two seemingly disparate topics are dynamically linked, as expressed in the following hypothesis: "The patient makes an unconscious equation between the control of thoughts and feelings and the control of bowel and bladder functions."

The working hypothesis one might hold regarding unconscious motives at play in this example could include a desire to expose herself in conflict with a wish to avoid humiliation based on the fear that her body is defective and her self, inferior. It is further assumed that these hypothesized possibilities are outside the patient's awareness at the beginning of treatment. The clinician would store these inferences in his or her memory and scan them periodically for their "fit" with other aspects of the evolving working model of the patient. If evidence emerged that these inferences were relevant to an understanding of the patient's core issues, the therapist could offer interpretations based on them. For example, "I notice that when you started getting teary just now you quickly tried to hold back your feelings. Recently you recalled how as a young girl you were afraid you might wet your pants if you were upset, and that if you did so, you would feel mortified. I wonder whether you're afraid that crying here would make you feel the same way." The nature of the patient's associations to such an interpretation, including what other childhood memories might be recalled, would be among the criteria a psychoanalytic clinician would use to evaluate the accuracy of the interpretation and its clinical utility.

It needs to be emphasized that this is merely an example of how a psychoanalyst might arrive at a particular clinical inference, which could become part of a dynamic formulation. We do not mean to suggest that this clinical hypothesis is necessarily a valid explanation for the contiguity of these two particular ideas in the patient's associations. Only further supportive, clinical material, uncontaminated by any suggestive interpretation of the kind offered previously, could increase one's confidence in the original hypothesis. It also should be noted that we are not implying that analysts are necessarily aware of the implicit "rules of clinical evidence" they are using but only that there is an underlying "clinical logic" to what might otherwise be seen as pure intuition or based on an arcane or mystical process.

In formulating a case, psychodynamically oriented clinicians use most or all of the working models described by Peterfreund (1976), usually on an implicit level. In so doing, they vary in terms of the quantity and quality of evidence they regard as necessary to support a case formulation. They also differ in how carefully they distinguish between observation and inference and the extent to which their formulations are theory-driven.

INCLUSION/EXCLUSION CRITERIA AND MULTICULTURAL CONSIDERATIONS

General Considerations

There are no exclusion criteria for a psychoanalytic case formulation. The approach described here can be used with all patients, although the richness, detail, and comprehensiveness of the formulation will depend on how self-disclosing the patient is willing and able to be. The patient's free associations as elicited in psychoanalytic sessions are the main source of information. The formulation, however, can also be based on interviews with someone who knows the patient, or on psychological test data.

The psychodynamically based case formulations also take into account other information about the patient. For example, in patients with organic or biological factors that contribute significantly to the patient's pathology, unconscious conflict will play a more modest role in the overall case formulation. Nonetheless, the psychoanalytic clinician will look carefully at the premorbid factors in such patients' psychological makeup that place a unique stamp on how their psychopathology is expressed. Thus, one will not rush to infer that the growing disorientation with regard to time, place, and sense of personal identity in a patient with Alzheimer's disease has dynamic meaning. At the same time, selective confusions and distortions often are understandable as reflecting long-standing conflicts and personality styles. At a similar stage of dementia, not all patients will express guilt over burdening their children or deny that they were ever married to their spouse of many years. Similarly, even if there is a genetic basis for schizophrenia or depression, it still leaves us with the necessity of explaining the particular content of the schizophrenic's delusional system or the psychotically depressed patient's view of his or her "sins." This way of looking at pathology has characterized psychodynamic approaches since Freud's observations of individual differences in reaction to traumatic events.

Multicultural Considerations

We now turn to multicultural considerations in psychoanalytic case formulation. To understand the multitude of factors that shape peoples' personality and contribute to the onset and maintenance of psychopathology, we need to situate our understanding of clients' current and past circumstances and stressors in the context of their cultural, ethnic, and religious background. For example, feelings of guilt over sexual impulses in someone who has had an extremely stern and religious upbringing may have a quite different meaning than similar feelings in a person who has been raised in a secular, liberal home. In understanding the meaning of an eating disorder, it is most helpful to know the cultural contributions to the problem, such as the societal attitude to thinness or ideal body type.

The study of attachment in different cultures provides a good illustration of the importance of the clinician being sensitive to cultural differences. Rothbaum, Weisz, Pott, Miyake, and Morelli (2000) compared American and Japanese children in attachment situations. They reported findings in Japan that differed from those found in the American samples, which pointed to the conclusion that the Western emphasis on autonomy and individuation did not apply in the same way in the Japanese children. This called into question the universality of some basic assumptions of attachment theory and the predictions one would make about later competence and social functioning. For example, relative to the United States the Japanese culture values group harmony and cooperation over individual accomplishments. Inhibition of hostile feelings is encouraged; assertive, autonomous strivings are seen as immature. Japanese mothers are more apt to react to the infant's need for social engagement than for individuation and to anticipate their infants' needs rather than waiting for signals of distress.

Findings such as these have important implications for attachment theory, which bears a close affinity to object relations theories. Cultural differences in attachment styles clearly have implications for case formulation and for the conduct of psychotherapy. As one instance, in Japan the avoidance of self-enhancement and an inclination to self-effacement is culturally normative as is the inhibition of hostility. Inferences about the patient's narcissistic issues, defensive styles, and core conflicts need to take into account these cultural differences. In the course of treatment, the therapist has to realize that strong filial piety is the culturally approved norm so that negative comments about one's parents likely would be made with greater difficulty and more guilt. Finally, Japanese therapists seem not to worry about gratifying the patient's dependency needs whereas American therapists are more concerned that such gratification would derail the patient's autonomous strivings. American therapists might need to soften this attitude when treating Japanese patients, particularly newly arrived immigrants.

Speaking more broadly, although we may regard separation, loss, and death as universal issues with which all human beings must cope, it is essential to appreciate the variety of ways in which different cultures are organized to cope with them. Assessing a person from a culture in which communication with the dead is a common belief should not automatically lead to the unwarranted conclusion that this is a manifestation of psychosis. Culture-bound psychiatric syndromes in general need to be assessed within the framework of the culture in question. An example of a culture-bound syndrome is "ataque de nervose," commonly found among Latinos in the Caribbean and in some Latin American countries. This culturally recognized idiom of distress, usually precipitated by a stressful event, includes a wide range of somatic symptoms, commonly accompanied by verbal and, sometimes, physical, aggression. The symptom picture overlaps with the symptoms of a panic attack and resembles some DSM-IV-TR categories but might or might not be indicative of the person having an actual mental disorder (Sue, 2004). The clinician who is aware of a Latino client's cultural background will be in a better position to evaluate the unconscious meanings of this syndrome. From a psychoanalytic perspective one would try to discern the unconscious wishes being expressed in the symptoms, the patient's ego strength, and the possible reasons for the current failure of the person's defenses (Lam & Sue, 2001; Okazaki, Kallivayalil, & Sue, 2002; Sue & Lam, 2002).

When evaluating a patient, the context of the evaluation is itself influential in determining the nature of the data that will be elicited. To illustrate: A 20-year-old African American, male college student was seen in a major urban city. His presenting complaint was that he often felt treated rudely and disrespectfully in this city compared with the polite treatment he had received in his small home town. In developing his case formulation the white clinician had to consider to what extent the prospective patient viewed his mistreatment by others as racially motivated and whether he might be probing to see whether he could expect to be treated respectfully by the therapist.

Our take-away point is that starting with the clinician–patient relationship, there are multiple, additional contexts including, but not limited to, the cultural one that the clinician needs to take into consideration in order to form an accurate understanding of the patient's inner world and current stressors. Because the traditional psychodynamic approach to case formulation is attuned to the implicit meanings of interpersonal communication and to issues of trust and the therapeutic alliance, it is a method that can be used with patients of different cultural and ethnic backgrounds. The clinician needs to be aware of what is normative for an individual from a particular cultural and ethnic heritage and how the individual experiences that heritage with respect to variables such as self-esteem, social values, and attitudes. This is particularly important when the patient is trying to adapt to a community or culture that does not share his or her cultural or socioeconomic background. Although it is undoubtedly wise for the psychoanalytic clinician to be sensitive to the issues outlined previously, what is stressed most in psychoanalytic practice are universal themes and issues with which we all must deal regardless of our particular cultural, racial, ethnic or religious background.

STEPS IN CASE FORMULATION

It should be apparent that there is no one, universally accepted method to construct a case study or formulation. Rarely is there any formal training in writing clinical narratives during graduate school, psychiatric residencies, or psychoanalytic training. Probably the closest approximation to such training occurs in psychodiagnostic testing courses taught from a psychodynamic perspective. In such courses, students generally are taught to organize test reports into major sections, such as "behavioral observations," "cognitive functioning," and "personality functioning" and to link observations in each section to an overall formulation of the person. This would include adaptive strengths, pathological features, diagnostic and prognostic considerations, and suitability for treatment. To this would be added, when writing psychotherapy summaries, a discussion of transference–countertransference issues. Thus, there are guidelines but no precise format or specific sequence to be followed in writing up a case. We urge students to avoid jargon and generalities such as "his defenses are strained under stressful conditions," and to construct a portrait of the individual that makes the person "come alive." We discourage excessive speculation and recommend that inferences be stated with a degree of conviction proportional to the strength of the clinical evidence.

Despite these caveats, there is enough commonality among psychoanalytically oriented psychotherapists to allow us to set out a framework of concepts typically drawn upon in case writeups, as well as to suggest how an interview should be conducted to elicit the information on which the formulation relies. This is followed by a case example illustrating how the theoretical concepts and the framework are applied in practice. Based on the previously described psychoanalytic concepts, we now outline how they are covered in a case formulation. In doing so, we have drawn on Friedman and Lister's (1987) useful format.

What Is Formulated

Structural Features of Personality

Structure refers to those aspects of psychological functioning that are fairly stable and enduring. There are four areas covered under this heading.

Autonomous Ego Functions. These include disruptions in basic biological, perceptual, motor, or cognitive functions, including language. Of special import here is the adequacy of the patient's reality testing.

Affects, Drives, and Defenses. This refers to the person's characteristic ways of experiencing impulses and feelings and containing them. Questions regarding drives and affects to be considered in the formulation include the following: Is the person able to tolerate a range of feelings without overly suppressing some or feeling overwhelmed by others? Is there one predominant affect that colors wide areas of the person's functioning? Are closely related affects—such as anger, hate, irritation, and jealousy—sufficiently differentiated or are they all subsumed under rage? How flexibly does the person respond on an emotional level to diverse circumstances?

Defenses are the intrapsychic mechanisms that allow us to manage difficult external events and internal turmoil. What are the characteristic defenses that the person employs? Are these successful in allowing the person sufficient emotional response without experiencing strong anxiety or depression? How mature or primitive are the defenses (e.g., intellectualization vs. denial or splitting)? Are the defenses interfering with or restricting the person's enjoyment of life?

Object-Related Functions. These refer to the person's basic modes of relating to others, including their internal representations of self and other and the links between self and other. Is the person able to be trusting, intimate, and, at the same time, autonomous? Can he or she sustain disappointment, disillusionment, and loss without becoming incapacitated? In relationships is the person overly controlling? too submissive? self-defeating? demanding?

Self-Related Functions. These refer to the person's ability to maintain the coherence, stability, and positive evaluation of the self. They also include issues of the individual's identifications, identity, ideals, and goals. Are the person's values stable? Do ambitions match desires and talents? Is the person overly susceptible to shame and humiliation, inflation of self or deflation of self? That is, how susceptible is the individual to precipitous drops in self-esteem?

Dynamic Features of Personality

"Just as the structural viewpoint examines the *form* of psychological functioning, the dynamic viewpoint examines its *content*. . . . The focus is consistently on meaning and motive" (Friedman & Lister, 1987; pp. 135–136). The psychoanalytic case formulation responds to the following questions in this sphere: What is the meaning of the symptom understood psychoanalytically? What motivates the person to act in particular ways? What are the person's major areas of conflict, be they intrapsychic or interpersonal? Within psychoanalytic theory, conflict and ambivalence are considered to be ubiquitous in human affairs.

What is the nature of the conflict among various motives such as wishes, fears, impulses, and needs? Does the patient effect some compromise among them which actually obscures the nature of the conflict? These wishes, fears, and conflicts are often of a sexual, dependent, or aggressive nature. For example, a woman may wish to enjoy sex more freely but feel morally remiss and guilty were she to do so. A man may wish to have an intimate relationship with a woman but, at the same time, fear being controlled or engulfed by her, or overly dependent on her. A woman may wish to speak up and express herself in a group but fear being shamed or humiliated. Any of these conflicts can lead to the formation of symptoms, anxiety, or inhibitions.

Sometimes the wishes are particularly disturbing, taking the form of homicidal fantasies, ego-alien sexual fantasies (e.g., of incest), or primitive urges to merge with the object. For example, a person may feel angry and want to express it but then fear losing control and having the anger emerge as murderous rage. Typically, there are layers of motive, meaning, and conflict, only some of which will be apparent in the initial interviews. In this part of the formulation, the object is to describe the various areas of motive and conflict, both intrapsychic and interpersonal, that may operate on conscious or unconscious levels.

Developmental Antecedents

Preceding and underlying the structural and dynamic facets of a patient's personality and psychopathology are earlier events that take on particular meaning depending on the developmental (or, in psychoanalytic parlance, "genetic") phase in which they occurred. These may include traumatic events such as physical or emotional abandonment, sexual or physical abuse, surgery, parental psychosis, or drug abuse or more moderate stresses such as the birth of a sibling, parental discord, school failure, and so forth. The meaning and impact of these events will be influenced by their timing, namely, the psychosexual and psychosocial stage of development that the person was going through when they occurred. In this way, the formulation takes into account the stages of infancy, childhood, and adolescence as these have affected patients' current psychological functioning.

Adaptive Features: Assets and Strengths

Because there tends to be an (understandable) emphasis in the case formulation on patients' deficiencies and maladaptive ways of interacting, it is important not to neglect noting their strengths. What are their accomplishments? Do they have intellectual strengths? mechanical aptitudes? artistic talents? Are they able to get along with others? Can they assert themselves appropriately? and so forth.

In recent years, there has been increasing recognition of biological determinants of behavior as well as the psychological sequelae of physical illnesses and limitations (McWilliams, 1999; Morrison, 1997; Summers, 2003). Among such factors are temperament (e.g., impulsivity), genetic endowment (e.g., intelligence), medical illness (e.g., multiple sclerosis and HIV/AIDS), perinatal conditions (e.g., fetal alcohol syndrome), the effects of substance abuse or head injury (e.g., cognitive impairment or confusion), and childhood psychiatric/neuorological conditions (e.g., Tourette syndrome). It is fitting to mention them here because, from a psychotherapy standpoint, the clinician's task is to help patients marshal their ego resources to adapt to a reality that often leaves little or no room for change in the basic condition. Nevertheless, recognizing such situations and enabling patients to talk about their fears, shame, or esteem issues surrounding the difficulties in an accepting atmosphere can be invaluable in increasing their ability to cope.

The Psychoanalytic Interview

The most usual source of information on which the case formulation is based comes from a skillfully conducted, psychoanalytically informed interview. In some settings, initial demographic information, or even more extensive descriptions of the person's complaints and background, are obtained by having the patient fill out a data sheet or life-history questionnaire. Objective tests such as the Minnesota Multiphasic Personality Inventory (MMPI) or the Millon scales, which are completed by the informant, may be used. In special circumstances, where the interview leaves considerable uncertainty regarding diagnosis and treatment recommendations, a full battery of tests is employed which includes projective techniques. The latter can be especially useful in addressing the structural and dynamic areas of the case formulation.

The interview can be thought of as having *content* and *process* features (MacKinnon & Michels, 1971), the first referring to the information to be gathered through the patient's words and cognitive style and the second, to the manner in which interviewer and patient relate to each other.

Content of the Psychoanalytic Interview

Identifying Information. This includes the patient's age, sex, ethnicity, socioeconomic status, education, marital status, occupation, means of referral, and living situation.

Chief Complaints/Symptoms. This is what the patient usually wants to talk about and it is important to get a clear picture of each symptom or complaint. What stresses or events precipitated the present episode? Were there previous occurrences, and, if so, under what circumstances did they occur and how were they resolved?

Personal and Family History. As time permits, one wants to get a history of each period of the person's life—infancy, childhood, adolescence, and adulthood. The object is to discern the personality patterns the person has developed in the process of responding to the environmental forces that have been formative. One may ask for the patient's earliest memories as these can often shed light on dynamic issues. One particularly notes difficulties that have arisen and instances of psychopathology that were apparent at any phase of development.

Family history includes a description of the parents and siblings in the patient's family of origin and the way he or she felt about and interacted with them in childhood and currently. Included are the names, ages, occupations, economic and social status, marital relationship, and history of physical and emotional illnesses of the most significant family members. One pays special attention to the occurrence of psychological problems such as depression, psychiatric hospitalization, suicide, alcoholism or other drug addiction, and mental retardation.

Optimally, one would conduct several interviews to be able to gather this much information and to observe the patient over a period of time. Typically, in the press of clinical practice, only one or two hours are available, and one must curtail the gathering of a full personal or family history, which are then combined in one section of the narrative. If the patient continues on to psychotherapy, one can then fill in the gaps as therapy proceeds.

Process of the Psychoanalytic Interview

Observing the Patient. In addition to gathering information from the patient, the interviewer notes the patient's behavior in the course of the interview. The traditional psychiatric way of referring to these observations is the *mental status* exam. This is a description of the patient's current emotions, behavior, thought processes, thought content, and perceptions. It includes appearance, general attitude (cooperative, withdrawn, seductive?), mood and affect (depressed, anxious, flat?), speech (coherent, relevant?), thought (grandiose, delusional, suicidal?), perceptions (hallucinations, derealization?), cognitive functions (memory, intelligence, judgment, and insight), and sensorium (orientation as to time, place, and person). This kind of information will also help establish a formal DSM-IV diagnosis.

It is important to observe in connection with what dynamic themes and what events the patient shows affect as these will tend to be the most significant. One also strives to follow patients' associations (i.e., to note the sequence in which themes are presented). This is in keeping with the psychoanalytic dictum that the order of a person's verbal production is partly determined by inferred underlying psychic forces, as described earlier.

One takes note of the development of transference, countertransference, and resistance. Patients may reveal, even in initial interviews, the way in which they regard the interviewer, based on their relationship to parental figures. There may be an exaggerated need for gratification of dependency needs, for example. The interviewer may experience a countertransference pull to gratify such needs, which alerts him or her to the nature of the transference. Regarding resistance, one notes how and when the patient expresses defense in sidestepping the recognition of certain feelings or thoughts, including those pertaining to the interviewer.

We turn now to a consideration of the general approach of the interviewer in obtaining the information on which the formulation is constructed.

Optimal Stance of the Interviewer. In the most general terms, the patient should be viewed as a partner in the interview, invited to struggle with contradictions, ambiguities, and puzzling aspects of his or her behavior . Although the clinical interviewer is an expert on human behavior, the patient is the more versed in the specifics of his or her functioning and, therefore, should be "engaged as thinker, synthesizer and co-creator of hypotheses" (Peebles-Kleiger, 2002, p. 55).

The interviewer should show an appreciation of the patient as a whole person, and not merely as an object of clinical focus. This includes attending to patients' assets as well as deficiencies. One is interested not solely in patients' diagnosis, symptoms, or complaints but in their total life functioning (work and love relations) in the context of their life history.

Even if one does not approve of what the patient does, it is important to try to accept the patient unreservedly. One attempts to maintain a certain degree of professional detachment, but this should not be construed as indifference. Nor should interviewers allow their own emotions to interfere with their judgment. Knowing their own emotional makeup and vulnerabilities will help them to predict those areas in which they are most likely to lose objectivity.

The clinical information should not be collected in a lockstep manner, but along the way where it seems to fit the flow of the individual's presentation. One line of thought often leads the patient to another and if one has the aforementioned format in mind, much information can be obtained without the interview becoming a question-and-answer session. In fact, one of the advantages of an interview over a paper-and-pencil questionnaire is that it allows the interviewer to observe the flow of information, affect, and behavior and to follow up on areas of special import. This contrasts with more structured interview formats such as the cognitive-behavioral one. We believe that psychoanalytic interviewing requires a more fluid listening process (an evenly hovering attention) to discern unconscious themes and issues that may take some time to learn and even more to master. These will go hand-in-hand with increasing knowledge of psychoanalytic theory and conducting, or being in, psychotherapy.

The most general guideline we can offer about the psychoanalytic interview is that one should try to listen without interrupting too frequently. Following are the circumstances in which the interviewer would want to intervene:

1. *One wants to know more about something than the patient is offering spontaneously.* One can simply lean forward expectantly, say "Uh-huh," "I see," or something similar. If this isn't sufficient, one can say "I'd like to hear more about that."

2. *The patient's anxiety level is too high or too low.* One can say, in the former case, "Go ahead, You're doing fine," or "Something makes it hard for you to talk to me about this matter. Can you tell me what it is?" In the case of low anxiety, one may need to be more probing and challenging to stir up some feeling.

3. *To encourage emotional expression.* Pressing patients for details of an emotion-laden event often gets them to relive it partially and can yield a clearer picture of the dynamics.

4. *To control irrelevance and chit-chat.* Because time is limited, one has to keep control of the interview and deflect patients from irrelevancies. One should also try to understand the defensive function served by excessive or trivial verbiage.

5. *To channel the interview.* One can ask questions that tactfully steer the patient back toward significant areas already touched on, or to matters that have not been brought forward. One should not confuse tact with timidity; that is, if one asks questions firmly, not hesitantly, one is more likely to get a useful answer.

The foregoing is a very condensed set of guidelines for the psychoanalytic interview. For a fuller exposition of content and process of the interview see Bocknek (1991), McWilliams (1999), Peebles-Kleiger (2002), and Sullivan (1954). For a broader psychoanalytic understanding of personality structure as it derives from the clinical process, we recommend McWilliams (1994).

CASE EXAMPLE

The case example below follows a template for organizing and presenting information gathered in the interview and for formulating that information within a psychoanalytic framework. The sequence of elements of the formulation may vary from case to case, although we prefer the logic of starting with the building blocks or structural elements of personality and psychopathology and then proceeding to the dynamic and adaptive features. We regard elements such as drive, ego, object, and self as complementary, each providing a different window on the patient. However, for some practitioners, more or most of a psychoanalytic formulation will fall into one or more of these domains.

Presentation of the Patient

Identifying Information

Jim is a 24-year-old, white, married, Catholic man in his first year of college, majoring in computer science. He is currently on leave from the U.S. Army which is financing his college education, upon completion of which he will owe 4 years of service as a computer programmer. He and his wife, Audra, to whom he has been married for 5 years, have recently returned from an army base overseas. Jim was self-referred to the college counseling center and this is his first contact with psychological services.

Presenting Problem: Chief Complaint and Symptoms

In taking an exam in a computer hardware course, Jim said he "blanked" out. Although the professor had a reputation for being tough, Jim had felt confident going into the exam. However, when he looked at the first question, he could not think clearly, got confused, and said to himself, "I can never do this. I don't know this." After he left the exam and sought the help of a tutor, it became clear that he did know the material and could have done well had he taken the exam.

Jim reported a similar sequence of events occurring twice before when he was taking college courses in the Army. In both cases, he knew the work well enough to have gotten a high grade had he followed through with the exam. He did not experience this specific problem taking exams in high school although he described himself as being perfectionistic about his work. For example, as a youngster he did excellent written and artistic work that the teachers admired but which he would crumple up and throw away as not being good enough. Although he could have had a career as a graphic artist, he prefers fields that are "sensible, logical, and orderly."

Personal and Family History

Jim's family consists of his father and mother and three younger siblings— Scott (22) who is 1 year younger, Michelle (21), 3½ years younger, and Warren (16), who is 8 years younger. They are living together in Arizona. Jim's father is an auto mechanic and his mother is an office administrator.

Jim described his father as a man who had a very difficult childhood due to his own father dying when he was 6 and having been left with his mother whom he described as "a bitch." In Jim's mind his father was "a madman" who could not tolerate his children's mistakes and would swear, scream, or smack them if their behavior did not meet his expectations. He broke furniture and dishes when he was in a rage. If Jim was visibly upset, his father would call him a baby or a girl. He forced his children to address him as "Sir" and stated, "I'm God and this house is my castle. You follow my laws."

When Jim was 7, he witnessed his father "lay out" a man who had tried to cheat him. The man cracked his head on the cement, and Jim had to clean up the blood. Jim decided at that moment that he would never fight his father and would always walk away from arguments. This resolution was reinforced on several other occasions when his father beat up other men. Jim handled his father's demands by saying "OK, Dad, whatever you say." He added that he hated his father and wanted to tell him to shut up, but held in his feelings, felt "totally tense," and kicked and punched walls instead (but not in his father's presence). He and Scott also rebelled silently by purposely not trying harder to improve their performance after father's scoldings and admonishments. When Jim was little he had looked up to his father who was affectionate to him, but after the age of 6, he never agreed with his father. His father was frequently unemployed and the family in debt, with father passing bad checks. He also stole money from the children that came from their newspaper routes, birthdays, and gifts from relatives.

Jim described his mother as warm, affectionate, and encouraging, and he believed himself to be her favorite child. As a young child, he would often get into bed with his parents, on his mother's side of the bed, and she would put her arm around him. His father brought an end to this when Jim was 6. Jim said there were times when his mother would sit with his father at the kitchen table and send Jim and Scott outside "like dogs." He always felt his father vied with him for his mother's attention "like another child," and it bothered him when she would attend to his father and shut him out. He had a recurrent dream from the age of 4 in which the family was away, leaving him alone with his mother who was dressed up as she would be to go out with his father. There were also times when his mother would say, "I wish I hadn't had you kids."

The relationship between his parents was stormy and the children asked their mother to divorce their father. When she would threaten to do so, Jim's father was contrite and cried, and "the whole matter blew over." She would say that she feared that if she left, his father would blow his brains out, which Jim believes would have been the case. His mother worked from the time Jim was 11, leaving him to care for his siblings. During this time, there was often no phone, electricity, or food in the house. Jim found respite in music, art, and books.

As a teenager, Jim hated all authorities such as principals, teachers, and policemen. He wrote sexual, angry, and violent poetry at this time. He said his sex education consisted of his father's saying, "If you want to fuck somebody, go jerk off." He was exposed to pornographic movies and magazines that his father left around the house, which Jim viewed while masturbating.

Jim's "breaking point" came at age 16 after his father broke Scott's nose when Scott had resisted being locked in the cellar for some minor misdemeanor. Jim began screaming and swearing at his father, telling him not to lay a hand on Scott. He said he was too angry to be scared and his father did not hit him. He told his father that he was leaving home and would never return. He then began spending his daytime hours at his girlfriend Audra's house, feeling close to her parents. He and Audra got engaged but broke the engagement briefly over fights about her being extremely possessive. They married 3 years later when she was 17 and he was 19. The last two times Jim saw his parents were at the wedding and a year later before he left for the service.

Jim described his wife in very positive terms, adding that although they fought while overseas, they argue very little now. While abroad, he came to feel that he had never been free to have responsibility for himself alone and considered leaving Audra. He felt pressure to be her ideal and discussed this with a close army friend, Bill, who told him to be who he wanted to be. When Jim and Bill were put on separate shifts, Jim encouraged Bill to use their house when he wasn't there. Bill then had an affair with Audra and, when Jim found out, they tried for several weeks to have an "open" marriage. Bill was told by a supervisor to stay away from Audra and she and Jim straightened things out. Jim felt betrayed by Bill and was afraid he would beat up Bill and kill him.

Currently, Jim feels good about his marriage, but he and Audra do have a conflict over his being turned on by pornography. They enjoy sex, but at times he is stimulated by sexual advertising, buys *Playboy* or *Penthouse* magazine and masturbates, or goes to porno houses and views movies.

So far Jim has been able to avoid any direct conflict with officers of higher rank, but he fears that he may one day react to an abuse of authority by, for example, laughing in the general's face during inspection. He hates what the army stands for, and hates the President who, he feels, does not "wish to take care of us, but only wants to go down in history." Jim would like to leave this country and live abroad or in the hills away from people.

Mental Status

Jim is an average looking man who came to one interview dressed neatly and to another looking wrinkled and unshaven. His affect was usually appropriate and wide ranging but he sometimes smiled while recounting upsetting events. In this connection, when asked to examine what he is experiencing, he backs off from his affect by minimizing, rationalizing, or focusing on others' feelings or motives. He does not appear depressed, nor is he suicidal, but there is a heaviness and seriousness to his mood. He is afraid of the intensity of his anger and will not fight for fear of hurting someone as his father did. He showed no evidence of thought disorder, severe acting out, or other serious psychopathology. He is very intelligent and has good judgment.

Case Formulation

In this case formulation, we draw only on the initial interviews because clinical cases are typically formulated at this juncture. Nevertheless, it is important to realize that a formulation may change as we learn more about the patient during the process of psychotherapy. In formulating a case, it is helpful to cover each of the inferential categories shown, although overlap among them is inevitable

Structural Features of Personality

Autonomous Ego Functions. When taking exams, Jim's cognitive functioning is severely hampered. He gets confused, blanks out, and is convinced that he is unable to proceed. That is, Jim's ego is overwhelmed by anxiety in this circumstance, leading to a highly dysfunctional response. Otherwise, his ego functioning, including reality testing, is largely unimpaired.

Expression of Drive and Affect and Defenses against Them. Jim has trouble containing and modulating the fierce anger he harbors against all authorities. He has managed to do so but at considerable cost in terms of psychic energy expended. That is, he needs to be constantly vigilant against the possibility that he will flout authority in some inappropriate way, such as laughing at the army general, or lashing out and even killing someone (as he felt he might do with Bill). One way he defends against the anxiety generated by this danger is by acting in an overly compliant manner with his perceived (and actual) attackers.

Jim not only has to struggle to contain his rage against authority but also to cover over and displace his sadness at not having received the nurturance and care he wished for. He does so by minimizing and rationalizing his own needs and projecting his despair of having his dependency needs met onto others (e.g., the President "who does not care for the people"). Another way in which he contains troubling feelings and impulses is by focusing on study and work areas that are "sensible, logical and orderly"—hence, his interest in computers where the messiness of feelings can be readily avoided. His effort is to keep in control at all costs. His drive/defense configurations are characteristic of an obsessive–compulsive personality, although they are not severe or pervasive enough to constitute a personality disorder.

Object–Related Functions. In relating to others, Jim tries to act as if everything is fine and compliantly to meet their expectations. He wants to look good and keep the peace, and this picture of a cooperative, helpful person constitutes his internal representation of self. His view of others is that they make demands to fulfill their own needs but not his or others and take advantage of him (professors who expect too much of their students; Bill and Audra who had an affair at his expense; his parents who mistreated him; the President who "doesn't care about us," etc.). Thus, the internalized relationship between self and other can be characterized as that of giver to taker or victim to victimizer.

Self-Related Function. Jim's sense of self is coherent and fairly stable, but also quite negative and, in some ways, false. It is negative insofar as he is subject to strong feelings of shame about his work or his actions and to lowered self-regard. It is false in that he tries to be the perfect son, husband, army man, and student but, in so doing, suppresses his own identity. Jim wants to be himself, speak up for himself, and take care of his own needs, but instead he feels that he lives at the whims of his wife, the army, and his professors. As such he is not a fully individuated person.

Dynamic Features of Personality

A central conflict for Jim, which is largely unconscious, is whether to obey authority slavishly or flout it defiantly. Currently, Jim either complies with others' standards, which he assumes to be as unreasonable as his father's, or he rebels in a passive way by doing what he wants to on the sly. For example, he turns to pornography, defying his wife's wishes, and satisfying his own sexual needs. He shows up at the college exam but rebels against the "tough" professor by blanking out and refusing to comply with the professor's implied demands that he perform, and perform well. The symptom of cognitive confusion is a compromise between a wish to go his own way by not even showing up at the exam and the contrary wish to be the good, obedient student who performs flawlessly. So he comes to take the exam but does not perform.

Jim evidences splits between good and bad internalized images of both parents. He says he hates his father but has internalized many of his father's standards and acknowledges still feeling some caring for him. He idealizes his mother, failing to recognize her rejection of him and his siblings as a burden and her failure to intercede on his behalf with his brutalizing father.

Several dynamic perspectives might be considered in understanding Jim's primary symptom of blocking during exams. Oedipal elements may

be interfering unconsciously with Jim's exam taking. His self-report and recurrent dream reveal a strong childhood wish to have mother to himself
and father out of the picture. That this is a sexualized wish may be hypothesized from the fact that, in the dream, his mother is dressed up as she
would be to go out with father, and that, until the age of 6, Jim cuddled
with mother in bed until extruded by father. He later acknowledged that
she kissed him in a way that made him uncomfortable. Was this experienced as a sexual, arousing incestuous wish followed by disgust? One
response to this Oedipal wish may be displacement of Jim's rageful and
competitive feelings toward father onto other authorities, such as the professor, whom Jim unconsciously wants to defeat even if it means bringing
the house down, Samson-like, on himself—that is, failing the exam. Another motive for Jim's blocking in exam-taking may be Oedipal guilt which
requires that he arrange to fail in order not to surpass his father. The wish
to have his mother to himself may represent both Oedipal elements and
early dependent longings and efforts to get the kind of nurturance he
needed to blossom. The concept of survivor guilt (e.g., Weiss, 1993) may
also be at play in his feeling that fate dealt harshly with his parents and that
he ought not do better in life than they, nor should he do better than he
"deserves." Not all these dynamic perspectives will prove to be accurate or
resonant in understanding Jim's symptoms and complaints, but more than
one may well apply in accordance with the psychoanalytic concept of the
multidetermination of symptoms. If Jim were to enter therapy, one would
seek further evidence to support or refute these hypotheses.

Developmental Antecedents

Jim was emotionally abused as a child by a domineering, controlling father and a seductive, immature mother who did not protect him from his
father's inappropriate demands. He hates them, yet longs for what he
missed out on as a child. Because of Jim's abrupt withdrawal from his
family during adolescence, he was never able to sort out his ambivalent
feelings toward his parents. The sudden loss has left him with a barely
acknowledged feeling of sadness, and there exists a lack of internal separation from them.

Adaptive Features: Assets and Strengths

Jim has considerable assets. He is bright, artistic, skilled with computers,
and recognized by others as such. He has found some contentment by escaping into art, music, and books. Even removing himself from a noxious
environment in adolescence speaks to his self-preservative abilities. He has
compassion for others, including his wife with whom he now has a reasonably good relationship. His defenses are flexible enough such that he can

access feelings without becoming overwhelmed. He also seems trusting of the interviewer and able to form a therapeutic relationship.

APPLICATION TO PSYCHOTHERAPY TECHNIQUE

Within a psychoanalytic framework, one use of a formulation is to determine suitability for an expressive, exploratory psychoanalytic therapy. The following criteria are important to consider: (1) the willingness to share personal thoughts and feelings with the interviewer; (2) access to, and an ability to experience and tolerate, dysphoric feelings such as anxiety, guilt, and sadness; (3) motivation for change; (4) psychological-mindedness, or the capacity for introspection; (5) flexibility of defenses; (6) the degree and intensity of fixation at the Oedipal versus pre-Oedipal stages; (7) a positive response to interpretation such as demonstrable affect, new associations, increased reflection, fresh memories; and so on. The formulation can help determine suitability for a range of approaches including brief psychodynamic therapy (when a clear focus is discernible), supportive therapy (when defense strengthening is necessary), group therapy (to help alleviate interpersonal problems), behavior therapy (e.g., for stress reduction), and so forth.

Another major use of the formulation is to set out goals and outcomes for therapy depending on the time and intensity of work possible. Here is a set of goals for Jim were he to enter an open-ended psychoanalytically oriented therapy:

1. *Autonomous ego functions: the symptom.* He will explore and understand the dynamics underlying his blanking out on tests, and gain symptomatic relief.

2. *Dynamic and self-related issues.* He will acquire a clearer sense of his wishes and needs and express more of who he is and what he wants. He will be less conflicted about complying versus rebelling, and will have a greater sense of freedom in choosing to act in either direction. His self-esteem will increase and will be less subject to buffeting by others.

3. *Affects, drives, and defenses.* Jim will be more able to face and accept his mixed feelings including anger, longing, deprivation, sadness, and guilt. He will have less need to escape, minimize, rationalize, or project feelings. He will be less inclined to act out violent feelings, and will be somewhat more relaxed and at peace with himself. He will work at expressing anger in a modulated way.

4. *Object relations: general.* In his relationships with others, he will come to feel less compelled to acquiesce automatically to fulfill others' needs and will ask appropriately to have his needs met. That is, he will not allow himself to be victimized or need to view the world according to the

sharp dichotomy of victimizer/victimized. In general, he will tend to be more open and comfortable with people.

5. *Object relations: parental introjects.* Jim will start to sort out his feelings about his parents and see them more realistically, with both their good and bad features. He will engage in a process of separating from them internally while feeling freer to visit them if he wishes.

6. *Object relations: marital interaction.* Jim will resolve his compulsion to view pornography by enjoying it without guilt or feeling less need for it, or both. The role it plays in his marital interaction will become clarified and at least partially resolved.

Broader aspects of a satisfactory therapeutic outcome are that the patient internalizes and comes to use the analyzing function initially supplied by the therapist and is able to arrive at a more integrated, self-accepting state. Although the formulation is not conveyed immediately or directly to the patient, its major elements would become clear as the therapy proceeds. The therapist's role is to act as a catalyst for the patient's self-exploration, using the case formulation as a road map for the journey. Thus, in addition to its role in prescribing the nature of the therapy and setting goals for it, the formulation serves like a ship's rudder, helping first the therapist and then the patient to steer a course which is most likely to result in reaching the desired shore.

In the case of Jim, the formulation served as a guide for the treatment, including goal setting. The case was formulated primarily in accordance with concepts highlighted in contemporary Freudian and object relations theory. Jim's major conflict was seen in impulse/defense terms as one between his wish to defy authority and to submit to it. One might expect this conflict to express itself in the way that Jim interacts with the therapist, namely, in a defiant and/or overly compliant manner. Interpretations in the therapy would address these themes, and the patient's responses would help to elaborate the case formulation. It was also noted that Jim longs for what he missed out on as a child, that he does not feel sufficiently separate from his parents, and that there are splits between the good and bad internalized images of both parents. These aspects of the formulation lend themselves more readily to interpretations that stem from object relations theory so that in this case concepts from different yet related analytic theories influence the therapist's interventions. For example, the formulation would lead us to expect that Jim will experience the therapist as someone whose nurturance he craves but from whom he expects to receive very little or by whom he expects to be mistreated. These enactments can turn out to be an obstacle to treatment or corrective emotional and interpersonal experiences.

Therapists vary in how much and at what level they share their developing working model of the patient. Most therapists offer a tentative, general, jargon-free formulation which points to the repetitive, ego-alien issues already somewhat familiar to the patient. In most instances the formulation presented by the clinician is more descriptive than explanatory and does not include interpretation of unconscious content. In fact, most psychoanalytic clinicians strive to create a therapeutic atmosphere in which the therapist and patient are coinvestigators and coauthors of a series of formulations that will emerge in the moment-to-moment interactions of the two participants. Thus, therapist and patient decide on the goals of psychotherapy collaboratively in the context of a frank discussion of the conditions of treatment. (See Wolitzky, 2003, for a more detailed exposition of the theory and practice of psychoanalytic therapy.)

TRAINING

To write a psychodynamic formulation, students need to have knowledge of developmental and adult psychopathology and various psychoanalytic theories. They also need to learn dynamic interviewing and psychotherapeutic skills to collect information necessary to construct the formulation. Thus, supervised exposure to intake interview material, therapy transcripts, psychodiagnostic test data, and their own therapy cases provide the clinical experience to complement students' theoretical knowledge. Psychoanalytic training programs often consider the student's own psychoanalytic therapy to be a vital source of knowledge in developing the clinical acumen necessary to create a complex dynamic formulation of the patient.

Our view is that training should illuminate the choice points for intervention as a function of the theory of pathology and change that one embraces. Thus, if one formulates that the patient suffers primarily from a disorder of the self stemming from failures in parental empathy, and that the amelioration of self-defects requires the opportunity to form idealizing and mirror transferences to compensate for the failure of the parents to function as idealizing and mirroring selfobjects, then one will want to act in ways most likely to facilitate these kinds of transferences. The specifics, however, will derive from the formulation.

A Kohutian supervisor would encourage the student to allow these kinds of transferences to blossom and to be careful lest the patient experience a retraumatization at the hands of the therapist. A Freudian supervisor, on the other hand, would be more inclined to point to the defensive functions of these kinds of transferences and to advise the student to begin to offer interpretations of the wishes and conflicts that presumably underlie the manifest clinical material, as presented in the case formulation. In fact, it has been shown that analysts of different theoretical persuasions can be distinguished on the basis of the interpretations that they are prepared to offer the patient (Fine & Fine, 1990). The relationship between theory and technique, however, is sufficiently loose to allow for considerable variation among practitioners of the same psychoanalytic approach, whether they are novices or experienced therapists.

RESEARCH SUPPORT FOR THE APPROACH

There is the danger that once made, a case formulation will become fixed in the clinician's mind, leaving him or her less open to other possibilities. For example, in a research project in which one of the authors participated several years ago (Dahl, 1983), clinicians weighted evidence in line with their own initial hypotheses more strongly than did other clinicians.

Involvement in the process of drawing inferences and making interpretations based on clinical material leads inevitably to a concern with the issues of reliability and validity. This topic is of vital importance with respect to the soundness of theory and the efficacy of treatment. Grünbaum (1984) has argued that data from the consulting room are "epistemologically contaminated." That is, the factor of suggestion carried in the therapist's interpretations, however inadvertent, prevents us from being in a position to validate core theoretical propositions within the context of the treatment situation. Grünbaum also argues that treatment outcome cannot be used to verify or disconfirm the accuracy of clinical interpretations. Others (e.g., Edelson, 1992), however, have taken issue with Grünbaum's conclusions.

To give one example of how the issue of reliability and validity can be framed and studied, Caston (1993, p. 493) has pointed out that psychoanalysis is as much endangered by overinflated agreement on stereotypical dynamic formulas as by lack of agreement. That is, even when there is good agreement among judges (and often there is not; see Seitz, 1966), it can be spurious if judges are using stereotypical inferences that are not particular to a given case. In a study designed to test this hypothesis, Caston and Martin (1993) used verbatim transcripts from the first five sessions of an audiorecorded psychotherapy. Their novel methodology included having some analysts make ratings *without benefit of reading the transcripts*. The authors demonstrated that in most domains of behavior, analysts agreed well among themselves and to a greater degree than would be expected if they were basing their judgments on theoretical stereotypes. In other words, they were responsive to the particulars of a given case.

On the other hand, using a different method of study, Collins and Messer (1991) have shown to what extent case formulations can be dependent on one's theoretical viewpoint. They found that two different research groups, guided either by Weissian cognitive–dynamic theory or by object relations theory, reliably endorsed different formulations of the same cases. This raised the question of whether adherence by the therapist to one or the other formulation had a differential effect on patient progress. To study this, Tishby and Messer (1995) compared the relationship between therapist interventions which were compatible with either a cognitive–dynamic or an object relations formulation and patient progress. They found that therapist interventions compatible with the object relations formulation were the better predictor of in-session patient progress in the middle phases of brief psychodynamic therapy for the two patients studied, as well as in the early phase for one of them. More such studies are needed in which the same cases are formulated from different perspectives and the relationship of such formulations to patient progress and outcome studied. It is these and other formal methods described in the chapters of this book that will be an important testing ground for the value of psychoanalytic case formulation.

As we noted earlier, there have been several efforts (e.g., McWilliams, 1999; Summers, 2003) to articulate the nature of traditional psychodynamic case formulation as it is practiced in a clinical, as opposed to a research, setting and to offer suggestions for how such formulations can be improved. However, a literature search from 1997 (when the first edition of this book appeared) through the first half of 2005 failed to uncover more than two or three research studies focused on the kind of psychodynamic case formulation that we have described. In contrast, there have been several recent research studies based on formal, quantitative methods of psychodynamic formulation (e.g., Luborsky's [Luborsky & Barrett, Chapter 4, this volume] and Perry's [1997] approaches).

It is unfortunate that there is such a dearth of empirical work on the nonquantitative, narrative style of case formulation used in routine clinical practice, as this is the context in which 99% of case formulations take place. The more formal methods, although useful for psychotherapy research, do not directly inform us about the validity or utility of case formulation as it is conducted in the typical clinical situation. It is our impression that the vast majority of psychodynamic clinicians continue to embrace the narrative tradition. They are not especially interested in applying more formal, systematic methods of case formulation on the grounds that these quantitative approaches fail to capture the richness, subtlety, and complexity of the clinical process.

As is common in all areas of research on psychodynamic approaches, there is an inevitable trade-off between richness of narrative or "thick description" and quantitative, systematic approaches. To their credit, investigators such as Luborsky (Luborsky & Barrett, Chapter 4, this volume) and Perry (1997) have made some inroads on minimizing the negative effects of this trade-off. Both make room for unconscious wishes in their scoring systems but avoid high levels of inference and, thus, unreliability. There is a downside, however. For example, masochism is a quality that Luborsky (1997) says should not be inferred because it cannot be scored reliably. He describes three levels of inference of which only the two lower levels are permissible in his system. Luborsky gives a concrete example in which the patient says, "So I don't even have unemployment coming in"; the wish that is inferred is "wants to get money" (p. 62). In formulating cases, psychodynamic clinicians do not want to be restricted to this level of inference and will gladly sacrifice reliability for complexity and subtlety.

Although Perry (1997) acknowledges that formulations of "dynamic patterns require clinical inference [his] rater-observers are required to support each assertion by listing the available evidence" (p. 142). While it is true that Perry's system also allows for inferences of unconscious wishes, one gets the impression that the requirement to cite evidence probably results mainly in the positing of conscious wishes. In fact, neither Luborsky nor Perry reports the percentage of inferred wishes that are assumed to be unconscious. For example, Perry, who works within an Eriksonian framework, lists wishes such as "Be comforted, soothed," "Be perfect, avoid shame," and "Attention from opposite sex." One assumes that most often the attribution of such wishes is based primarily on manifest content.

Our remarks are intended less as criticism of Luborsky's and Perry's work than at explaining why most psychodynamic clinicians do not make greater use of it. However, because Luborsky and his colleagues have been able to show that interpretation of the CCRT is correlated with therapy outcome (Crits-Christoph, Cooper, & Luborsky, 1988), the onus is on psychodynamic clinicians to show that interpretations of unconscious or deeper material are at least as effective in promoting positive therapeutic change.

It appears that aside from the formal methods of case formulation described in the chapters in this volume, virtually all the other recent empirical work on case formulation has been conducted by Eells (e.g., 1997) as described in Chapter 1 (this volume). Most relevant for our purposes is his unsettling finding that novice and experienced clinicians did not differ in the quality of their case formulations (Eells, Lombart, Kendjelic, Turner, & Lucas, 2005), although experts performed better than either novice or experienced clinicians. The experts, however, were a small, select group who were particularly interested in the issue of case formulation. They were either nationally recognized for their work on case formulation, had developed a method for case formulation, or had published or conducted workshops on the topic—hardly a typical group of clinicians.

These results are consistent with the fact that there rarely is any rigorous, sustained training in the construction of case formulations. In an earlier study, Eells, Kendjelic, and Lucas (1998) reported that when relatively inexperienced clinicians (psychiatric residents, social workers, and a psychiatric nurse) were asked to make case formulations based on brief vignettes, fewer than half included inferences about the causes of the patient's problems and, in general, used only very low level inferences.

Eells (1997) advises that a case formulation "should serve as a blueprint guiding treatment, as a marker for change" (p. 2). However, if inexperienced clinicians construct case formulations that are primarily descriptive (Eells et al., 1998) and if experienced clinicians are no better than novices at case formulation (Eells et al., 2005), one wonders how reliable and valid such formulations are as a "blueprint guiding treatment" when constructed by individual clinicians in the context of their routine clinical practice. One limitation of these studies, however, was that the clinical material was brief and perhaps lacked the richness to allow complex inferences. One reason that psychodynamic clinicians prefer open-ended, unstructured initial interviews is to create a more detailed database for case formulation. Despite having sounded these cautionary notes, we nevertheless favor further attempts to study case formulation empirically and to relate it to the process and outcome of psychotherapy.

ACKNOWLEDGMENTS

We express our appreciation to Nancy McWilliams, Katherine Parkerton, and Jamie Walkup for their helpful suggestions.

NOTES

1. It could be argued that the reference to three major models neglects Sullivan's interpersonal approach, the neo-Freudian schools such as Jung, Horney, and Adler, and the disciples of Klein (e.g., Schafer, 1994). Nor does this categorization give adequate consideration to theorists who have attempted to integrate two models such as Kernberg's (1980) effort to combine traditional Freudian and ego-psychological theory with object relations concepts. Nevertheless, the present classification is sufficient for our present goal of explicating the nature of, and the issues involved in, psychodynamic case formulation. Also note that, for present purposes, we use the terms "psychoanalytic" and "psychodynamic" interchangeably.

2. The postmodern sensibility in contemporary culture not only is seen in literary criticism and in the humanities but has influenced psychoanalysis as well. As Leary (1994) notes, a key feature of postmodernism is that there is no "truly objective" knowledge of the "real order" of things. As applied to psychoanalytic discourse, this view suggests that meanings are generated or created in a dyadic context; they are a coauthored narrative based on the interaction of two subjectivities. That is, whereas in Freud's day there were meanings to be discovered, in the postmodern view there are no "essential meanings" to be unearthed. In keeping with Freud's archaeological metaphor, one could dig into deeper and deeper layers of the unconscious and find important pieces of the individual's past history that were living on in the present. Even if the idea that recall of a traumatic event would cause the symptom to disappear had to be abandoned, one could fall back on the notion that interpretations that "tally with what is

real" would alleviate symptoms. When it became evident that one could not reliably demonstrate any kind of cause-and-effect relationship between interpretations with specific content and symptom remission, the door was open to the theoretical pluralism that characterizes contemporary psychoanalytic thought.

REFERENCES

Bocknek, G. (1991). *Ego and self in weekly psychotherapy.* Madison, WI: International Universities Press.

Brenner, C. (1973). *An elementary textbook of psychoanalysis* (rev. ed.). New York: International Universities Press.

Brenner, C. (1982). *The mind in conflict.* New York: International Universities Press.

Breuer, J., & Freud, S. (1955). Studies on hysteria. In J. Strachey (Ed. and Trans.), *The standard edition of the complete psychological works of Sigmund Freud* (Vol. 3, pp. 1–305). London: Hogarth Press. (Original work published 1893–1895)

Caston, J. (1993). Can analysts agree? The problems of consensus and the psychoanalytic mannequin: I. A proposed solution. *Journal of the American Psychoanalytic Association, 41,* 493–512.

Caston, J., & Martin, E. (1993). Can analysts agree?: The problems of consensus and the psychoanalytic mannequin: II. Empirical tests. *Journal of the American Psychoanalytic Association, 41,* 513–548.

Collins, W. D., & Messer, S. B. (1991). Extending the Plan Formulation Method to an object relations perspective: Reliability, stability and adaptability. *Psychological Assessment: A Journal of Consulting and Clinical Psychology, 3,* 75–81.

Crits-Christoph, P., Cooper, A., & Luborsky, L. (1988). The accuracy of therapist's interpretations and the outcome of dynamic psychotherapy. *Journal of Consulting and Clinical Psychology, 56,* 490–495.

Dahl, H. (1983). On the definition and measurement of wishes. In J. Masling (Ed.), *Empirical studies of psychoanalytic theories* (pp. 39–67). Hillsdale, NJ: Erlbaum.

Edelson, M. (1992). Telling and enacting stories in psychoanalysis. In J. Barron, M. Eagle, & D. L. Wolitzky (Eds.), *Interface of psychoanalysis and psychology* (pp. 99–124). Washington, DC: American Psychological Association.

Eells, T. D. (1997). Psychotherapy case formulation: History and current status. In T. D. Eells (Ed.), *Handbook of psychotherapy case formulation* (pp. 1–25). New York: Guilford Press.

Eells, T. D., Kendjelic, E. M., & Lucas, C. P. (1998). What's in a case formulation? Development and use of a content coding manual. *Journal of Psychotherapy Practice and Research, 7,* 144–153.

Eells, T. D., Lombart, K. G., Kendjelic, E. M., Turner, L. C., & Lucas, C. P. (2005). The quality of psychotherapy case formulations: A comparison of expert, experienced, and novice cognitive-behavioral and psychodynamic therapists. *Journal of Consulting and Clinical Psychology, 73,* 579–589.

Fairbairn, W. R. D. (1952). *Psychoanalytic studies of the personality.* London: Tavistock & Routledge & Kegan Paul.

Fine, S., & Fine, E. (1990). Four psychoanalytic perspectives: A study of differences in interpretive interventions. *Journal of the American Psychoanalytic Association,* 38, 1017–1041.

Freud, S. (1953). The interpretation of dreams. In J. Strachey (Ed. and Trans.), *The standard edition of the complete psychological works of Sigmund Freud* (Vols. 4 & 5). London: Hogarth Press. (Original work published 1900)

Friedman, R. S., & Lister, P. (1987). The current status of psychodynamic formulation. *Psychiatry, 50,* 126–141.

Greenberg, J., & Mitchell, S. A. (1983). *Object relations and psychoanalytic theory.* Cambridge, MA: Harvard University Press.

Grünbaum, A. (1984). *The foundations of psychoanalysis: A philosophical critique.* Berkeley: University of California Press.

Guntrip, H. (1971). *Psychoanalytic theory, therapy and the self.* New York: Basic Books.

Kernberg, O. (1980). *Internal world and external reality: Object relations theory applied.* New York: Jason Aronson.

Klein, M. (1948). *Contributions to psychoanalysis, 1921–1945.* London: Hogarth Press.

Kohut, H. (1971). *The analysis of the self: A systematic approach to the psychoanalytic treatment of narcissistic personality disorders.* New York: International Universities Press.

Kohut, H. (1977). *The restoration of the self.* New York: International Universities Press.

Kohut, H. (1984). *How does analysis cure?* Chicago: University of Chicago Press.

Lachmann, F. M., & Lichtenberg, J. (1992). Model scenes: Implications for psychoanalytic treatment. *Journal of the American Psychoanalytic Association, 40,* 17–132.

Lam, A. G., & Sue, S. (2001). Client diversity. *Psychotherapy: Theory, Research, Practice, Training, 38,* 479–486.

Leary, K. (1994). Psychoanalytic "problems" and postmodern "solutions." *Psychoanalytic Quarterly, 63,* 433–465.

Luborsky, L. (1997). The Core Conflictual Relationship Theme: A basic case formulation method. In T. D. Eells (Ed.), *Handbook of psychotherapy case formulation* (pp. 58–83). New York: Guilford Press.

MacKinnon, R. A., & Michels, R. (1971). *The psychiatric interview in clinical practice.* Philadelphia: Saunders.

McWilliams, N. (1994). *Psychoanalytic diagnosis.* New York: Guilford Press.

McWilliams, N. (1998). Relationship, subjectivity, and inference in diagnosis. In J. W. Barron (Ed.), *Making diagnosis meaningful* (pp. 197–226). Washington, DC: American Psychological Association Press.

McWilliams, N. (1999). *Psychoanalytic case formulation.* New York: Guilford Press.

Messer, S. B., Sass, L. A., & Woolfolk, R. L. (Eds.). (1988). *Hermeneutics and psychological theory: Interpretive perspectives on personality, psychotherapy and psychopathology.* New Brunswick, NJ: Rutgers University Press.

Messer, S. B., & Warren, C. S. (1995). *Models of brief psychodynamic therapy: A comparative approach.* New York: Guilford Press.

Morrison, J. (1997). *When psychological problems mask medical disorders: A guide for psychotherapists.* New York: Guilford Press.

Okazaki, S., Kallivayalil, D., & Sue, S. (2002). Clinical personality assessment with

Asian Americans. In J. N. Butcher (Ed.), *Clinical personality assessment: Practical approaches* (2nd ed., pp. 135–153). London: Oxford University Press.

Peebles-Kleiger, M. J. (2002). *Beginnings: The art and science of planning psychotherapy.* Hillsdale, NJ: Analytic Press.

Perry, J. C. (1997). The idiographic case formulation method. In T. D. Eells (Ed.), *Handbook of psychotherapy case formulation* (pp. 137–165). New York: Guilford Press.

Perry, S., Cooper, A. M., & Michels, R. (1987). The psychodynamic formulation: Its purpose, structure, and clinical application. *American Journal of Psychiatry, 144,* 543–550.

Peterfreund, E. (1976). How does the analyst listen?: On models and strategies in the psychoanalytic process. In D. P. Spence (Ed.), *Psychoanalysis and contemporary science* (Vol. 4, pp. 59–101). New York: International Universities Press.

Pine, F. (1990). *Drive, ego, object, and self: A synthesis for clinical work.* New York: Basic Books.

Prince, M. (1905). *The dissociation of a personality.* London: Longmans Green.

Rapaport, D., & Gill, M. M. (1959). The points of view and assumptions of metapsychology. *International Journal of Psycho-Analysis, 40,* 153–162.

Rothbaum, F., Weisz, J., Pott, M., Miyake, K., & Morelli, G. (2000). Attachment and culture: Security in the United States and Japan. *American Psychologist, 55,* 1093–1104.

Schafer, R. (1976). *A new language for psychoanalysis.* Oxford, UK: Yale University Press.

Schafer, R. (1992). *Retelling a life: Narration and dialogue in psychoanalysis.* New York: Basic Books.

Schafer, R. (1994). The contemporary Kleinians of London. *Psychoanalytic Quarterly, 63,* 409–432.

Seitz, P. F. D. (1966). The consensus problem in psychoanalytic research. In L. A. Gottschalk & A. H. Auerbach (Eds.), *Methods of research in psychotherapy* (pp. 209–225). New York: Appleton-Century-Crofts.

Silverman, D. (1986). A multi-model approach: Looking at clinical data from three theoretical perspectives. *Psychoanalytic Psychology, 3,* 121–132.

Slap, J., & Slap-Shelton, L. (1991). *The schema in clinical psychoanalysis.* Hillsdale, NJ: Analytic Press.

Sue, S. (2004). *Ethnocultural psychotherapy.* Washington, DC: American Psychological Association.

Sue, S., & Lam, A. G. (2002). Cultural and demographic diversity. In J. C. Norcross (Ed.), *Psychotherapy relationships that work: Therapist contributions and responsiveness to patients* (pp. 401–421). London: Oxford University Press.

Sullivan, H. S. (1954). *The psychiatric interview.* New York: Norton.

Summers, R. F. (2003). The psychodynamic formulation updated. *American Journal of Psychotherapy, 57,* 39–51.

Tishby, O., & Messer, S. B. (1995). The relationship between plan compatibility of therapist interventions and patient progress: A comparison of two plan formulations. *Psychotherapy Research, 5,* 76–88.

Weiss, J. (1993). *How psychotherapy works: Process and technique.* New York: Guilford Press.

Winnicott, D. (1965). *The maturational process and the facilitating environment.* New York: International Universities Press.

Wolitzky, D. L. (2003). The theory and practice of traditional psychoanalytic treatment. In A. S. Gurman & S. B. Messer (Eds.), *Essential psychotherapies: Theory and practice* (pp. 24–68). New York: Guilford Press.

Chapter 4

The Core Conflictual Relationship Theme

A Basic Case Formulation Method

LESTER LUBORSKY
MARNA S. BARRETT

HISTORICAL BACKGROUND OF THE APPROACH

An old goal of personality assessment—to devise a reliable measure of the central relationship pattern—began to be developed in the mid-1970s. Detailed examinations of treatment sessions were conducted to look for ways in which a central pattern of relating was revealed. Early papers dealing with the idea of a central relationship pattern (Luborsky, 1976, 1977) were found to include the essentials of the Core Conflictual Relationship Theme (CCRT) method (Luborsky, 1998a, 1998b).

Advances in both CCRT scoring and empirical studies with diverse clinical populations have been large enough to require a new CCRT guide (Luborsky & Crits-Christoph, 1990, 1998) and an updated review of its usefulness. Our aim in revising this chapter for this edition was (1) to present a clearer and more organized set of rules for measuring the central relationship pattern evident in psychotherapy sessions, and (2) to show how the CCRT can serve as a model for detailed examination and understanding of the patient–therapist exchange.

CONCEPTUAL FRAMEWORK

Psychotherapy now has a sound measure for study of the central relationship pattern in psychotherapy sessions—the CCRT. The central principle of the CCRT method is that repetition across relationship narratives is good for assessing the central relationship pattern. It reflects an underlying schema of each person's partly conscious and partly unconscious knowledge structure of how to conduct relationship interactions.

Starting in 1973, Luborsky retraced the cues that led him to infer a central relationship pattern: (1) the relationship pattern of patients focuses on narratives about wishes and responses in relationships with others and with the self; and (2) the central relationship pattern was best defined by the combination of the most frequent wishes, the responses from others, and the responses of the self across relationship episodes. In other words, the CCRT represents a complex interaction of wishes and responses, in combination with the pervasiveness of each of these components. For instance, in Case 2, Ms. Roberts describes an interaction with a coworker in which the following exchange was reported:

> // In fact a girl called me crazy today//. And I wanted to cry// I wanted to tell her I think you need to go see a psychiatrist yourself // and sometimes people do act crazy. I told her // I wasn't ashamed of it. //

This relationship episode includes wishes (to be assertive and accepted), the response of other (to criticize), and the response of the patient (to be angry, not hurt). By examining several of these relationship exchanges with different people, patterns emerge such that the therapist can recognize the central theme that defines relationship conflicts for the patient.

Whereas reductions in distress or other measures of symptomatic improvement indicate a beneficial outcome to therapy, treatment benefits can also be identified through changes in the CCRT. For instance, benefits can be evidenced by (1) changes in the CCRT patterns (Crits-Christoph & Luborsky, 1998a), (2) reductions in the pervasiveness of CCRT components (Cierpka et al., 1998), (3) increases in the accuracy of interpretation, (Crits-Christoph, Cooper, & Luborsky, 1998), and (4) mastery of the central relationship patterns (i.e., emotional self-control and intellectual self-understanding) (Grenyer & Luborsky, 1996).

In using the CCRT method to guide clinical case formulations, four basic assumptions are made. First, the unit of text to be scored is the narrative told during sessions about relationship episodes. The narrative includes wishes, the response from other people, and/or the response of self. Second, the CCRT can be reliably extracted from identified relationship episodes. A third assumption is that the CCRT is based on pervasiveness, which is the frequency of each relationship component divided by the number of relationship episodes examined. Fourth, the CCRT is a central pattern that is evident across a variety of relationship interactions.

From a theoretical perspective, each of the assumptions of the CCRT method is consistent with an object relations perspective on interpersonal and intrapersonal conflicts. In other words, conflicts with others and with self are defined by early patterns of relating. Moreover, the CCRT offers an operational measure of what Freud (1912/1958a, 1912/1958b) conceived of as the "transference template."

INCLUSION/EXCLUSION CRITERIA AND MULTICULTURAL CONSIDERATIONS

When people describe relationship episodes they provide material for assessment of their CCRT. All people, as Freud (1912/1958) said, have "a stereotype plate (or several such)" (p. 100). Our experience in using the CCRT method suggests that the formulation can be applied to people across all levels of psychiatric severity and ethnic and cultural groups with a nearly unique pattern for each person. For instance, although we have standard categories and clusters into which the wishes and responses of most people would fall, early work in developing the CCRT found considerable variability among patient narratives. In fact, the first two editions of the CCRT (Crits-Christoph & Demorest, 1988; Luborsky, 1986) recognized this variability and allowed for additional "tailor-made" categories for individual patient responses.

Although a number of studies have included men and women as well as individuals of varying ethnicity, relatively few studies have directly examined differences between these groups in terms of CCRT categories. One of the only studies of gender (Staats, May, Herrmann, Kersting, & König, 1998) examined the relationship patterns of men and women over the course of group therapy. Although some gender stereotypes persisted in narratives (e.g., women reported more negative responses suggesting the need to be cared for) and the number of negative responses given by men increased (perceiving that wishes are blocked and they are no longer in control), these differences were not related to symptom changes. These findings, although limited, suggest that stereotypical gender responses or increased negative responses may not reflect maladaptive interpersonal patterns but expected gender differences.

The research on racial and cultural differences in CCRT patterns is even less clear-cut than that for gender. Although the CCRT method has been used in research studies with German, Mexican, Italian, and Latin American populations (Albani, Blaser, Hölzer, & Pokorny, 2002; Charlin et al., 2001; Contiero et al., 2002; Hinojosa Ayala, 2005), the findings tell us little about potential differences in CCRT narratives that would influence clinical practice. For instance, the CCRT components in narratives from 32 German female psychotherapy patients were more reliable than that found in U.S. populations (Albani, Blaser, Körner, et al., 2002) suggesting the stability of wishes and responses across people. In contrast, in an Italian sample, judges had such poor agreement on assignment of CCRT categories that the authors concluded that "linguistic and cultural meanings" of words from different languages and different peoples need to be considered in using the CCRT with different cultural groups (Dazzi et al., 1998).

Thus, we encourage caution when using the standard categories in patients from non-U.S. cultures, but note that use of "tailor-made" categories may be quite helpful especially when developed in conjunction with the patient (see Luborsky, 1986). Moreover, despite the lack of data we would speculate that any interpersonal dynamic that is unique to a culture would, in general, affect CCRT formulations. For example, among many Asian cultures there is a strong sense of interdependence between the individual and cultural community and a reticence to discuss problems outside the family. Thus, one might expect that such characteristics would result in narratives with generally fewer responses, few negative components in the wishes and responses, and CCRT patterns that may be more reflective of the cultural group than the individual.

In an effort to demonstrate possible racial differences, we have selected case examples that involve a Caucasian woman and an African American woman. However, as can be seen from the CCRT formulation for these women (Tables 4.2 and 4.3), racial differences did not seem to alter the main relational themes. This finding may suggest that within an American sample, differences are only evident at the component level (i.e., a specific wish or response). However, research studies with large numbers of patients are needed to fully address potential race, culture, and gender differences in CCRT patterns.

STEPS IN CASE FORMULATION

The CCRT is at the heart of each case formulation. The CCRT procedures for scoring relationship episodes are provided below as well as in the clinical guide by Book (1998). There are two different settings in which a CCRT is extracted: (1) *during the session*, when the patient tells narratives to a therapist and the therapist uses them in the session to make formulations, or (2) *after the session*, when an evaluator or researcher reviews the narratives, usually from transcripts, then scores the CCRT.

Identifying a Relationship Episode

There are two main phases in scoring a CCRT: during "phase A" the relationship episodes are identified and during "phase B" the CCRT is extracted from the relationship episodes. By far the most usual source of relationship episodes is psychotherapy sessions (see below for additional sources of relationship episodes). These episodes are almost always spontaneously told, with an average of about four relationship episodes per session. These episodes are defined as the part of a session in which there is an explicit narrative about relationships with others, or at times, with the self.

In the course of the narratives, each relationship episode (RE) describes an interaction between the patient and a main other person. It is part of the judge's (or therapist's) job to determine the main other person and the boundaries of the episodes (i.e., where a relationship episode begins and ends). These episodes tend to be easily recognized because they have a typical narrative structure, with a beginning, middle, and ending. Also, just before a narrative begins, the intention to tell a narrative is often introduced by some usual signs, such as a pause, followed by a direct statement introducing the narrative. For example, after a pause the patient might introduce a narrative with the statement "I met Joe today and we had a chance to talk it out." In this example the naming of another person with whom an event has occurred is an indication of the beginning of a narrative.

If the CCRT is scored using a transcript, the boundaries of each relationship episode are identified on the session transcript by an independent experienced judge. The components of the episodes are then scored by trained CCRT judges. Although each relationship episode is scored independently, the CCRT scoring is done with knowledge of the other narratives in the context of the session. This "in-context-of-the-session" scoring is important in guiding the scorer to the most accurate assessment.

It should be noted that some practice is needed to become proficient at identifying and scoring CCRTs during a session. However, proficiency can be obtained in a relatively short time by scoring several transcripts outside therapy, making note of the RE in-session, and keeping a list of component categories handy for review.

The Relationship Anecdote Paradigms Interview

The Relationship Anecdote Paradigm (RAP) interview is a method specifically designed to increase the frequency of narratives by having the interviewee tell several relationship episodes. Directly requesting narratives about relationships broadens the sources of data for the CCRT and is particularly useful in research (Luborsky, 1998c). Each narrative is an actual event in which there is a specific interaction with a specific person. The interview generally takes 30–50 minutes during which the interviewee generates about 10 narratives. Current research suggests that CCRTs from RAP narratives yield results similar to CCRTs from session narratives (Barber, Luborsky, Crits-Christoph, & Diguer, 1995).

The CCRT Self-Report Questionnaire

In addition to the traditional CCRT method, a questionnaire form of the CCRT was developed by Crits-Christoph (1986) that asks patients to rate on a 1–5 scale how typical each of a number of wishes and responses are of their relationships (see also Barber, Foltz, & Weinryb, 1998; Dahlbender, Albani, Pokorny, & Kächele, 1998). The self-report questionnaire also asks patients to write a sentence or two about their main conflicts. The CCRT questionnaire has demonstrated significant intercorrelations within component categories (Crits-Christoph & Luborsky, 1998b) and has shown negative correlations with measures of repressive style (Luborsky, Crits-Christoph, & Alexander, 1990). However, correlations with RAP-generated CCRTs were generally low (Crits-Christoph & Luborsky, 1998b) and no study has yet compared the CCRT questionnaire with CCRT formulations from psychotherapy sessions.

The Self-Interpretation of the CCRT

Another method for learning about the degree to which patients understand their own central relationship pattern is through the use of a self-interpretation procedure (Luborsky, 1965). In this procedure patients/subjects are either given a transcript of their narratives from a session or are asked to review their RAP narratives (see Crits-Christoph, 1986). In response to each narrative, individuals rate each of a number of wishes and responses on the degree to which they apply to the behavior of the individual in the identified RE. Patients/subjects also describe what conflict, if any, was present in each interaction. Research on the self-interpretation of the CCRT found reasonably high internal consistency for wishes (i.e., same themes identified across several REs) with patient-identified wishes consistent with ratings by clinicians (Crits-Christoph & Luborsky, 1998b).

Scoring Methods

Scoring Units

Having noted each relationship episode, the judge/therapist now identifies the components in each episode that are able to be scored, that is, the wishes (W), response of others (RO), and response of self (RS). The components to be scored are underlined or identified by slash marks (///) before and after the component in the episode (see examples that follow).

Standard Categories

Each component of a relationship episode is scored according to a uniform set of categories that have been established through previous research and are detailed in Table 4.1 (Barber, Crits-Christoph, & Luborsky, 1998; Crits-Christoph & Demorest, 1988; Luborsky, 1986). The most recent version of the categories (Barber, Crits-Cristoph, & Luborsky, 1998) are relatively easy to use and are based on cluster analysis techniques that yielded eight categories of W (34 statements), eight categories of RO (30 statements), and eight categories of RS (30 statements).[1]

Although a complete assessment should include a listing of all categories that fit the statement, at a minimum two ratings should be made. The category that "best fits" the component statement is listed first. The second number listed is the next best-fitting category. A line under a number means it is an exact fit to a category in the list; a question mark means the "fit" is questionable. Although each of the component categories is relatively distinct, patients may also distinguish ROs that are *expected* to happen from ROs that have already *happened*. Those that are expected should be scored as "RO-expected" so that comparisons can be made with ROs that have happened to see whether these have a different significance.

The Most Desirable Range of Inference for Proper Scoring

When scoring each component statement, some degree of inference may be required in selecting the appropriate category. For instance, patient statements may fit directly into a standard category so that almost no inference is required. On the other hand, a moderate level of inference may be required when the statement does not directly fit a category, as in the following: "*So I don't even have 'unemployment'* (money) *coming in.*" When a category is to some extent inferred, the component is noted with surrounding parentheses, such as a (W), as in the previous example of an inferred wish for money/security.

The Intensity of Each Type of Component

The intensity of each component refers to the degree of affect reflected in the statement. Either the affect is directly experienced by the patient or the experience of affect is inferred from the statement. Intensity is rated from 1 for "little or none" to 5 "very much." For example, the statement "*that irritated me*" would be rated 4 as an RS; in contrast, "*I wish to assert this*"

TABLE 4.1. Standard Categories for Scoring CCRT Components

Edition 3 (clusters)	Edition 2
Wishes	
1. To assert self and be independent	21. To have self-control
	28. To be my own person
	34. To assert myself
	23. To be independent
2. To oppose, hurt, and control others	18. To oppose others
	16. To hurt others
	19. To have control of others
3. To be controlled, hurt, and not responsible	15. To be hurt
	20. To be controlled by others
	29. To *not* be responsible/obligated
	13. To be helped
	27. To be like others
4. To be distant and avoid conflicts	17. To avoid conflicts
	14. To not be hurt
	10. To be distant from others
5. To be close and accepting	4. To accept others
	5. To respect others
	9. To be open
	6. To have trust
	8. To be opened up to
	11. To be close to others
6. To be loved and understood	33. To be loved
	3. To be respected
	1. To be understood
	2. To be accepted
	7. To be liked
7. To feel good and comfortable	30. To have stability
	31. To feel comfortable
	32. To feel happy
	24. To feel good about self
8. To achieve and help others	22. To achieve
	25. To better myself
	12. To help others
	26. To be good
Responses from other	
1. Strong	24. Strong
	23. Independent
	24. Happy
2. Controlling	26. Strict
	20. Controlling
3. Upset	16. Hurt
	22. Dependent
	28. Anxious
	27. Angry
	19. Out of control
4. Bad	8. Not trustworthy
	25. Bad

TABLE 4.1. (*continued*)

Edition 3 (clusters)	Edition 2
5. Rejecting and opposing	7. Don't trust me
	6. Don't respect me
	2. Are not understanding
	4. Rejecting
	10. Dislike me
	12. Distant
	14. Unhelpful
	17. Oppose me
6. Helpful	15. Hurt me
	13. Are helpful
	18. Cooperative
7. Likes me	30. Loves me
	5. Respects me
	9. Likes me
	21. Gives me independence
8. Understanding	11. Open
	1. Understanding
	3. Accepting

Responses of self

1. Helpful	7. Am open
	1. Understand
	9. Am helpful
2. Unreceptive	2. Don't understand
	8. Am not open
	6. Dislike others
3. Respected and accepted	28. Feel comfortable
	29. Feel happy
	30. Feel loved
	4. Feel respected
	3. Feel accepted
	5. Like others
4. Oppose and hurt others	11. Oppose others
	10. Hurt others
5. Self-controlled and self-confident	14. Self-controlled
	15. Independent
	18. Self-confident
	12. Controlling
6. Helpless	13. Out of control
	17. Helpless
	19. Uncertain
	16. Dependent
7. Disappointed and depressed	21. Angry
	20. Disappointed
	22. Depressed
	23. Unloved
	24. Jealous
8. Anxious and ashamed	27. Anxious
	26. Ashamed
	25. Guilty

would be rated 3 as a W. These ratings may be more easily made when the CCRT formulation is determined within the session because affect can be directly observed.

It is also useful to indicate whether the scored component is toward or against the satisfaction of W (see gender issues). If the component is in support of W, the component is considered positive and preceded by a P (PRO). If the component is against satisfaction of W, the component is considered negative and is preceded by an N (NRS).

A CCRT Scoring Method Based on Sequences of Components

Noting the sequence of the W, RO, and RS within each relationship episode can offer additional insight into the patient's typical relationship patterns. Whereas the usual CCRT method relies on the highest frequency of each type of CCRT component regardless of sequence, the sequence-of-components method focuses only on sequences of components in the RE (Luborsky, 1998b; Dahlbender et al., 1998). The sequence-of-components method has identified CCRTs similar to that derived using the standard CCRT method (Luborsky, Barber, Schaffler, & Cacciola, 1998). Moreover, sequences involving a higher percentage of interactions with people were associated with better psychological health (Mitchell, 1995).

Time Required for Scoring the CCRT

A formulation of the CCRT *during* a psychotherapy session takes no extra time as it is done in the session. The therapist identifies relationship episodes as they are described by the patient and listens for evidence of W, ROs, and RSs. Once familiar with the CCRT, the therapist periodically organizes what the patient says into the CCRT framework.

However, when using a session transcript to identify the CCRT, it can take 45 minutes to 1 hour to read the transcript, identify the REs, and score each component. Although experience can certainly shorten the time needed, it should be recognized that a typical session has about 4 REs and each episode may have several W, ROs, and RSs to be scored, thus requiring a fair amount of time. Regardless, the time required for using the CCRT scoring method is less than that required for other available transference-related measures.

APPLICATION TO PSYCHOTHERAPY TECHNIQUE

Help in Understanding

In most forms of psychotherapy, and certainly in dynamic psychotherapies, the therapist tries to make an accurate formulation of the patient's main conflicts (Luborsky, 1994). Accurate formulations will lead to accurate CCRT interpretations, as well as limiting the countertransference expressed in the interpretations (Singer & Luborsky, 1977). The steps in making accurate formulations and interpretations in supportive–expressive psychotherapy have been described for patients in general (Luborsky, 1984) as well as patients with depression (Luborsky, Mark, Hole, Popps, Goldsmith, & Cacciola, 1995); generalized anxiety disorder (Crits-Christoph, Crits-Christoph, Wolf-Palacio, Fichter, & Rudick, 1995), and substance abuse (Grenyer, Luborsky, & Solowij, 1995; Luborsky, Woody, Hole, & Velleco, 1995; Mark & Luborsky, 1992; Mark & Faude, 1995).

To formulate the CCRT during a session the therapist listens for the redundant components across the narratives that the patient tells. The CCRT is formulated by keeping track of the number of the most redundant Ws, the most redundant ROs, and most redundant RSs.

Help with Shaping Interpretations

As a general principle, the shorter the time limit of the treatment, the more a consistent focus of interpretations on the CCRT is useful. The CCRT pattern provides more impetus for the patient's recognition of the CCRT and gradually stimulates the patient's growth through mastering conflicts in the pattern.

Because the CCRT is a complex formulation, it is unusual for the therapist to present the entire CCRT in one interpretation. Instead, the following guidelines will help in deciding how to present the CCRT piecemeal so that the patient builds up a concept of a main pattern and attends to the mastery of the problems within it.

1. Begin with the aspects of the CCRT that the patient is most readily able to handle, such as those that are most familiar to the patient or occur most frequently across REs. Also, choose interpretations involving the W and the RO, as there is more empirical support for the use of these components in interpretations (Crits-Christoph et al., 1998).

2. Fashion some interpretations with CCRT components that contain the symptom. In this way the patient will begin to form a concept of the context in which the symptom appears. As with Ms. Smyth (Case 1), the therapist's repeated statements can be reduced to a single main unit, "*You want to be helped but feel rejected and so become depressed.*"

3. Because significant emotional reactions often accompany negative interpersonal exchanges and attending to such exchanges can advance treatment, it is especially helpful to concentrate interpretations on negative components. However, it should be noted that attention to emotionally charged interpersonal episodes risk potential ruptures in the therapeutic alliance that may hinder the progress of treatment.

4. Choose a style of interpretation that strengthens the alliance and does not provoke resistance. For example, Wachtel (1993) suggests that any tinge of a blaming, confrontational manner in providing interpretations may stimulate resistance. In contrast, presenting interpretations in a way that demonstrates interest, attention, and collaboration is likely to enhance the alliance and increase acceptance.

5. Where needed, ask the patient to describe more fully some parts of an event or an experience. Such elaboration can be helpful to the therapist in formulating a CCRT thereby helping the patient as well. For example, a patient described "*an experience of feeling little, almost fainting and having an adrenaline rush.*" The therapist asked for more information about that experience and finally was able to say, "*So I hear you better now, you are feeling very little and helpless in relation to me and that scares you and depresses you.*"

Help with the Treatment Atmosphere

In short-term hospital settings the CCRT has a special value. When the initial evaluation team includes a CCRT and then uses it to set treatment goals, the atmosphere of the residential setting becomes more treatment-oriented and less custodially oriented (Luborsky, Van Ravenswaay, et al., 1993).

Case Examples

The patients presented in the following examples were both treated in supportive–expressive (SE) psychotherapy for depression (Luborsky, Mark, et al., 1995) according to the assigned research protocol. The therapists were females and had more than 10 years of clinical experience. These examples are designed to illustrate (1) the formation of a helping alliance, (2) the use of identified relationship episodes to derive a CCRT (Luborsky, 1998b), and (3) the use of the CCRT as a focus for interpretations (Luborsky, Popp, Luborsky, & Mark, 1994).

Example I

Ms. Sandy Smyth was a 32-year-old single woman, a recovering alcoholic, who came for treatment of depression. In addition to her long-term dysthymia (chronic depression) she became severely depressed (major depression) when she failed a training course. Her DSM-III-R diagnosis based on the initial evaluation was major depressive disorder with Dysthymia.

The therapy began inauspiciously when Ms. Smyth came half an hour late for her first appointment and then said she was unable to schedule the next appointment. The therapist was angry but contained it and used her own awareness to understand and empathize with Ms. Smyth's behavior in their interaction. When Ms. Smyth said she was afraid of "sabotaging herself," the therapist indicated that Ms. Smyth was correct to be afraid. Although Ms. Smyth continued to have difficulty keeping appointments she nevertheless responded to treatment remarkably well, much to the surprise of the therapist. In fact, in her final report the therapist noted that she "had not expected that someone with such severe depression and who already was making full use of self help via therapeutic groups, such as AA, could have resolved her depression without the use of psychopharmacology."

In the termination interview Ms. Smyth said she was feeling good and "everything is a lot better." She was less pessimistic and more confident and hopeful. She felt better able to care for herself and no longer showed the disorganized pattern she demonstrated during the initial evaluation. Ms. Smyth was working regularly in a clerical job and had set up a stable living arrangement with a female roommate.

At 6 months posttermination Ms. Smyth's depression was in remission; her Beck Depression Inventory was 9. She continued to work full time at the same job. Since the termination of treatment Ms. Smyth learned that she was pregnant by the man she had been dating for 11 months. Ms. Smyth wants to marry her boyfriend but he is less certain. This situation has left her feeling angry and anxious but able to handle whatever happens. They have entered weekly couple therapy and she plans on keeping the baby.

A helping relationship in psychotherapy appeared to come about through (1) communication of the therapist's intention to be helpful and caring about Ms. Smyth's welfare and (2) the therapist's interpretative focus around Ms. Smyth's continuing involvement in self-defeating relationships with a boyfriend and others who fail to provide the care and help she needs. Although the therapist was surprised at Ms. Smyth's good response to treatment, it is not uncommon that a good alliance forms as a consequence of the therapist's being accurate and helpful.

The Therapist's During-the-Session CCRT Formulation

The following transcript is taken from session 3 of Ms. Smyth's treatment and includes four relationship episodes. The CCRT as the therapist formulated it during the session and a sample of accurate interpretations based on the CCRT are provided in Table 4.2. In formulating the CCRT, the therapist examined the relationship episodes with each of the main people who were the subject of the narratives. The interpretations are presented to illustrate the use of the CCRT to help the patient become aware of the relationship context in which depression appears. Special prominence is given to

TABLE 4.2. CCRT Summary for Case 1, Ms. Sandy Smyth, Session 3

Relationship episodes (other person)	CCRT components in each episode		
	Wish	Response from other	Response of self
RE1: Therapist	W1: I want treatment	RO1: Will not give treatment without money	RS1: Unhappy, Depression
RE2: Ex-employer	W1: I want job and help	RO1: Discharges me	RS2: Helpless; RS1: Depression, Discouragement
RE3: Brother	W1: I want care	O1: Treats me badly	RS3: Get angry; Discouragement RS1: Depression
RE4: Boyfriend	W1: I want him to care	RO1: Gives no support	RS1: Crying, sad; RS3: Anger

CCRT formulation by the therapist during the session

W1:   4REs: To get care and support
RO1: 4REs: Rejects
RS1:   4REs: Discouragement and depression
RS2:   1RE: Helplessness
RS3:   2REs: Anger

A sample of "accurate" interpretations based on the CCRT

Interpretation: "I see you get depressed after you deal with people who won't give you what you need."
Interpretation: "You could see me as one of those people."

---

the symptom (i.e., depression) by including it in the context of the relationship conflicts. For example, in one interpretation the therapist said, "*I see you get depressed after you deal with people who won't give you what you need.*"

Ms. Sandy Smyth, Session 3

CCRT scoring   Relationship episodes

RE 1: Ex-employers, completeness rating 2.5

NRS: Can't get money (17, 20)   P: //^{RS}I cannot collect unemployment//
NRO: Stop me from money (14, 4) ^{RO}because the ex employers who put in a big stink, //
(W) Wants help to get money (13, 23)^{W}so I don't even have unemployment coming in.//
NRO: Fired me (4, 17)   P: //^{RO} The ex employers who fired—
W: Asked for help (13, 34)   //^{W} I went on appeal //

NRO: Cut off help (14, 4)	^{RO} and then the employers (clears throat) are denying
NRS: Helpless (17, 19)	me unemployment,// ^{RS} I mean I really don't know—
NRS: Depressed (22, 20)	what move to take. //^{RS} (pause) It's horrible.

RE 2: Ex-employers, completeness rating 4.0

NRO: Rejected for job (4, 14)	//^{RO}And then the other job was ah, they didn't even give me a chance. // I was supposed to work on this computer and the computer wasn't hooked up and they said, well you don't have to work it. // We're replacing you with some-body else. // So I was replaced with
NRS: Anger (21, 20?)	somebody else. //^{RS}It really pissed me off //
NRS: Have no job, nothing (17, 20?)	^{RS}(pause) cause I gave up another job to get this job and I ended up with nothing at all, no unemployment, no
NRS: Horrible state (22, 20)	nothing. // ^{RS}It's horrible. //
W: I want job (help) (13?, 22)	^WI call 'em every day, // but they always say we don't have anything. // It's just terrible. //
NRS: Helpless (19, 17)	^{RS}Because I don't know what I'm going to do.
NRS: Discouraged (22, 20)	//(Pause) ^{RS}It's really discouraging. // It's so hard to get out and—get the door slammed in my face constantly. (pause)//

RE 3: Brother and sister-in-law, completeness rating 4.5

(W): To get out of bad rel. (28, 23)	//^WAnyway, I want to move out of Bob and Jane's (brother and sister-in-law) house as soon as possible.
NRO: Rejecting (6, 4)	//^{RO}Treated like a second rate citizen there.
NRS: Feel bad about self (26, 22)	//^{RS}It's not very good for my self-esteem. // Like they're both addicts and they have the personality of addicts. //
W: To be in good rel. (25?, 14?)	^WI guess—I, I much rather be around sober people. // Yeah. The old tapes start running and it's just real bad. //
NRS: Feel bad (22?, 26?)	^{RS}I mean I start thinking negatively as soon as I'm
NRO: Negative (25, 10)	around them, //^{RO} 'cause they're both negative. //
NRO: Dishonest (8,15)	^{RO}They're dishonest.

NRO: Put me down (4, 15)

//^{RO}They're acting like they're doing me a big favor//, but I'm paying half the rent there, for their apartment // and I have this tiny little room, no closet, and their junk's in the room and uh I have to work around their lives. //

NRS: Dislikes others (6, 21)

^{RS}(pause) So, I ah just can't stand them.//

RE 4: Boyfriend, completeness rating 5.0

PRS: Stop a bad rel. (14, 15)

^{RS}Yeah, I've, and I've stopped speaking to that

NRO: Rejecting (4, 10?)

married guy //^{RO}cause he got to be a real a_____.

PRS: Assertive against negative rel. (15, 11)

about stopping, bad//^{RS}I mean I'm not taking any s_____—from anybody this year—for the rest of my life

NRO: Stop talking to me (4, 10)

//^{RO}and uh, he just sort of stopped talking to me and uh, he didn't contact me, //he didn't even—where was I going to move to this week. //He didn't contact me //

NRS: Anger (21, 6)

^{RS}so screw him, //

NRS: I stop contact with him (11, 21)

^{RS}I'm not going to contact him not at all either . . . // it just makes me mad. //

W: Reject other (18, 23)

^WI really don't want anything at all to do with him.

NRS: Lonely, crying (23, 22)

//Never again will I—^{RS}Christmas eve I spent alone in church crying my eyes out cause it was an intensely

W: Not to feel isolated (32, 24)

lonely feeling. //^Wand I said no way am I ever gonna feel

NRS: Isolated (23, 20)

that bad again. No way. // ^{RS}I'm isolated from my friends and family because of this guy I wanted—this married guy. // It's just a conflict between honesty and dishonesty. // . . . I just ah, he pissed me off. //

PRO: Friends gave support (13, 9)

^{RO}All my other friends gave me all kinds of

moral support, even some financial support for this horrible

NRO: Gave no support (14, 4)

dilemma I'm in right now. //^{RO}He didn't do s_____—. //He didn't buy me a Christmas present or a card, or a birthday—.//

Example 2

Ms. Ann Beth Roberts is a married black woman, age 42 years, with two adult children. She was diagnosed with chronic depression (DSM-III-R) and treated with 20 sessions of psychotherapy following the treatment protocol associated with the study in which she participated (Luborsky, Barber, et al., 1993). She attained a high school education and at the start of treatment worked as a store clerk. Although employed full time, Ms. Roberts was concerned about a potential dismissal due to her constant tardiness. As an adolescent she was diagnosed with dyslexia and reported being afraid of others finding about this difficulty and judging her negatively. She was extremely concerned with being liked by others and apparently used her lateness and her coworkers' concerns about it as a tool to gain their affection. Ms. Roberts was quite clear in communicating her thoughts and she and her therapist agreed to begin treatment focusing on her problem with tardiness.

During treatment, Ms. Roberts separated from her husband. She blamed herself for the separation and made attempts to compromise in order to feel loved by him. The anger she feels for her husband tends to push her into the depressed moods. As a result of the separation, she now lives with her adult son, who is in drug treatment, and her adult daughter who attends school.

Ms. Roberts's father is a recovering alcoholic who, during her childhood, was abusive to her mother, also an alcoholic. Because of this situation, Ms. Roberts was sent to live with her grandmother who raised her. Although Ms. Roberts continues to be uncertain about her mother's love for her, another focus of treatment has been her desire to develop a better relationship with her mother.

By session 17, Ms. Roberts was consistently on time for work. Her depression was in partial remission and showed significant improvement subjectively and on objective measures of outcome (i.e., the Hamilton Rating Scale for Depression decreased from 15 to 3 and the Beck Depression Inventory moved from a rating of 21 to 10). She reported feeling more competent and confident about her ability to control her depressed mood. In fact, she stated, "*I see myself more clearly now . . . I feel better about myself.*"

The Therapist's During-the-Session CCRT Formulation

The second example is taken from session 17 of Ms. Roberts's treatment and includes five relationship episodes. The CCRT as the therapist formulated it during the session and a sample of accurate interpretations based on the CCRT are provided in Table 4.3. Using methods similar to Case 1, the

TABLE 4.3. CCRT Summary for Case 2, Ms. Ann Beth Roberts, Session 17

Relationship episodes (other person)	CCRT components in each episode		
	Wish	Response from other	Response of self
RE1: Girl in programming	W1: I want to be respected/liked W3: I want to assert myself	RO2: Anger RO1: Dislikes me	RS2: Assert self RS1: Depression RS4: Anger
RE2: Girl in programming	W1: I want to be respected/liked W4: I want to be helped	RO2: Anger RO1: Dislikes me	RS1: Depression RS2: Helps
RE3: Boss	W3: I want to help	RO4: Grateful	RS2: Assert self RS2: Helps
RE4: Work-people	W1: I want to be respected/liked	RO1: Dislikes me	RS2: Assert self RS5: Respects
RE5: Coworker	W1: I want to be respected/liked	RO2: Anger RO1: Dislikes me	RS1: Depression

CCRT formulation by the therapist during the session

W1:   2REs: To be respected/liked
RO1: 4REs: Dislikes you
RS1: 2REs: Depression
RS4: 1RE: Angry
RS5: 1RE: Respects

A sample of "accurate" interpretations based on the CCRT:

Interpretation: "Could it be that sometimes when that happens somebody disappointed you in some kind of way? And then you get that sadness without thinking it consciously?"
Interpretation: "You really want everybody to like you, don't you?"

therapist formulated the CCRT by examining the relationship episodes with each of the main people who were the subject of the session's narratives.

Ms. Ann Beth Roberts, Session 17

CCRT scoring   **Relationship episodes**

RE 1: Girl in programming, completeness rating 2.0

NRO: Criticize (15, 27)   //^{RO}In fact a girl called me crazy today//. And I

NRS: Angry (21, 10)   wanted to c_____ //$^{RS,\ (W)}$I wanted to tell her I think

(W): Assert (34, 14)

(W): To be accepted (2, 1)

PRS: Not hurt (14, 15)

you need to go see a psychiatrist yourself //
^(W)and sometimes people do act crazy. I told her
//^{RS}I wasn't ashamed of it//

RE 2: Girl in programming, completeness rating 3.0

NRO: Angry (27, 10)

// . . . ^{RO}this particular girl, she kind of resents it that I get paid more money than she does //. And she has the capabilities to do a lot of different jobs and she does do it so she thinks that she's overworked. //

NRO: Angry (27, 10)

^{RO}So kind of resents me because, I, I'm just not smart enough to do a lot of different things that she does.//

NRO: Dislike (10, 27)

^{RO}So this programmer from another department came and gave me a job to do and um, she just got, just didn't like.// She was just thinking about her position all over again. So I think it was just that she don't like, //

NRO: Jealous (10, 27)

^{RO}she thought it was special treatment being shown me//and also she thought all of the other jobs that do. And so I told her I said well tomorrow //

W: Be helped (13, 25)

W: To better herself (25, 12)

^Wif you show me how to do one of the jobs
//^{W,RS}I'll try to do it.// Well one reason why the

PRS: Helps (9, 7)

supervisor hasn't put me on that job, it's doing the mail, is that she's afraid that I'll make a mistake. And I have made mistakes in the past doing that metering.

PRS: Helps other (9, 7)

//^{RS}But I don't mind going on and trying again.//

NRS: Sad (22, 20)

^{RS}So I felt a little bit sad about that.
T: *You really want everybody to like you don't you?*
P: (sighs) I have to think about that. You said that before. I don't know. I guess, I gotta think what that—what I—

NRS: Disappointed (20, 22)

cause it's just like, // ^{RS}it was just so unnecessary for her to act like that.// I don't know if it was that I wanted her to like

NRS: Don't understand (2, 20)

me or I just thought that //^{RS}she had no reason to get angry whereas she wasn't so much angry with me as she was angry with all of her workload and I just got some of that anger thrown at me. I don't know. You've gotta tell me how it is that I might, might, might want her to like me.

RE 3: Boss, completeness rating 2.0

W: To help (12, 26)

PRS: Assert (15, 9)
PRO: Grateful (29, 9)
PRO: Appreciates (5, 19)

//^{W}And so I, I told administration why don't you just buy Mr. Beckner a coffee maker //cause I went and got you know, well didn't go get it. Virginia went and got it but //^{RS}I talked her into getting it. // ^{RO}So he just, he came and thanked me. // ^{RO}He said if it weren't for me he wouldn't have got that coffee because nobody had ever bought him a coffee pot . . .

RE 4: Work people, completeness rating 1.5

NRO: Critical (27, 10)

(W): To be respected (3, 17)

PRS: Asserts (15, 11)
PRS: Respects (5, 7)
PRS: Grateful (30, 16)

//^{RO}And some people just accused me of brown nosing the boss. //$^{(W), RS}$I said I'm not brown nosing him you know.

//^{RS}He's the president.
//^{RS}If it weren't for him I wouldn't have a job.

RE 5: Co-worker, Completeness rating 2.5

PRS: Excited (29, 3)

NRS: Depressed (22, 17)
NRS: Helpless (17, 22)
NRO: Angry (10, 27)

NRS: Depressed (22, 17)

NRO: Critical (4, 10)

W: To be respected (3, 7)

//And then at one time in administration the lady who was the head of administration she left and he was gonna offer me the position as head of administration. //^{RS}And I was all excited but that was I felt—// ^{RS}I really started to get depressed again // ^{RS}because I realized I couldn't handle that job. // ^{RO}That somebody had accused me of being a sex pot and in front of him, that's why he was offering me the job. // ^{RS}And that made me depressed. And that brought me way down.//$^{RO, W}$ You know, that they would say something like that. That I couldn't do the work. All I could do was just be really cutesy for him.// And he's always been a perfect gentleman and he's never like said or did anything but that's why they say he offered me a job. Anyway I didn't get it.

Postsession Formulation of the CCRT

Researchers and other assessors have an advantage over therapist "in-the-session" CCRT formulation in that decisions can be made about which REs are appropriate to score. The steps to be followed for postsession CCRT formulation are summarized below:

1. *Use only reasonably complete REs and only on scorable thought units.* Using typed transcripts of the session, a judge first identifies appropriate REs then divides each one into thought units, which are indicated by double slashes. For thought units determined to be W, ROs, or RSs, the judge notes the component to be scored just above the start of the thought unit. For example, a thought unit representing an RS would be noted as— //^{RS}I cannot collect unemployment//. Because narratives about relationship episodes may vary widely in the details (i.e., ranging from a brief personal reference to discussion of an event, including the W, the RO, the RS, and the outcome), the RE judges have the task of determining which REs are complete enough to make judgments about the CCRT. Relying on the Likert 5-point completeness scale (Luborsky, 1998b), only REs having a completeness rating of 2.5 or greater should be scored.

2. *Score the same thought units by all CCRT judges.* Following the initial determination of RE components to be scored, the CCRT judge scores each thought unit in terms of standard categories. All scores are recorded in the left margin of the transcript. In selecting standard categories, two options are suggested. A judge can either choose the two best-fitting standard categories for a component or rate all the standard categories for each thought unit. The score for each category would then be the highest mean ratings of the categories (as illustrated in Luborsky, Luborsky, et al., 1995).

3. *Compare judges' agreement by weighted kappas.* If the two best-fitting standard categories for a component are used in scoring, agreements between pairs of CCRT judges are computed according to the weighting system of Luborsky and Diguer (1998) based on Cohen's (1968) weighted kappa.[2]

4. *Summarize the results.* Once categories have been assigned for each component across all REs, a summary of the main category is determined. For example, in Case 1 the CCRT summary includes the Wish, "*to get care and support*" which is present in all four REs.

TRAINING

In order to use the method during psychotherapy sessions, therapists need only learn the basics of the CCRT method. With some practice, identification of REs can be done during the session and periodically examined for component patterns comprising the CCRT. In contrast, use of the CCRT method in research requires considerably more knowledge and training since the goal is to be as complete and comprehensive as possible in identifying and scoring all REs.

Regardless of the setting for use of the model, the initial step in training is to become familiar with the general descriptions of the CCRT method (see Luborsky, 1998b). Having learned the components of the CCRT, identification of an RE, and scoring procedures, the next step is to begin scoring transcripts with thought units and component indicated. On such a transcript, the text of the RE is given on the right side of the page with each thought unit indicated with brackets. The component scoring is placed to the left of the text. To gain skill in scoring, a beginning judge (or therapist) should cover the scoring on the left, score the text, and then compare the two scorings. Only score the parts of the text with thought units that begin with a notation of the component. After several practice cases are scored and compared, agreement with other judges should be calculated (in reliability studies, a correlation of .70 or greater should be achieved).

REs can typically be identified after relatively little practice (often as few as two to three sessions). However, identifying categories and using them to formulate the CCRT requires more practice—particularly for a novice in psychodynamic formulations. Even with this caveat, though, most individuals can become adept at CCRT formulations after four to five sessions (approximately 20–25 REs). Identifying REs during a therapy session and scoring the components postsession can facilitate familiarity with the list of categories and ease in-session development of the CCRT. It may also be useful to audiotape sessions such that REs and component scoring can be done more accurately. As with any other case formulation, the CCRT may need to be revised as additional information is shared or uncovered. This is one of the strengths in using the CCRT; that is, it allows for quick assessment and reformulation of relational patterns within the session such that accurate interpretations can be offered.

RESEARCH SUPPORT FOR THE APPROACH

Reliability of Scoring the CCRT

The reliability of the CCRT is generally good (Luborsky & Diguer, 1998). Reliability ratings from six studies did not differ markedly between eight samples, nor did they differ from component to component. For example, there was a high level of agreement for completeness of the relationship episode ($r = .68$), main other person in the RE (97% agreement), and location of the RE (85% agreement).[3] In a comparison of the CCRT for session versus RAP narratives, reliability ratings were somewhat better for the session transcripts (weighted kappas of .64 to .81 vs. .60 to .68 for RAP narratives). This relatively good reliability was obtained although the samples used few if any of the currently recommended procedures for achieving adequate reliability (Luborsky & Diguer, 1998), which are detailed below.

Recommendations

1. An independent judge prepares the session transcript for scoring by the CCRT judges. These preliminary judges identify the thought units (marked off by slashes) and the type of component to be scored in each unit.

2. The CCRT judges score the two top-ranking categories for each component although the most comprehensive picture can be obtained if all the categories are scored.

3. Prior to selecting CCRT judges, potential raters are asked to make component ratings for all REs across several session transcripts. Those raters reaching an acceptable level of agreement (around .70) with the other CCRT judges are appropriate for inclusion.

4. To make the most accurate assessments of reliability it is important that each CCRT judge rate the entire sample rather than only a small part.

5. As was previously suggested (see *postsession formulation of the CCRT*), the similarity of scoring between the judges should be measured by a weighting system. In such a system different weights are assigned to different degrees of similarity based on the two best-fit categories for each component.

Validity of the CCRT

Comparisons of the CCRT with Other Measures of Central Relationship Patterns

Measures of central relationship patterns are relatively new (within the last two decades) and vary considerably in their reliability and validity. Although the CCRT has set the standard and is among the most advanced psychometrically, there are other measures of relationship patterns that are of significance: the Structural Analysis of Social Behavior (Benjamin, 1979), Plan Diagnosis (Weiss, Sampson, & Mt. Zion Psychotherapy Research Group, 1986), Frame (Dahl & Teller, 1994), Check Lists of Psychotherapy Transactions and Interpersonal Transactions (Kiesler, 1987), and the Quantitative Analysis of Interpersonal Themes (Crits-Christoph, Demorest, Muenz, & Baranackie, 1994). These measures, though diverse, have commonalities in their basic categories as well as unique aspects as demonstrated in several recent comparison studies (Horowitz, Luborsky, & Popp, 1991; Luborsky & Barber, 1994; Luborsky, Popp, & Barber, 1994).

Given the commonalities across measures of central relationship patterns, what are the key characteristics of the CCRT and what advantages does this measure have over other similarly robust measures? In an effort to address these questions we have compiled a list of central characteristics of the CCRT and its applicability in various settings.

Characteristics of the CCRT

1. *Narratives about relationship episodes are routinely told in psychotherapy sessions.* The average number of relationship episodes per session in the Penn Psychotherapy Study was 4.1, with a range of one to seven complete narratives (Luborsky et al., 1998; Luborsky, Barber, & Diguer, 1992). The length of each narrative, measured as the number of typed lines of speaking, was 51.1 lines for early sessions and ranged from 7 to 207 lines across all sessions (Luborsky, Crits-Christoph, Mintz, & Auerbach, 1988).

2. *Similar CCRTs appear in different states of consciousness.* An examination of the degree of similarity between dream and narrative CCRT formulations found that for each of the three CCRT components moderate agreement between judges was obtained (Popp et al., 1996).

3. *The most usual types of CCRTs have been established.* This evaluation demonstrated that the most frequent W was *"to be close and accepting,"* the most frequent RO was *"rejecting"* and *"opposing,"* and the most frequent RSs were *"disappointed,"* *"depressed,"* and *"angry."*

4. *Consistency of narratives.* Significant similarity and consistency has been shown for CCRT narratives relating REs outside therapy with CCRT narratives derived from early psychotherapy sessions (Barber et al., 1995).

5. *Consistency of CCRTs over the course of treatment.* The pervasiveness of the CCRT from beginning to end of psychotherapy shows moderate consistency, with the W component most consistent (Crits-Christoph & Luborsky, 1998a). Wilczek, Weinryb, Barber, Gustavsson, and Asberg (2004) found that even though the main CCRT did not change substantially after a period of long-term psychotherapy (3 years), patients showed an increased flexibility in their use of different W, ROs, and RSs in the REs described.

6. *Consistency in CCRTs over the lifespan.* Some degree of consistency of the CCRT across ages has been demonstrated. For example, the CCRT of children has been found to be relatively constant from ages 3–5 years (Luborsky, Luborsky, et al., 1995). More recently, using RAP narratives to examine CCRT changes during adolescence, relative stability of CCRT components were found across ages 14–18 years (Waldinger et al., 2002).

7. *Consistency of CCRTs across different relationships.* Consistent with Freud's (1912/1958a) observation that the transference template tends to be a general pattern across multiple relationships, we found a fairly simi-

lar pattern within a person's narratives across relationships with different people. For instance, in a sample of 35 patients the CCRT for the relationship with therapist was significantly similar to the CCRT with other people (Fried, Crits-Christoph, & Luborsky, 1992).

8. *Differences in CCRTs for different diagnoses.* A few examples are worth mentioning. Comparing patients with and without dysthymia, Luborsky et al. (1998) found that those with dysthymia were more likely to wish *"to oppose, hurt, or control others,"* see others as *"less upset,"* and see themselves as more *"responsive."* In a study of patients with borderline personality disorder (Chance, Bakeman, Kaslow, Farber, & Burge-Callaway, 2000), the relational pattern most often described by participants was a wish *"to be loved and understood,"* experiencing others as *"rejecting,"* and responding with *"depression and disappointment,"* which is similar to that reported for depressed patients (see also Drapeau & Perry, 2004). In another study of neurotic, psychotic, and borderline personality organizations (Diguer et al., 2001) more similarities than differences were found although the psychotic group had the least negative responses and the lowest narrative complexity.

9. *Associations of the CCRT with defenses.* Because the CCRT offers general patterns of relating it has been postulated that the defensive structure of an individual would relate to the CCRT. Indeed, researchers (DeRoten, Drapeau, Stigler, & Despland, 2004; Luborsky et al., 1990) have found significant associations between defenses, defensive functioning and the CCRT.

10. *Greater pervasiveness of CCRT components in narratives is associated with greater psychiatric severity.* CCRT pervasiveness, which represents the frequency of conflicts across the REs, has been suggested to relate to the severity of symptoms. Indeed, Cierpka et al. (1998) have shown that greater pervasiveness of CCRT components across narratives is associated with greater psychiatric severity, such that greater distress was associated with fewer positive RSs (see Crits-Christoph & Luborsky, 1998a).

ACKNOWLEDGMENTS

This chapter was supported in part by Research Scientist Award No. MH 40710-22, National Institute on Drug Abuse (NIDA) Grant No. 5U18 DA07085, and NIDA Research Scientist Award No. 2KO5 DA00168-24 (to Lester Luborsky).

NOTES

1. Cohen's (1968) weighted kappa statistic, a measure of agreement between judges, was significant for all categories (.60 to .71 for each of the 24 response categories).

2. Rosenthal (2006) argues that Pearson correlations are a more accurate assessment of agreement than a weighted kappa since a kappa based on tables larger than 2 × 2 may not give accurate judgments of reliability.
3. The weighted kappas ranged from .60 to .71.

REFERENCES

Albani, C., Blaser, G., Hölzer, M., & Pokorny, D. (2002). Emotionen und Beziehung— zum Beziehungsaspekt emotionaler Äußerungen. Eine Validierungsstudie der Methode zur Klassifikation verbalisierter Emotionen nach DAHL et al. (Emotions and relationships—the relationship aspect of verbalized emotions. A validation study of the method of classification of verbalized emotions according to Dahl). *Zeitschrift für Klinische Psychologie, Psychiatrie und Psychotherapie, 50,* 29–46.

Albani, C., Blaser, G., Körner, A., König, S., Marschke, F., Geißler, I., et al. (2002). Zum zusammenhang yon bindungsprototypen und zentralen beziehungsmustern (Connections between attachment prototypes and relationship patterns). *Psychotherapie Psychosomatik Medizinische Psychologie, 52,* 521–525.

Barber, J. P., Crits-Christoph, P., & Luborsky, L. (1998). A guide to the CCRT standard categories and their classification. In L. Luborsky & P. Crits-Christoph (Eds.), *Understanding transference: The Core Conflictual Relationship Theme method* (2nd ed., pp. 43–54). Washington, DC: American Psychological Association Books.

Barber, J. P., Foltz, C., & Weinryb, R. M. (1998). The Central Relationship Questionnaire: Initial report. *Journal of Counseling Psychology, 45,* 131–142.

Barber, J. P., Luborsky, L., Crits-Christoph, P., & Diguer, L. (1995). A comparison of core conflictual relationship themes before psychotherapy and during early sessions. *Journal of Consulting and Clinical Psychology, 63,* 145–148.

Benjamin, L. S. (1979). Use of structural analysis of social behavior (SASB) and Markov chains to study dynamic interactions. *Journal of Abnormal Psychology, 88,* 303–319.

Book, H. (1998). *How to practice brief psychodynamic psychotherapy: The Core Conflictual Relationship Theme method.* Washington, DC: American Psychological Association Books

Chance, S. E., Bakeman, R., Kaslow, N. J., Farber, E., & Burge-Callaway, K. (2000). Core conflictual relationship themes in patients diagnosed with borderline personality disorder who attempted, or who did not attempt, suicide. *Psychotherapy Research, 10,* 337–355.

Charlin, R., Larrea, V., Florenzano, R., Valdes, M., Serrano, T., & Roizblatt, A. (2001). Modelo de entrevista en adolescentes: Aplicación del CCRT de Luborsky (Adolescent interview model based in Luborsky's CCRT). *Acta Psiquiatrica y Psicologia de America Latina, 47,* 333–339.

Cierpka, M., Strack, M., Benninghoven, D., Staats, H., Dahlbender, R., Pokorny, D., et al. (1998). Stereotypical relationship patterns and psychopathology. *Psychotherapy and Psychosomatics, 67,* 241–248.

Cohen, J. (1968). Weighted kappa: Nominal scale agreement provision for scaled disagreement or partial credit. *Psychological Bulletin, 70,* 213–220.

Contiero, L., Calloni, S., Gatti, M., Giussani, S., Pastori, M., Rodini, C., et al. (2002). Individuazione Focus Terapeutico e Verifica Dell'Esito Di Una Psicoterapia a Tempo Definito A Indirizzo Psicodinamico "Supportivo-Espressivo": Uso Dell'Intervista R.A.P. Con Codifica C.C.R.T. e S.A.S.B (Individualized therapeutic focus and verification of a time-limited, expressive-supportive psychodynamic psychotherapy: Use of the RAP interview with CCRT and SASB coding). *Ricerca in Psicoterapia, 5*, 57–74.

Crits-Christoph, P. (1986). *Assessing conscious and unconscious aspects of relationship themes from self-report and naturalistic data.* Paper presented at the MacArthur Workshop on Person Schemata, Palo Alto, CA.

Crits-Christoph, P., Cooper, A., & Luborsky, L. (1998). The measurement of accuracy of interpretations. In L. Luborsky & P. Crits-Christoph (Eds.), *Understanding transference: The Core Conflictual Relationship Theme method* (2nd ed., pp.197–211). Washington, DC: American Psychological Association Books.

Crits-Christoph, P., Crits-Christoph, K., Wolf-Palacio, D., Fichter, M., & Rudick, D. (1995). Supportive-expressive dynamic psychotherapy for generalized anxiety disorder. In J. P. Barber & P. Crits-Cristoph (Eds.), *Dynamic therapies for psychiatric disorders: Axis I* (pp. 43–83). New York: Basic Books.

Crits-Christoph, P., & Demorest, A. (1988). *A list of standard categories (Edition 2).* Unpublished manuscript, University of Pennsylvania, Philadelphia.

Crits-Christoph, P., Demorest, A., Muenz, L., & Baranackie, K. (1994). Consistency of interpersonal themes for patients in psychotherapy. *Journal of Personality, 62*, 499–526.

Crits-Christoph, P., & Luborsky, L. (1998a). Changes in CCRT pervasiveness during psychotherapy. In L. Luborsky & P. Crits-Christoph (Eds.), *Understanding transference: The Core Conflictual Relationship Theme method* (2nd ed., pp. 151–163). Washington, DC: American Psychological Association Books.

Crits-Christoph, P., & Luborsky, L. (1998b). The perspective of patients versus that of clinicians in the assessment of central relationship themes (MacArthur conference proceedings of the program on conscious and unconscious mental processes, March 1986, Palo Alto, CA). In L. Luborsky & P. Crits-Christoph (Eds.), *Understanding transference: The Core Conflictual Relationship Theme method* (2nd ed., pp. 221–231). Washington, DC: American Psychological Association Books.

Dahl, H., & Teller, V. (1994). The characteristics, identification, and applications of FRAMES. *Psychotherapy Research, 4*, 253–276.

Dahlbender, R., Albani, C., Pokorny, D., & Kächele, H. (1998). The Connected Central Relationship Patterns (CCRP): A structural version of the CCRT. *Psychotherapy Research, 8*, 408–425.

Dazzi, N., De Coro, A., Ortu, F., Andreassi, S., Cundari, M., Ostuni, V., et al. (1998). Il CCRT in un campione italiano di psicoterapie: Uno studio della relazione tra categorie su misura e categorie standard (The CCRT in an Italian psychotherapy sample: A study on the relation of measured categories and standard categories). *Ricerca in Psicoterapia, 1*, 205–223.

De Roten, Y., Drapeau, M., Stigler, M., & Despland, J. (2004). Yet another look at the CCRT: The relation between Core Conflictual Relationship Themes and defensive functioning. *Psychotherapy Research, 14*, 252–260.

Diguer, L., Lefebvre, R., Drapeau, M., Luborsky, L., Rousseau, J., Hébert, É., et al.

(2001). The core conflictual relationship theme of psychotic, borderline, and neurotic personality organizations. *Psychotherapy Research, 11,* 169–186.

Drapeau, M., & Perry, J. C. (2004). Interpersonal conflicts in borderline personality disorder: An exploratory study using the CCRT-LU. *Swiss Journal of Psychology—Schweizerische Zeitschrift für Psychologie-Revue Suisse de Psychologie, 63,* 53–57.

Freud, S. (1958a). The dynamics of the transference. In J. Strachey (Ed. and Trans.), *The standard edition of the complete psychological works of Sigmund Freud* (Vol. 12, pp. 99–108). London: Hogarth Press. (Original work published 1912)

Freud, S. (1958b). Recommendations to physicians practicing psycho-analysis. In J. Strachey (Ed. and Trans.), *The standard edition of the complete psychological works of Sigmund Freud* (Vol. 12, pp.111–120). London: Hogarth Press. (Original work published 1912)

Fried, D., Crits-Christoph, P., & Luborsky, L. (1992). The first empirical demonstration of transference in psychotherapy. *Journal of Nervous and Mental Disease, 180,* 326–331.

Grenyer, B. F. S., & Luborsky, L. (1996). Dynamic change in psychotherapy: Mastery of interpersonal conflict. *Journal of Consulting and Clinical Psychology, 64,* 411–416.

Grenyer, B. F. S., Luborsky, L., & Solowij, N. (1995). *Treatment manual for supportive–expressive dynamic psychotherapy: Special adaptation for treatment of cannabis (marijuana) dependence* (Technical Report 26). Sydney, Australia: National Drug and Alcohol Research Centre.

Hinojosa Ayala, N. A. (2005). Transference and relationship: Technical implications in the psychoanalytic process with a borderline patient. *International Forum of Psychoanalysis, 14,* 36–44.

Horowitz, M. J., Luborsky, L., & Popp, C. (1991). A comparison of the Role Relationship Models Configuration and the Core Conflictual Relationship Theme. In M. J. Horowitz (Ed.), *Person schemas and maladaptive interpersonal patterns* (pp. 213–219). Chicago: University of Chicago Press.

Kiesler, D. J. (1987). *Check List of Psychotherapy Transactions—Revised (CLOPT-R) and Check List of Interpersonal Transactions—Revised (CLOIT-R).* Richmond: Virginia Commonwealth University.

Luborsky, L. (1965). Clinical manual for the self-interpretation of the TAT. In M. Kornrich (Ed.), *Psychological test modifications* (pp. 242–265). Springfield, IL: Thomas.

Luborsky, L. (1976). Helping alliances in psychotherapy: The groundwork for a study of their relationship to its outcome. In J. L. Claghorn (Ed.), *Successful psychotherapy* (pp. 92–116). New York: Brunner/Mazel.

Luborsky, L. (1977). Measuring a pervasive psychic structure in psychotherapy: The core conflictual relationship theme. In N. Freedman & S. Grand (Eds.), *Communicative structures and psychic structures* (pp. 367–395). New York: Plenum Press.

Luborsky, L. (1984). *Principles of psychoanalytic psychotherapy: A manual for supportive–expressive (SE) treatment.* New York: Basic Books.

Luborsky, L. (1986). *A set of standard categories for the CCRT (Edition 1).* Unpublished manuscript, University of Pennsylvania, Philadelphia.

Luborsky, L. (1994). The benefits to the clinician of psychotherapy research: A clinician–

researcher's view. In P. F. Talley, H. H. Strupp, & S. F. Butler (Eds.), *Psychotherapy research and practice: Bridging the gap* (pp. 167–180). New York: Basic Books.

Luborsky, L. (1998a). The early life of the idea for the Core Conflictual Relationship Theme Method. In L. Luborsky & P. Crits-Christoph (Eds.), *Understanding transference: The Core Conflictual Relationship Theme method* (2nd ed., pp. 3–14). Washington, DC: American Psychological Association Books.

Luborsky, L. (1998b). A guide to the CCRT method. In L. Luborsky & P. Crits-Christoph (Eds.), *Understanding transference: The Core Conflictual Relationship Theme Method* (2nd ed., pp. 15–42). Washington, DC: American Psychological Association Books.

Luborsky, L. (1998c). The Relationship Anecdotes Paradigms (RAP) interview as a versatile source of narratives. In L. Luborsky & P. Crits-Christoph (Eds.), *Understanding transference: The Core Conflictual Relationship Theme method* (2nd. ed., pp. 109–120). Washington, DC: American Psychological Association Books.

Luborsky, L., & Barber, J. P. (1994). Perspectives on seven transference-related measures applied to the interview with Ms. Smithfield. *Psychotherapy Research, 4,* 152–154.

Luborsky, L., Barber, J. P., Binder, J., Curtis, J., Dahl, H., Horowitz, L. M., et al. (1993). Transference-related measures: A new class based on psychotherapy sessions. In N. Miller, L. Luborsky, J. P. Barber, & J. Docherty (Eds.), *Psychodynamic treatment research: A handbook for clinical practice* (pp. 326–341). New York: Basic Books.

Luborsky, L., Barber, J. P., & Diguer, L. (1992). The meanings of the narratives told during psychotherapy: The fruits of a new operational unit. *Psychotherapy Research, 2,* 277–290.

Luborsky, L., Barber, J. P., Schaffler, P., & Cacciola, J. (1998). The narratives told during psychotherapy and the different types of CCRTs within them. In L. Luborsky & P. Crits-Christoph (Eds.), *Understanding transference: The Core Conflictual Relationship Theme method* (2nd ed., pp. 135–150). Washington, DC: American Psychological Association Books.

Luborsky, L., & Crits-Christoph, P. (1990). *Understanding transference: The Core Conflictual Relationship Theme method.* New York: Basic Books.

Luborsky, L., & Crits-Christoph, P. (1998). *Understanding transference: The Core Conflictual Relationship Theme method* (2nd ed.). Washington, DC: American Psychological Association Books.

Luborsky, L., Crits-Christoph, P., & Alexander, K. (1990). Repressive style and relationship patterns—Three samples inspected. In J. Singer (Ed.), *Repression and dissociation: Implications for personality theory, psychopathology and health* (pp. 275–298). Chicago: University of Chicago Press.

Luborsky, L., Crits-Christoph, P., Mintz, J., & Auerbach, A. (1988). *Who will benefit from psychotherapy? Predicting therapeutic outcomes.* New York: Basic Books.

Luborsky, L., & Diguer, L. (1998). The reliability of the CCRT measure: Results from eight samples. In L. Luborsky & P. Crits-Christoph (Eds.), *Understanding transference: The Core Conflictual Relationship Theme method* (2nd ed., pp. 97–107). Washington, DC: American Psychological Association Books.

Luborsky, L., Graff, M., Pulver, S., & Curtis, H. (1973). A clinical–quantitative examination of consensus on the concept of transference. *Archives of General Psychiatry, 29,* 69–75.

Luborsky, L., Luborsky, E. B., Diguer, L., Schmidt, K., Dengler, D., Schaffler, P., et al. (1995). Extending the core relationship theme into early childhood. In G. Noam & K. Fisher (Eds.), *Development and vulnerability in close relationships* (pp. 287–308). New York: Erlbaum.

Luborsky, L., Mark, D., Hole, A. V., Popp, C., Goldsmith, B., & Cacciola, J. (1995). Supportive–expressive (SE) dynamic psychotherapy of depression: A time-limited version. In J. P. Barber & P. Crits-Christoph (Eds.), *Dynamic therapies for psychiatric disorders (Axis I)* (pp. 13–42). New York: Basic Books.

Luborsky, L., Popp, C., & Barber, J. P. (1994). Common and special factors in different transference-related measures. *Psychotherapy Research, 4,* 277–286.

Luborsky, L., Popp, C., Luborsky, E., & Mark. D. (1994). The Core Conflictual Relationship Theme. In L. Luborsky, J. P. Barber, C. Popp, & D. Shapiro (Eds.), Seven transference-related measures: Each applied in an interview with Ms. Smithfield [Monograph]. *Psychotherapy Research, 4,* 172–183.

Luborsky, L., Van Ravenswaay, P., Ball, W., Steinman, D., Sprehn, G., & Bryan, C. (1993). Come centrare il trattamento in ambiente psichiatrico: Uso del metodo CCRT-FIT (Trattamento ospedaliero centrato) [How to focus psychiatric hospital treatment: Use of the CCRT-FIT method (Focused Inpatient Treatment) method]. *Prospettive Psicoanalitiche nel Lavoro istituzionale, 11,* 9–16.

Luborsky, L., Woody, G., Hole, A. V., & Velleco, A. (1995). Supportive–Expressive dynamic psychotherapy for treatment of opiate dependence. In J. P. Barber & P. Crits-Christoph (Eds.), *Dynamic therapies for psychiatric disorders (Axis I)* (pp. 131–160). New York: Basic Books.

Mark, D., & Faude, J. (1995). Supportive–expressive therapy of cocaine abuse. In J. P. Barber & P. Crits-Christoph (Eds.), *Dynamic therapies for psychiatric disorders (Axis I)* (pp. 294–331). New York: Basic Books.

Mark, D., & Luborsky, L. (1992). *A manual for the use of supportive–expressive psychotherapy in the treatment of cocaine abuse.* Unpublished manuscript, University of Pennsylvania, Philadelphia.

Mitchell, J. (1995). Coherence of the relationship theme: An extension of Luborsky's Core Conflictual Relationship Theme method. *Psychoanalytic Psychology, 12,* 495–512.

Popp, C., Diguer, L., Luborsky, L., Faude, J., Johnson, S., Morris, M., et al. (1996). Repetitive relationship themes in waking narratives and dreams. *Journal of Consulting and Clinical Psychology, 64,* 1073–1078.

Rosenthal, R. (2006). Conducting judgment studies: Some methodological issues. In J. A. Harrigan, R. Rosenthal, & K. R. Scherer (Eds.), *The new handbook of methods in nonverbal behavior research: Series in affective science* (pp. 199–234). New York: Oxford University Press.

Singer, B., & Luborsky, L. (1977). Countertransference: The status of clinical vs. quantitative research. In A. Gurman & A. Razin (Eds.), *The therapist's handbook for effective psychotherapy: An empirical assessment* (pp. 433–451). New York: Pergamon Press.

Staats, H., May, M., Herrmann, C., Kersting, A., & König, K. (1998). Different patterns of change in narratives of men and women during analytical group psychotherapy. *International Journal of Group Psychotherapy, 48,* 363–380.

Wachtel, P. (1993). *Therapeutic communication: Principles and effective practice.* New York: Guilford Press.

Waldinger, R., Diguer, L., Guastella, F., Lefebvre, R., Allen, J.P., Luborsky, L., et al. (2002). The same old song?—Stability and change in relationship schemas from adolescence to young adulthood. *Journal of Youth and Adolescence, 31,* 17–29.

Weiss, J., Sampson, H., & Mount Zion Psychotherapy Research Group. (1986). *The psychoanalytic process: Theory, clinical observations, and empirical research.* New York: Guilford Press.

Wilczek, A., Weinryb, R. M., Barber, J. P., Gustavsson, J. P., & Asberg, M. (2004). Change in the Core Conflictual Relationship theme after long-term dynamic psychotherapy. *Psychotherapy Research, 14,* 107–125.

Chapter 5

Configurational Analysis

States of Mind, Person Schemas, and the Control of Ideas and Affect

MARDI J. HOROWITZ
TRACY D. EELLS

The systematic method we propose answers several important questions about a psychotherapy: What are desirable changes? How can these occur? And, after a time in or after therapy, what is it that did change? In other words, configurational analysis is a useful tool for therapists to use in initial evaluations, to use during the process of therapy, and to assess its outcome. It is based on clinical research about what clinicians can observe and infer in the same way, that is, on studies of reliability and validity summarized in books such as *Person Schemas and Maladaptive Interpersonal Patterns* (Horowitz, 1991) and *Cognitive Psychodynamics: From Conflict to Character* (Horowitz, 1998), as well as *Formulation as a Basis for Planning Psychotherapy Treatment* (Horowitz, 1997).

Configurational analysis is a method of explanation that starts on the surface by stating what phenomena, often signs and symptoms or problems, are to be explained. Then it examines states in which these do or do not occur, noting especially both mood and control of emotion in each state. The first steps are thus (1) phenomena listing and (2) states of mind, including cycles of states or state configurations (desired states, dreaded states, and defensive compromise states). The third step examines the unresolved topics that should be examined, and the control processes that may impede working them through. The fourth and most inferential step deals with the self and other role relationship models that organized the different play of these emotional topics as the patient may cycle through different states of mind.

Configurational analysis (CA) is a flexible tool that can be applied to difficult patients presenting with mixed-symptom disorders and personality problems, as well as with less complex patients or those with well-circum-scribed problems for which a brief psychotherapy is indicated. CA was originally introduced by Horowitz in 1979 (see also Horowitz, 1987) and has recently been updated as a system for understanding psychotherapy change (Horowitz, 2005).

CA is a biopsychosocial system of formulation. At each step one considers what one can of each level of causation, as well as interactive explanations. For example, one cause of an intensely fearful and out-of-control state can be biological exhaustion or a lesion discovered in the amygdala, another cause could be stigmatization and victimization of the person by a prejudiced mob, yet another contribution could be a recent similar state of terror caused by evocation of a traumatic memory.

HISTORICAL BACKGROUND OF THE APPROACH

CA is an integrative approach to case formulation in the sense of attempting a theoretical synthesis (Norcross & Newman, 1992) of psychodynamic and cognitive-behavioral concepts into a new theory, which we call "person schemas theory" (Horowitz, 1987, 1988, 1989, 1991, 1997; Horowitz, Merluzzi, et al., 1991). CA is rooted in psychodynamic theory, especially its emphases on conflict in intrapsychic and interpersonal relationships. It organizes personal meanings according to wish–fear–compromise configurations. These configurations focus on multiple schemas of self and of others, and on the control of associational linkages among schemas in order to manage stress and conflict.

Horowitz's (1986) work on individuals with posttraumatic stress disorder provided him with insights as to how these individuals adaptively and maladaptively attempt to process the memories and fantasies associated with the traumatic events. CA is also influenced by cognitive science, primarily information-processing models of mind–brain activities. The influence of information processing on CA is seen in the assumption of CA that mental representations mediate thought, feeling, and behavior. Our focus on these mental representations, or schemas, is consistent with demonstrations by cognitive psychopathologists that schemas appear to mediate major depressive disorder and anxiety disorders (e.g., Andersen & Limpert, 2001; Hope, Rapee, Heimberg, & Dombeck, 1990; Segal, Truchon, Horowitz, Gemar, & Guirguis, 1995; Williams, Mathews, & MacLeod, 1996). Our use of the schema concept reaches beyond what has been reliably demonstrated in research. We feel justified in doing so, however, due to the heuristic and practical value of our concepts and because we recognize that CA is only an initial step toward bridging gaps between theoretical and empirical findings emerging from cognitive science laboratories and the practical demands of busy day-to-day clinical work.

Eric Berne's (1961) transactional analysis has also played a role in its emphasis on multiple self-states and transactions among them. Berne's is an attractive and deceptively simple theory about how individuals engage in social maneuvers ("games") and play out unconscious life plans ("scripts") that often deprive them of longed for self-esteem and intimacy. Berne proposed a triad of ego states—parent, adult, and child—that compete for dominance in personality. For example, the "parental" role is often harshly judgmental and offers only conditional affection. In CA, this may correspond to a schema of an internal critic, or introject, as a "harsh and critical parent."

CA has also been influenced by circumplex-based interpersonal theories (Kiesler, 1996) and by Luborsky's Core Conflictual Relationship Theme (CCRT; Luborsky & Crits-Christoph, 1990; see Luborsky & Barrett, Chapter 4, this volume), particularly its focus on wish–wish and wish–fear conflicts.

CONCEPTUAL FRAMEWORK

There are four classes of information that are formulated in CA: significant clinical phenomena; states of mind; schemas of self, other, and relationships; and the control of ideas and affect. The CA formulation process moves stepwise from attending to observations about a patient to making inferences about a patient's personal meaning system.

Clinical Phenomena

These include the patient's presenting symptoms and list of problems, as well as any other observable or near-surface events occurring in the consultation room or reported by the patient as occurring elsewhere. Phenomena might include unusual gestures, facial expressions, manner of speech, topics discussed, and style of managing emotion. The clinician tries to pay close attention to the patient without his or her observations being overly influenced by a priori theoretical considerations or by where the patient may try to direct the clinician's attention. These phenomena provide the material to be explained by the remaining classes of information in CA.

States of Mind

States of mind are recurrent, coherent complexes of affect, thought, experience, and behavior. They are assumed to limit the accessibility of certain ideas and affect. To illustrate, *Jill,* who entered treatment after the death of her father, seemed to alternate between *depressed and helpless* and *excitedly working* states of mind. When in the *depressed and helpless* state, *Jill* felt unable to generate the energy, interpersonal skills, or positive self-concept that accompanied the *excitedly working* state of mind. It was as if the latter state never existed. Similarly, when in the *excitedly working* state, she avoided any thoughts of her father as if thinking of him would precipitate her *depressed and helpless* state and its accompanying tears and fear of loss of control. The concept of a state of mind is similar to that of mood but is more inclusive because mood usually refers only to an emotion that is sustained through time and does not directly reference accompanying cognition, behaviors, gestures, expressions, and the like.

In addition to describing states in adjectival terms, as just illustrated, the clinician can classify them into one of the four broad categories shown in Table 5.1. As indicated there, undermodulated states are those in which intense and poorly controlled emotions are expressed; in well-modulated states, the individual readily accesses and integrates a variety of emotional and ideational expressions; overmodulated states involve excessive control of behavior; and shimmering states are those in which the individual appears to fluctuate rapidly between two states of mind or to experience them simultaneously. Table 5.2 shows how a variety of states of mind can fit into these broad categories.

Schemas of Self, Others, and Relationships

At the heart of CA lies the assumption that individuals possess a repertoire of person schemas. Schemas are relatively stable knowledge structures that help organize an individual's self-concept, concept of others, and dominant self-with-other relationship patterns (Singer & Salovey, 1991). They result from overlearned and generalized interpersonal experiences—as well as from constitutional, genetic, and intrapersonal sources—that become ingrained into an individual's psychological makeup. Schemas are not consciously experienced, but they influence conscious experiences. They can increase the efficiency of information processing by focusing attention on particular elements of one's intrapersonal and interpersonal world and by enabling one to readily anticipate their meaning. Social cognition researchers have also posited multiple selves as a possible cognitive model of personality, social, and cultural functioning (e.g., Kihlstrom & Cantor, 1984; Kihlstrom et al., 1988; Markus, 1990; Markus & Nurius, 1986; Unemori, Omoregie, & Markus, 2004).

Role Relationship Models

Role relationship models (RRMs) are diagrams that organize core interaction patterns, or relationship schemas. As shown in Figure 5.1, an RRM has three components: a self schema, schema of other, and a relationship

TABLE 5.1. Major States of Mind and How They Are Experienced by the Patient and Observers

State of mind	Definition	Experience of patient	Experience of observers
Undermodulated	Dysregulation of emotional expression.	Intense sobbing, impulsive outbursts of anger; impulsivity; feeling out of control. Sharp increases in the intensity of verbal expressions may appear as the patient experiences emotional surges or pangs.	Empathic emotional surges; an urge to intervene to help the patient regain control. "Freezing" in response to attacking outbursts of anger.
Well-modulated	A relatively smooth flow of ideas and affective expression.	Affective displays are experienced as genuine, and thoughts as freely flowing and spontaneous. The individual feels a sense of poise, regardless of the intensity of affective or ideational expression.	Subjective interest and empathy; feels connected to an individual engaged in an organized communication process without major discords between verbal and nonverbal modes of expression.
Overmodulated	Excessive control of expressive behavior.	Constricted, stiff; enclosed, anxious, or walled-off. There is a narrowing of experience to verbal expression; affect seems forced or feigned; the person feels false.	A feeling of disconnection, boredom, or difficulty, paying attention. The observer appraises the individual as distant.
Shimmering	Rapid shifting between, or simultaneous experience of, under- and overcontrolled states of mind.	Excited, distracted; drawn toward and away from a topic; alternately undercontrolled and overcontrolled.	Puzzlement, confusion, caught up in patient's excitement.

script. The script includes the following: (1) an anticipated action, emotion, wish or motivation of the self; (2) the expected response of the other; (3) the reaction of the self to the response of the other; (4) a self-appraisal of these reactions; and (5) the expected other's appraisal of these reactions. The first three often suffice.

As shown in Figure 5.2, mental working models combine an individual's perception of an actual situation with a priori person schemas. The largest box in Figure 5.2 symbolizes the social transactions between self and other. The large circle to the left represents the self and its contents,

TABLE 5.2. **Dictionary of States of Mind Organized by Degree of Modulation and Emotional Coloration**

Emotional coloration	Degree of modulation		
	Undermodulated	Well-modulated	Overmodulated
Sadness	Distraught Out-of-control crying Demoralized and deflated Desperately overwhelmed	Quietly needy Crying Struggle against crying Poignantly empathic Unhappily vulnerable	As if sad Phony poignancy As if remorseful
Fear/anxiety	Bodily panic Panicky emptiness Frightened vulnerability Panicky helplessness	Fearful worry Apprehensive vigilance Mixed rage/fear Nervously irritable	As if anxious Numbing from fear
Self-disgust/ shame/guilt	Shameful mortification Revolted self-disgust Intrusive guilt Panicky guilt	Ashamed disgrace Bashfully shy Remorseful Angry self-disgust	As if self-disgust Shame/guilt
Anger	Explosive fury Panicky rage Self-righteous rage Grandiose bellicosity Tantrum Defiance Shame/rage/fear	Angry Bitter Resentful Annoyed, skeptical Sniping Whining	As if angry Blustering Cutely angry
Tension	Excitedly disorganized Confused Overwhelmed and pained Hypervigilant Anxious and withdrawn Distracted	Tentative engagement Struggle with vulnerability	As if strained
Dullness	Foggy withdrawal Listless apathy Fugue or coma Hurt and unengaged	Bored Meandering	Coldly remote
Communication	Pressured confusion Pressured dumping Frenzied activity	Assured, productive Compassionate Composed, authentic Earnest activity	Rigid reporting Technical display As if bold Pontification Controlled documentarian
Engagement	Giddy engagement Foolishly excited	Composed, authentic Earnest activity Elated and poised Shining (smiling, beaming)	As if bold Pontification Social chitchat Snide sociability As if lighthearted (*continued*)

TABLE 5.2. (*continued*)

Emotional coloration	Degree of modulation		
	Undermodulated	Well-modulated	Overmodulated
Emotional affection	Foolishly enthralled Overawed	Tender Assured compassion	As if illuminated
Creative excitement	Excited hyperactivity Frenzied creativity Shining (smiling, beaming)	Oceanic Illuminated Creative flow	As if illuminated
Joy	Foolishly enthralled Foolishly excited, histrionic	Cheerful Sharing	As if lighthearted
Sexual excitement	Enthralled love Flooded with eroticism Sexually titillated	Flirtatious pleasure Eroticized sensuality	As if eroticized

symbolizing mental processes of perceiving, thinking, emotion, schematizing, and action planning. The working model of the relationship between self and other is partially organized through perceptual activity directed into the interpersonal world and partially by information from enduring schemas about how transactions unfold. From this repertoire of organized meaning structures, one schema may dominate the template of the working model, as shown by the heavy arrow. Enduring schemas of a type may also have layers of more progressive or regressive forms.

Enduring schemas may not accord with the real properties of self and other in the transaction situation. Nonetheless, they may so affect the inner working model of that situation that transference reactions occur. That is, the person repeats an earlier schematized pattern that is currently "erroneous" in some way.

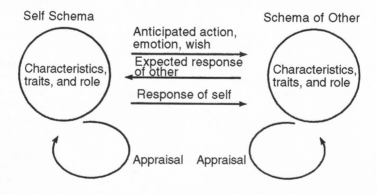

FIGURE 5.1. Format for a role relationship model (RRM).

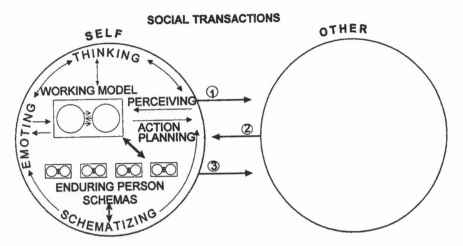

FIGURE 5.2. RRMs as working models, and enduring person schemas, of current social transactions. The circled numbers indicate a sequence of actual interpersonal expressions.

Role Relationship Model Configurations

Role relationship model configurations (RRMCs) are organizations of RRMs into a wish–fear–compromise format. As shown in Figure 5.3, the bottom half of an RRMC comprises desired and dreaded RRMs. The desired RRM organizes states of satisfaction. The dreaded RRM organizes states of intense suffering and loss of control. The top half of the RRMC comprises the compromise RRMs, which organize states of greater control. Compromise RRMs are divided into more and less adaptive versions.

As shown in Figure 5.3, self-schemas are arrayed within a circle at the center of the RRMC format. These multiple self-schemas may or may not be forged into the supraordinate self-organization suggested by this circle. The reader may also note that schemas with negative emotional potential are to the left of an RRMC and those with positive emotional potential to the right. Several RRMCs can be constructed for complex cases, classifying RRMs into sets according to type of relationship or type of self-schemas. See Horowitz (1997) and Horowitz, Merluzzi, et al. (1991) for further details on constructing RRMCs and clinical examples.

A filled-in RRMC for the case example discussed later in this chapter is shown in Figure 5.4. Although patients may initially offer information that would be placed in a problematic compromise RRM, we have found that for narrative purposes RRMCs are best read beginning at the desired quadrant, moving to the dreaded quadrant, then to the protective compro-

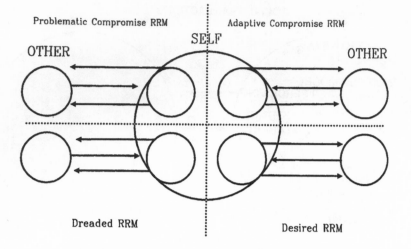

FIGURE 5.3. Format for configurations of RRM.

mise, and finally to the problematic compromise. Figure 5.4 can be summarized narratively as follows:

> *Desired quadrant.* This patient wishes to be an adoring daughter who admires her idealized father and is supported and admired by him.
>
> *Dreaded quadrant.* This wish for mutual admiration is obstructed by a view of herself as an overly trusting girl in relationship to a cold and selfish father figure who tricks her; she responds by remaining loyal but is then scorned and suppresses her rage rather than display out-of-control emotions as her mother did. This scenario leaves her feeling ashamed and guilty.
>
> *Protective compromise quadrant.* To escape this wish–fear conflict and as a consequence of it, the patient feels worthless and dissociates herself from important male figures; she is uncommunicative, but when encouraged she has the capacity to restore a concept of self as worthwhile and to guardedly engage in productive work with men.
>
> *Problematic compromise.* Alternatively, the patient may respond to her wish–fear conflict by viewing herself as worthless and degraded by critical others; she withdraws but still feels attacked, so she develops a "counteridentity" as a compensation for feelings of worthlessness and to avoid feeling too depressed.

As this example illustrates, the information in an RRMC is quite condensed. For this reason, we have found the RRMC to be a helpful format for efficiently and succinctly conveying a large amount of information; nev-

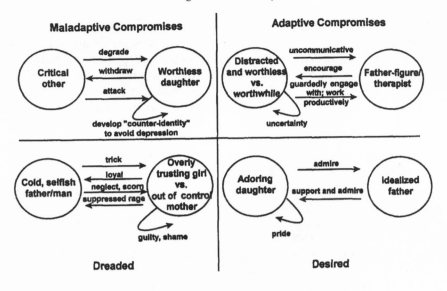

Maladaptive Compromises   **Adaptive Compromises**

FIGURE 5.4. RRMC of Connie.

ertheless, the clinician may elect instead to summarize the same information in a narrative format, as we have just done.

Control of Ideas and Affect

The concept of defense mechanisms remains a controversial one in psychology (Singer, 1990). Although consensus has not been reached about the existence of defense mechanisms (Holmes, 1990), the concept is one of the most resilient in clinical psychology and has probably been one of the most useful for those who practice psychotherapy.

Although many mechanisms of defense have been proposed, all rest on the assumption that three preconditions of mental functioning must be met for defensive operations to occur (Horowitz, Markman, Stinson, Fridhandler, & Ghannam, 1990). The first precondition is the presence of a motivational force aimed at conscious representation or action. Second is a capacity to process the motives into forms accessible to conscious representation. Third is the capacity to anticipate the consequences of conscious representation or action. The third precondition is problematic, however, because it leaves open the question of how it is possible to anticipate (and then ward off) the consequences of a conscious representation without that representation itself existing in consciousness.

Information-processing theory suggests two possible answers. First, the consequences of conscious representation might be anticipated in unconscious information processing without any conscious representation.

Horowitz et al. (1990) suggest that memory traces of past associations and sensitizations might operate entirely in unconscious information processing. A second possibility is that small amounts or periods of conscious representation could occur, but with feedforward inhibitions as a result of assessing these episodes. Both of these possibilities assume a "smart" unconscious (Loftus & Klinger, 1992), that is, one capable of assessing threats and selecting control operations likely to reduce the threat. Regardless of which "answer" one prefers, it is useful to think of the regulation of thought and affect in terms of three categories: purposes, outcomes, and processes (Horowitz, 1988; Wallerstein, 1983).

Control Purposes

The concept of a *control purpose* provides a motivational component to CA. Control purposes include a person's wishes, goals, hopes, and intentions; they do not assume conscious awareness of these purposes. Purposes may be categorized broadly as adaptive or maladaptive. Adaptive purposes are those that facilitate personal growth and development, the satisfaction of emotional needs, interpersonal relationships, and the like. Maladaptive purposes are those that inhibit growth and development, narrow the individual's life and range of experience, fail to meet emotional needs, and inhibit the development of healthy interpersonal relationships.

Readers might note that the concepts "defense mechanism" and "coping style" are similar in that both are marshaled to manage threatening ideas and feelings. Although some theorists characterize defenses as maladaptive and coping mechanisms as adaptive, we agree with Vaillant (1992) that there are conceptual advantages to viewing certain defensive outcomes as adaptive and others as maladaptive. Furthermore, we believe that both coping and defensive mechanisms can involve unconscious regulatory processes (Horowitz & Stinson, 1995; Horowitz, Znoj, & Stinson, 1996).

Control Outcomes

Outcomes are the resultants of the regulatory purposes and processes involved in managing conflictual ideas and affect that aim at conscious representation. They reflect varying degrees of deflections from awareness of these ideas and affect. Thus instead of thinking, "I hate my deceased spouse," a person may deflect this idea into "I idealize my deceased spouse" (reaction formation), "He had his reasons for being hateful" (rationalization), or "My feelings about my deceased spouse are unimportant" (minimization). A standard list of defense mechanisms such as that found in the appendices of DSM-IV (American Psychiatric Association, 1994) can serve as a list of control outcomes.

Control Processes

Processes lie between purposes and outcomes. They are analogous to the various paths that individuals might follow to a given destination. There are many routes to the same destination, but the route can affect the meaning of arriving at a destination. For example, a grieving person might rationalize the thought "I hate my deceased spouse" into "My feelings about my spouse don't matter" by any of the following processes or combinations of them: (1) switching topics; (2) decreasing arousal level; or (3) shifting from a multimodal representational set (i.e., the ability to access information in the form of images, words, smells, and tactile memories) to a unimodal set (e.g., only words).

For present purposes we refer to a control process as any of a variety of ways in which incipient thoughts and feelings might be inhibited, facilitated, or otherwise regulated. We distinguish three categories of control processes. These are the regulation of *mental set, schemas,* and *topic selection avid* flow. We briefly summarize these categories here. Readers wishing a more elaborated discussion of them are referred to Horowitz and Stinson (1995), Horowitz (1997), and Horowitz et al. (1996); see also Table 5.3.

Control of Mental Set

Mental set is the most basic level of a control process. It is a "state of preparedness for processing a constellation of ideas and emotions" and includes "a determination of the next theme for conscious representation and how this theme will be processed" (Horowitz et al., 1990, p. 66). Mental set refers to an individual's present capacity to contemplate and adaptively manage a theme once it enters consciousness, as well as one's readiness to permit entry of a stressful theme into consciousness. Some of the parameters that are determined by the notion of a mental set are the following: (1) the setting of an "intentional hierarchy," reflecting one's capacity to select one from among a set of themes for contemplation; (2) "temporal set," or the expanse of time one is able to take into account when processing a theme (short term vs. long term); (3) "sequential set," which address one's problem-solving style, for example, systematic and orderly, through reverie, or chaotically and randomly; (4) "representational set," or the mode in which ideas and feelings take form, including words, images, and behavior, either in isolation or in concert; (5) locus of attention (either toward thought or action); and (6) level of arousal.

TABLE 5.3. Control Purposes, Processes, and Outcomes in Configurational Analysis

Control process	Control outcome/control purpose	
	Adaptive	Maladaptive
Control of mental set		
Intentional hierarchy	Dosing	"Forgetting"
Temporal set	Telescoping to gain perspective, close examination to gain understanding	Continual focus on crises, denial, or avoiding examination of episodic memories
Sequential set	Planning, generation of positive imagery	Chaotic, haphazard
Representational set	Verbal dominant, other modes accessible via dosing	Numbing, denial, intrusion of images, acting out
Locus of attention	Toward thought, toward action	Easily distractible, dissociated
Level of arousal	Alert, attentive	Suppression, somnolence
Control of schemas		
Altering self schemas	Flexible adaptation	Reaction formation, turning against the self, regression
Altering schemas of others	Flexible adaptation	Projection, passive aggression
Altering relationship schemas	Sublimation, succorance, nurturance, altruism	Role reversal, projective identification, devaluation, splitting, excessive idealization
Control of topic selection and flow		
Control of representations by: Facilitation of associations	Working through	"As if" working, intellectualization, rumination
Inhibition of associations	Dosing to adaptive modulation	Denial, repression, suppression, disavowal, undoing, minimization, somatization
Sequencing ideas by: Seeking information	Working through, understanding, learning	Intellectualization, displacement
Switching concepts	Facilitative associations, smooth transitions, affect and thought concordance	Isolation of affect, rationalization, undoing, reaction formation
Altering meanings	Humor, wisdom, appreciation of irony	Narcissistic devaluation, exaggeration, lying, omnipotent control

(continued)

TABLE 5.3. (*continued*)

Control process	Control outcome/control purpose	
	Adaptive	Maladaptive
Hierarchical arrangement of ideas	Purposeful discourse, self-control	Paranoia, suspiciousness, rigidity
Revision of working models	Empathy, compassion for the self, self-control	Projection, externalization, blaming
Practicing new modes of thinking and acting	Self-efficacy	Regression, acting out

Note. Adapted from Horowitz (1988).

Control of Schemas. These controls regulate processes associated with an individual's sense of identity and self, as well as how he or she thinks, feels, and acts in relationships. As shown in Table 5.3, one might control the flow of ideas and affect into consciousness by altering self-schemas, schemas of others, and relationship schemas.

Control of Topic Selection and Flow. This category of controls includes those governing how individuals select topics for contemplation and how these topics are organized, consciously represented, and presented to others. Individuals might control the flow of representations either by facilitating or inhibiting associations. The sequencing of ideas might be described by seeking information or by topic switching. Other controls in this category are altering meanings, the hierarchical complexity or simplicity of information, revision of working models, and enacting new modes of thinking and feeling. Table 5.3 presents adaptive and maladaptive outcomes for each of these processes.

These thoughts about the control of conflictual ideas and affect provide a language close to signs observed during psychotherapy. Our clinical experience tells us that these control purposes, processes, and outcomes are often habitual patterns adopted by patients, operating largely outside awareness.

INCLUSION/EXCLUSION CRITERIA AND MULTICULTURAL CONSIDERATIONS

CA is appropriate for any individual regardless of culture undergoing a course of psychotherapy in which interpersonal relationships and concepts of self and others play an important role, or when one of the goals of therapy is to alter the patient's system of interpersonal meanings. CA is not restricted to any psychotherapy modality but is applicable to therapies as diverse as psychodynamic, cognitive, interpersonal, experiential, or behavioral. A CA formulation may offer an especially fresh perspective to therapists practicing in nondynamic modalities who may not accept the entire theory from which CA grew. Control process theory, for example, may illuminate obstacles to treatment success based on cognitive-behavioral principles. As noted previously, however, CA is particularly appropriate in the treatment of individuals with DSM-IV Axis II diagnosis or those seeking to change long-standing interpersonal problems.

Consideration of multiple concepts of self and other, and attendant values, is especially valuable in considering the influence of culture on individual psychotherapy. A male client may have been taught by his father that men of his clan do not cry and by his mother that his father is too strict in his beliefs and that in her community sensitive men express their feelings. Obviously these cultural differences affect issues of control over feelings and how they may be expressed as they occur in treatment. The patient and therapists, with such aspects of formulation, may then be in a position to clarify the value differences in therapy in a way that leads the patient to make his own personal assessment of his own principles and to change certain attitudes about his own identity now and as a future parent.

STEPS IN CASE FORMULATION CONSTRUCTION

There are four basic steps in CA case formulation. These steps should be done at evaluation and then repeated during phases of therapy process: The goal is revision, correction, and utilization in flexible ways to guide technique. The goal of these steps is to proceed systematically from readily observable material exhibited by a patient to a set of inferences that the therapist can use to better understand and treat the patient. Each step moves toward a greater level of inference and builds on what is learned in the previous steps. The four steps are as follows: (1) describing clinically relevant phenomena; (2) identifying the patient's repertoire of states of mind; (3) identifying and organizing the patient's central relationship schemas and schemas of self and other; and (4) labeling unresolved emotional themes and defensive control processes. Table 5.4 summarizes these steps. Materials to use are intake assessments, process or progress notes, and the clinician's recall of therapy sessions. In research, we use audiovideo recordings or transcripts of therapy sessions. Readers interested in more details are referred to book-length treatments by Horowitz (1987, 1997, 2005).

Step 1: Describe Clinically Relevant Phenomena

In this first step, the clinician simply makes a list of significant signs and symptoms observed in therapy or reported by the patient to occur outside therapy. In day-to-day clinical practice, this step can take place in the context of usual preliminary evaluations and updated as new information emerges.

TABLE 5.4. Steps in Configuration Analysis Case Formulation and Their Application to Treatment Planning

Phenomena

Select and describe symptoms, problem list, and noteworthy signs.

States of mind

Describe states in which the selected phenomena occur and do not occur. Describe patterns of state cycles. Refer to Tables 5.1 and 5.2 to select state descriptors.

Schemas of self and other

Describe the roles, beliefs, and scripts of expression and action that organize each state. Describe wish–fear dilemmas in relation to desired and dreaded RRMs. Infer how control processes and compromise RRMs may ward off such dangers. Identify dysfunctional attitudes and how these are involved in maladaptive state cycles.

Control of ideas and emotion

Describe themes of concern during problematic states. Describe how expressions of ideas and emotions are obscured. Infer how avoidant states may function to ward-off dreaded, undermodulated states. (Use Table 5.3 and Appendix X of DSM-IV; American Psychiatric Association, 1994)

Therapy technique planning

Consider the interactions of phenomena, states, controls, and RRMs. Plan how to stabilize working states by support, how to counteract defensive avoidances by direction of attention, and how to alter dysfunctional attitudes by interpretation, trials of new behavior, and repetitions; integrate psychological plan with biological and social plans, when indicated.

Note. Adapted from Horowitz (1997). Each step can also include social and biological levels as well as past developmental contributors to the current situation.

There is no effort at inference in Step 1. Instead, the clinician notes what any observant and interested individual would see. Information the clinician might list includes presenting symptoms and problems, posture, affective style, unusual verbalizations or gestures, any idiosyncratic mannerisms, salient traits, the style in which information is organized and presented, topics discussed, and the patient's pattern of shifting topics or of avoiding some topics altogether. The therapist should also be alert to what the patient is not saying. If a patient talks for several minutes about her mother, then shifts to siblings, then to work problems with a male supervisor, the therapist might wonder why the patient did not mention her father.

"Behavioral leakage" is particularly important to note at this stage of the formulation process. Behavioral leakages are signs exhibited by a patient that may suggest unexpressed affect or significant themes. Examples are perspiration that is out of context to the current topic, a reddening of the eyes that appears and then disappears as if the patient were about to cry but then suppressed the tears, fidgetiness, or a change in the patient's usual style of eye contact.

The therapist should also be alert to his or her reaction to the patient. One assumption of CA is that patients unwittingly cast therapists into roles that conform to interpersonal expectations, goals, and fears based on previous experiences with important others. Therefore, the therapist should also note his or her own behaviors, thoughts, and feelings—in particular those that deviate from the usual.

At the completion of Step 1, the clinician should have a list of observations, some of which may be clinically significant, some of which may not be. The goal of the following steps is to select those that might be significant, and then test them in the psychotherapy.

Step 2: Identify Patient's Repertoire of States of Mind

The clinician begins to label states of mind by grouping the phenomena observed in Step 1 into sensible patterns. If a patient becomes angry while discussing his being passed over for a promotion, says *"Nothing ever works out for me,"* then *goes silent,* the therapist might label these phenomena (indicated in italics) as an "angry powerlessness" state of mind. (The clinician may be helped in choosing state names by consulting Table 5.2.) Terminology from Benjamin's (1993) Structural Analysis of Social Behavior (SASB) is also useful in labeling states of mind.

The following suggestions are offered to assist therapists further in identifying states of mind:

1. Common indications of states include changes in facial expression, speech intonation and inflection, the content of verbal reports, degree of self-reflective awareness, overall level of awareness, and experienced capacity for empathy.

2. Be alert to the degree of control associated with a state. Assessing the level of control prepares the way for inferring control maneuvers used to avoid undermodulated states.

3. States can also be labeled "positive" or "negative." Positive states of mind are those that the patient probably experiences as more pleasurable than displeasurable. Conversely, negative states of mind are those that are experienced with displeasure or which include negative appraisals. In Step 3, this labeling will be used to classify self, other, and relationship schemas.

4. Notice the sequence in state shifts. Is there a pattern of moving from one state to another? For example, a patient may enter a state in which she challenges the therapist to do more for her, then shift to a self-deprecating state, and subsequently become remote and seemingly indifferent to the therapist. The therapist should also be attentive to any external events that trigger a state shift, such as the telephone ringing, a seemingly innocuous comment, starting a session late, or seeing another patient in the waiting room. At the end of Step 2 the therapist has a list of states, each

tentatively labeled "positive" or "negative" and "undermodulated," "over-modulated," or "well modulated." These states may not initially seem to cohere well. The list may be long or short, although the usual range is from three to seven.

Step 3: Identify Self, Other, and Relationship Schemas

The third step in CA case formulation is to use the list of states of mind to identify a patient's recurrent views of self and other. The following guidelines are helpful:

1. Note expressions such as "I am the sort of person who . . ., " "I always . . ., " and "My husband (friend, parent) is a very . . . person."

2. Be particularly attentive to narratives told by patients. The clinician can keep an RRM format in mind to aid in inquiry. For example, if a patient says, "I felt stupid when the professor called on me" (self schema), the therapist may ask, "What do you imagine was going through the professor's mind when she called on you?" in an effort to elicit a schema of other.

3. If a patient repeatedly describes him- or herself as shy with friends or relates stories that indicate this, one might include "shy friend" as a role of the self. Similarly, if the patient describes friends as better than he or she is, "superior friend" may be included as a role of the other.

4. Action sequences, which include communications about intentions, judgments, and emotions, are listed in an RRM as transaction scripts. These can be noted in verb–adverb pairs, as in "approach tentatively," "feels disparaged," and "withdraws." A dictionary of RRM scripts published elsewhere may also be helpful (Horowitz, Merluzzi, et al., 1991).

5. Organize self and other schemas into RRMs, as shown in Figures 5.1 through 5.4.

6. Include memories and fantasies about the past to show how the patient's current schematic and motivational structure developed.

7. Tentatively label schemas as desired, dreaded, protective compromises, or maladaptive compromises. Arrange them into RRMs and RRMCs, as shown in Figures 5.1 and 5.2.

Step 4: Identify Control Purposes, Processes, and Outcomes

Because several controls might operate in a single session, we recommend focusing on one part of a session at a time, perhaps a narrative told by the patient. After a section has been identified, first note the patient's "mental set." Consider the following questions: Do ideas flow easily and naturally or in a constricted manner? Do multiple ideas compete for expression, or does the patient have difficulty finding ideas? Can the patient shift from generalizations to episodic memories and vice versa? What structure does the patient impose on his or her narratives? Are these narratives relatively coherent or disorganized? How complete are they? Is the patient alert and attentive or sleepy, distant, and distracted? Do thoughts and feelings appear concordant or discordant?

Using the foregoing information to estimate the patient's mental set, consider next how concepts of self and other are presented. Notice different roles into which the self and others are cast. Observations of this type help the therapist determine the extent to which the patient alters schemas of self and other to avoid potentially painful information. To what extent are these roles consistent or inconsistent across narratives? Does the patient describe others in a stereotypical way or in away that permits the therapist to formulate an image of a unique human being? How are themes of power and affiliation portrayed in narratives? Are distinct roles assigned to self and other, or do these roles tend to blend into each other?

Finally, a detailed consideration of topic selection and flow can aid in identifying control processes. Focusing again on specific narratives, consider whether the patient engages in genuine, focused self-examination that aims at increasing self-understanding or, whether there is an "as if" quality or an intellectualized tone to the patient's expressions. Does the patient make assertions, then qualify, retract, or otherwise deflect meaning from the original content? Does the patient downplay the significance of clearly important life events? It is also helpful to contrast how a range of topics are communicated. Ideas, states, and emotions associated with some topics may be "welcomed" into awareness, whereas those associated with other topics may be experienced only with difficulty.

Once the therapist has completed these steps, the formulation can be transposed into a narrative or can remain as an RRMC and a worksheet with formulation components completed.

APPLICATION TO PSYCHOTHERAPY TECHNIQUE

We do not typically share the entire formulation with the patient in one intervention. Doing so would inevitably produce an unwieldy intervention and might overwhelm the patient. Instead, parts of the formulation are tested through simple and to-the-point interventions. The therapist also attempts to maximize the therapeutic impact of a formulation-based intervention by timing it appropriately, as relevant topics and themes arise.

Each of the four aforementioned steps generates information that can contribute to psychotherapy process and content, as well as to the evaluation of treatment success. Identifying noteworthy phenomena can help increase a patient's self-awareness, capacity for self-observation, and sense of control and self-mastery. For example, an overcontrolled and emotionally constricted patient seen by Eells struggled for months to change a destructive interpersonal pattern in which he demeaned family members, then felt guilty for his aggressive behavior. A turning point seemed to be reached after the therapist pointed out how sad it was that the patient was perpetuating a pattern with his own children that was inflicted on him as a child. The patient's face reddened, signifying behavioral leakage. When attention was called to his flushed face, the patient initially indicated a lack of awareness but then began to feel sad and tears welled in his eyes for the first time in therapy.

It is also useful therapeutically to label major states of mind or to help the patient to do so. This activity helps patients realize the impermanent nature of these states, which in itself can aid the goals of therapy. In addition, pointing out patterns of state shifts helps a patient avert entry into undermodulated states or into self-impairing repetitive patterns and interpersonal relationships.

The self and other schemas depicted in RRMs and RRMCs also provide a practical way to help the patient understand contradictions within identity, and the different, sometimes competing patterns that may come up in different states within relationships.

Finally, a greater awareness of control processes can help a patient more fully recognize patterns of avoiding important ideas and feelings.

CASE EXAMPLE

Death of a Parent

Connie was a 28-year-old single Caucasian woman with a college degree who, when entering therapy, was supporting herself on unemployment assistance while retraining for a more fulfilling career. She had recently broken off a live-in relationship with a man and moved in with other friends. Connie came self-referred with complaints of crying spells and depression that began after the death of her father 5 weeks earlier.

Step 1: Clinically Significant Phenomena

Connie complained of intrusive crying spells, which she criticized and attempted to suppress. During conversations with others, she was unable to follow the thread of meaning and instead became dazed. After the death of her father, her creative work stopped. She was frightened by these symptoms because they seemed to lead into states in which she had less and less control over herself. She was preoccupied with thoughts of death, experienced sudden outbursts of sadness, and felt that her life lacked purpose and direction.

Connie's problems in living included frequent disruptive love affairs. She selected men she saw as cold and remote and vainly tried to teach them about love. Connie was also unable to achieve an adult understanding of her relationship with her father, an issue exacerbated by his death.

Problematic topics included Connie's inability to understand the meaning of various episodes in which her father had rejected her. She was unable to experience any resentment toward him for rejecting her, without having to distort the meaning of the good relationship she remembered. This led to feelings of confusion about who she was, who he was, and how she should respond to his death appropriately. This problem was intensified by Connie's inability to know where she stood with her mother, except for a relatively imperative need to be different from her. Connie, her father, and her siblings all shared a view of the mother as a person who gave way to messy, out-of-control episodes of rage and depression.

Step 2: States of Mind

The most upsetting problematic state was characterized by *uncontrolled and intrusive crying.* There were other states used to avoid painful crying, primarily increased *sleeping* and feeling *dazed and distracted.* Connie also experienced a high-pressured state in which she felt *as if she were going crazy.*

Step 3: Self and Relationship Schemas

Connie was vulnerable to concepts of herself as defective, especially regarding her vocational identity. Like her father, she earned a college degree in business and found work in banking. Connie felt that her career was at a dead end, however, and her lack of more advanced skills left her feeling worthless. She quit her job in order to reorient her values and develop new skills. She was in the midst of this development when her father died. His death meant the interruption of her plan in which he would come to see that she was a worthwhile person, revise a rejection she had felt for the past 5 years, and so restore an early adolescent relationship of mutual admiration. Five years earlier, her father divorced her mother, and Connie sided with him. Soon after the divorce, however, she experienced her father as remote and rejecting. During this time, he married a woman much younger than himself and they had a baby, which Connie also experienced as rejection.

Her father's rejection of her perplexed and troubled Connie even before his death. When she last saw him, Connie had tried to regain the positive attachment of her earlier adolescence or at least to find out the reasons for his neglect and remoteness. At times, she saw her father as a cold, selfish man who had tricked and used her in his eventual divorce from her mother, then neglected and no longer needed her when he remarried. She experienced scorn and then felt herself to be either defective or unfairly rejected. Connie interpreted her father's death as a final rejection because it meant the impossibility of his ever reendorsing her worth. She also felt that his death might be his way of punishing himself for rejecting her. That is, the early and unexpected stroke was seen as a psychosomatic response to his recognition that he had destroyed a meaningful attachment.

Connie was unable to identify with her mother, although she had lost some of the basis for her identification with her father and her projections of what she ought to be. Her father wanted the divorce supposedly because of her mother's episodic, out-of-control rages and crying spells. Connie feared that by expressing reactive anger, fear, and sadness after his death, she would appear to be too much like her mother. These concepts of self and other are depicted in an RRMC format in Figure 5.4.

Step 4: Control of Ideas and Affect

The death of Connie's father set in motion a train of thought that would ideally lead to a greater understanding of her past relationship with him. Achieving this understanding appeared to be obstructed, however, by Connie's unwillingness to experience resentment, anger, and hurt toward her father. When these impulses arose she inhibited them for fear of losing control or feeling too guilty or ashamed. If her efforts at suppression were not entirely successful, she was prone to entering the previously mentioned distracted and dazed state of mind. Another significant control was idealization of her father, which also served to inhibit a view of him as cold and rejecting.

Formulation of Therapy Processes

Connie underwent a 12-session psychotherapy that aimed at relieving her symptomatology, at increasing feelings of self-efficacy, and at enhancing her understanding of her relationship with her father, thus laying a foundation for greater satisfaction in future intimate relationships.

States of Mind

Connie experienced *intrusive crying* with an evaluation interviewer but suppressed crying while talking with the therapist. The therapist detected her inhibition and blinking back of beginning tears. He told her that he would not feel critical of her if she did cry. She gradually became able to engage in *open crying*. As she worked through themes of mourning and of resentment toward her father, she was increasingly able to engage in a *working* state, expressing her emotions with fear of losing control.

Because the therapist was helpful and concerned, she could see him as an ideal father reestablishing the lost ideal relationship. During some episodes, she exhibited a *shining* state, which was like one previously referred to as mutual admiration with her father.

Although most of the time in therapy was spent by both persons working productively together, there were early episodes in which Connie began the interview in a *distracted* state, not knowing what to say.

Self and Relationship Schemas

A therapeutic alliance was established quickly, facilitated by Connie's intense need, and her symptoms decreased rapidly over the first few sessions. Subsequently however, Connie appeared skeptical and challenged the therapist, as if testing whether he would reject her, whether he could tolerate her resentment, and whether meaningful communication could take place.

A critical emerging issue was whether the therapist would see Connie as worthwhile or worthless because some of her attitudes might run counter toy his presumed cultural stance of conformity and conservatism. These counterculture attitudes were also revealed to be "counterfather" attitudes. As she found that the therapist did not refute or degrade her values, she herself tended to feel them as more authentic and an increase in self-esteem resulted. As her self-esteem increased, she was more willing to accept the challenge of further exploration of her ideas and feelings.

Control of Ideas and Affect

The main theme explored during therapy was the need to understand the meaning of her father's rejection of her. It appeared that Connie deflected feelings of resentment and hurt toward her father through self-distraction, suppression of crying, and idealization. As the therapist labeled these controls, Connie was gradually able to get in touch with feelings of resentment, weakness, and degradation in connection with her father. Immersion in early experiences with her parents, especially with her father, during the first few sessions led to an increased focus on her current life. One of the important themes interpreted by the therapist was Connie's tendency to repeat the relationship with her father in her selection of men whom she could idealize but who were older, cold, and remote. It seemed that the death of her father also created a pivotal point at which she might reject men altogether as persons who were incapable of returning love and care. Another version of this theme was the need to rescue men and some remorse that she had failed to rescue her father from what she saw as a psychosomatic illness.

Formulation of Outcome

States of Mind

Three months after the termination of therapy, Connie no longer had episodes of *intrusive crying*. She was less depressed and felt generally more purposeful and able to have long periods in which she was in a *working* state.

Self and Relationship Schemas

Connie felt an increased self-worth, which she viewed as a return to how she felt before her father's death rather than a new development. At the follow-up, she was engaged in reviewing the meaning of her father's death and accepting the mourning process without fear or blocking. She was considering new relationships and had embarked on one that she felt might be potentially long lasting.

Control of Ideas and Affect

The major change in the status of ideas was the creation of a concept of the development and meaning of her relationship with her father. She integrated various self-images and relationship models so that she now had a central view of him not as cold and rejecting but as presenting multiple self-images: as needing her while standing aloof and expressing an absence of need, and as telling her to be independent while covertly telling her to be tied to his views and person. She was able to differentiate her fear of weakness, sadness at loss, resentment of scorn, and remoteness from "messy emotions," and also to develop a more complex, less stereotyped view of her mother. The premise that she could not feel angry with her father for being neurotically conflicted was altered so that she believed it acceptable to express anger with him and with related male figures. Because of these changes, she could allow herself to progress through waves of grief work characteristic of mourning. She was aware in part of her inhibitory operations, but little if any alteration of this habitual style occurred.

TRAINING

Because it is a relatively complex method of psychotherapy case formulation, CA requires a commitment of time and effort to learn. Those familiar with psychodynamic concepts, particularly object relations theory and self psychology, will probably find CA easier to learn than those working in other modalities. A first step is to become familiar with concepts and terminology such as states of mind, multiple schemas, and control processes. After working with these terms for a while, they will become second nature. A second step, one that can be taken concurrently with the first, is simply to try out the method on a patient—new or not new—and see for oneself whether one has gained a better understanding of the patient. Third, it may be helpful to read more published case studies of individuals formulated with CA and compare one's own formulation with those of the authors (see Horowitz, 1997, 2005).

RESEARCH SUPPORT FOR THE APPROACH

Two studies have been completed assessing the reliability of the person schemas components of CA (Horowitz & Eells, 1993; Eells, Horowitz, et al., 1995). Horowitz and Eells (1993) demonstrated that trained clinical judges could correctly match RRMCs to videotapes of psychotherapy session of patients for whom the RRMCs had been constructed. Eells, Horowitz, et al. (1995) showed that two groups of clinicians were able to construct similar RRMCs when working from the same set of psychotherapy transcripts.

Reliability of state descriptions has also been established (Horowitz, Ewert, Milbrath, & Sonneborn, 1994). Preliminary data on the reliability of control purposes, processes, and outcomes are promising (Horowitz et al., 1996), especially because many researchers have had difficulty measuring defenses reliably (Vaillant, 1992).

The validity of a case formulation method can be established in different ways. In a study by Horowitz, Luborsky, and Popp (1991), convergent validity of the RRMC was measured by qualitatively comparing it with the CCRT method of case formulation (Luborsky & Crits-Christoph, 1990; see Luborsky & Barrett, Chapter 4, this volume). The results were that the methods identified similar core emotional and interpersonal conflicts, that the CCRT was easier to perform, but that the RRMC yielded more information about defense processes. In another study (Horowitz, Fells, Singer, & Salovey, 1995), RRMCs constructed early in a long-term therapy were compared with psychotherapy transcripts in the second and third thirds of the psychotherapy. Findings were that key interpersonal, emotional, and defensive themes identified early in therapy were still the focus of attention at later points in the therapy. This might be considered a form of predictive validity. Other approaches showing validity have compared the RRMC approach to those from multidimensional scaling using repertory grid-type ratings of adjectives as applied to self and significant others. These are reported in detail elsewhere (Tunis, Fridhandler, & Horowitz, 1990; Eells, 1995; Eells, Fridhandler, & Horowitz, 1995; Hart, Stinson, Field, Ewert, & Horowitz, 1995; Merluzzi, 1991).

CONCLUSION

CA is a systematic approach to case formulation. It has a good level of complexity: It permits one to examine multiple states of mind in terms of multiple self and other concepts that may organize emotional themes differently. In addition, CA facilitates an examination of how a patient copes with external stressors and attempts to control potentially disturbing feelings and thoughts. The advantage of the "good level of complexity" is that it avoids static, unitary, oversimplified inferences that fit the patient only some of the time.

CA proceeds from surface to depth. It cannot be completed in a single interview, but a good start can be made and followed up by additions and revisions. The levels can be done sequentially: phenomena, states, person schemas, and controls. But one can also make inferences from any level, then move back and forth to see if these inferences illuminate other facets of one's formulation. Sometimes really clear self-concepts are revealed as irrational aspects of a patient's identity, and these then clarify how to label a state of mind or infer a defensive distortion.

CA also points to technique: What phenomena are key problems to address first? What therapist interventions might increase well-modulated states and protect the patient from dreaded out-of-control states? Which dysfunctional attitudes about self and others can be changed at this point in treatment? What countermeasures are available to modify maladaptive control processes yet help the patient to tolerate strong emotions in more realistic ways? Individualized answers to such questions may emerge as the formulation is clarified.

REFERENCES

American Psychiatric Association. (1994). *Diagnostic and statistical manual of mental disorders* (4th ed.). Washington, DC: Author.

Andersen, S. M., & Limpert, C. (2001). Future-event schemas: Automaticity and rumination in major depression. *Cognitive Therapy and Research, 25,* 311–333.

Benjamin, L. S. (1993). *Interpersonal diagnosis and treatment of personality disorders.* New York: Guilford Press.

Berne, E. (1961). *Transactional analysis in psychotherapy.* New York: Ballantine Books.

Eells, T. D. (1995). Role reversal: A convergence of clinical and quantitative evidence. *Psychotherapy Research, 4,* 297–312.

Eells, T. D., Fridhandler, B., & Horowitz, M. J. (1995). Self schemas and spousal bereavement: Comparing quantitative and clinical evidence. *Psychotherapy, 32,* 270–282.

Eells, T. D., Horowitz, M. J., Singer, J., Salovey, P., Daigle, D., & Turvey, C. (1995). The Role-Relationship Models method: A comparison of independently derived case formulation. *Psychotherapy Research, 5,* 154–168.

Hart, D., Stinson, C., Field, N., Ewert, M., & Horowitz, M. (1995). A semantic space approach to representations of self and other in pathological grief: A case study. *Psychological Science, 6,* 96–100.

Holmes, D. S. (1990). The evidence of repression: An examination of sixty years of research. In J. L. Singer (Ed.), *Repression and dissociation: Implications for personality, psychopathology, and health* (pp. 85–102). Chicago: University of Chicago Press.

Hope, D. A., Rapee, R. M., Heimberg, R. G., & Dombeck, M. J. (1990). Representations of the self in social phobia: Vulnerability to social threat. *Cognitive Therapy and Research, 14*(2), 177–189.

Horowitz, M. J. (1979). *States of mind.* New York: Plenum.

Horowitz, M. J. (1987). *States of mind: Configurational analysis of individual psychology* (2nd ed.). New York: Plenum Press.

Horowitz, M. J. (1988). *Introduction to psychodynamics: A new synthesis.* New York: Basic Books.

Horowitz, M. J. (1989). Relationship schema formulation: Role-Relationship Models and intrapsychic conflict. *Psychiatry, 52,* 260–274.

Horowitz, M. J. (1991). *Person schemas and maladaptive interpersonal patterns.* Chicago: University of Chicago Press.

Horowitz, M. J. (1997). *Formulation as a basis for planning psychotherapy treatment.* Washington, DC: American Psychiatric Press.

Horowitz, M. J. (1998). *Cognitive psychodynamics: From conflict to character.* New York: Wiley.

Horowitz, M. J. (2001). *Stress response syndromes* (4th ed.). Northvale, NJ: Aronson.

Horowitz, M. J. (2005). *Understanding psychotherapy change.* Washington, DC: American Psychological Association.

Horowitz, M. J., & Eells, T. D. (1993). Role-Relationship Model Configurations: A method for psychotherapy case formulation. *Psychotherapy Research, 3,* 57–68.

Horowitz, M. J., Eells, T. D., Singer, J., & Salovey, P. (1995). Role Relationship Models for case formulation. *Archives of General Psychiatry, 52,* 625–632.

Horowitz, M. J., Ewert, M., Milbrath, C., & Sonneborn, D. (1994). *American Journal of Psychotherapy, 151,* 1767–1770.

Horowitz, M. J., Luborsky, L., & Popp, C. (1991). A comparison of the Role-Relationship Models Configuration and the Core Conflictual Relationship Theme. In M. J. Horowitz (Ed.), *Person schemas and maladaptive interpersonal patterns* (pp. 213–220). Chicago: University of Chicago Press.

Horowitz, M. J., Markman, H. C., Stinson, C. H., Fridhandler, B., & Ghannam, J. H. (1990). A classification theory of defense. In J. L. Singer (Ed.), *Repression and dissociation* (pp. 61–84). Chicago: University of Chicago Press.

Horowitz, M. J., Merluzzi, T. V., Ewert, M., Ghannam, J. H., Hartley, D., & Stinson, C. H. (1991). Role-Relationship Models Configuration. In M. J. Horowitz (Ed.), *Person schemas and maladaptive interpersonal patterns* (pp. 115–154). Chicago: University of Chicago Press.

Horowitz, M. J., & Stinson, C. H. (1995). Consciousness and processes of control. *Psychotherapy Research, 4,* 123–139.

Horowitz, M. J., Znoj, H., & Stinson, C. (1996). Defensive control processes: Use of theory in research, formulation, and therapy of stress response syndromes. In M. Zeidner & N. Endler (Eds.), *Handbook of coping* (pp. 532–553). New York: Wiley.

Kiesler, D. J. (1996). *Contemporary interpersonal theory and research: Personality, psychopathology, and psychotherapy.* Oxford, UK: Wiley.

Kihlstrom, J. F., & Cantor, N. (1984). Mental representations of the self. *Advances in Experimental Social Psychology, 17,* 1–4.

Kihlstrom, J. F., Cantor, N., Albright, J. S., Chew, B. R., Klein, S. B., & Niedenthal, P. M. (1988). Information processing and the study of the self. *Advances in Experimental Social Psychology, 21,* 145–178.

Loftus, E., & Klinger, M. R. (1992). Is the unconscious smart of dumb? *American Psychologist, 47,* 761–765.

Luborsky, L., & Crits-Christoph, P. (1990). *Understanding transference: The Core Confictual Relationship Theme method.* New York: Basic Books.

Markus, H. (1990). Unresolved issues of self-representation. *Cognitive Therapy and Research, 14,* 241-253.

Markus, H., & Nurius, P. (1986). Possible selves. *American Psychologist, 41,* 954–969.

Merluzzi, T. V. (1991). Representation of information about self and other: A multidimensional scaling analysis. In M. J. Horowitz (Ed.), *Person schemas and maladaptive interpersonal patterns* (pp. 155–166). Chicago: University of Chicago Press.

Segal, Z. V., Truchon, C., Horowitz, L. M., Gemar, M., & Guirguis, M. (1995). A priming methodology for studying self-representation in major depressive disorder. *Journal of Abnormal Psychology, 104,* 205–241.

Singer, J. L. (Ed.). (1990). *Repression and dissociation: Implications for personality theory, psychopathology, and health.* Chicago: University of Chicago Press.

Singer, J. L., & Salovey, P. (1991). Organized knowledge structures and personality. In M. J. Horowitz (Ed.), *Person schemas and maladaptive interpersonal patterns* (pp. 33–79). Chicago: University of Chicago Press.

Tunis, S., Fridhandler, B., & Horowitz, M. J. (1990). Identifying schematized views of self with significant others: Convergence of quantitative and clinical methods *Journal of Personality and Social Psychology, 59,* 1279–1286.

Unemori, P., Omoregie, H., & Markus, H. R. (2004). Self-portraits: Possible selves in European-American, Chilean, Japanese and Japanese-American cultural contexts. *Self and Identity, 3,* 321–328.

Vaillant, G. E. (Ed.). (1992). *Ego mechanisms of defense: A guide for clinicians and researchers.* Washington, DC: American Psychiatric Press.

Wallerstein, R. (1983). Defenses, defense mechanisms, and the structure of the mind. *Journal of the American Psychoanalytic Association, 31,* 201–225.

Williams, J. M. G., Mathews, A., & MacLeod, C. (1996). The emotional Stroop task and psychopathology. *Psychological Bulletin, 120,* 3–24.

Chapter 6

Cyclical Maladaptive Patterns
Case Formulation in Time-Limited
Dynamic Psychotherapy

HANNA LEVENSON
HANS H. STRUPP

HISTORICAL BACKGROUND OF THE APPROACH

Time-limited dynamic psychotherapy (TLDP) is an interpersonal, time-sensitive approach for patients with chronic, pervasive, dysfunctional ways of relating to others. Its goal is to modify the way a person relates to him- or herself and others. The focus is not on the reduction of symptoms per se (although such improvements are expected to occur) but, rather, on changing ingrained patterns of interpersonal relatedness or personality style.

While the framework of TLDP is psychodynamic, it incorporates current developments in interpersonal, object relations, and self psychology theories, as well as cognitive-behavioral and system approaches. The type of formulation we discuss in this chapter—the cyclical maladaptive pattern—is structured to inform the therapist about the patient's present mode of relating, the goals for the work, and how to keep the therapy attuned to these goals.

TLDP makes use of the relationship that develops between therapist and patient to kindle fundamental changes in the way a person interacts with others and him- or herself. Its premises and techniques are broadly applicable regardless of time limits. However, its method of formulating and intervening makes it particularly well suited for the so-called difficult patient seen in a brief or time-limited therapy. Its particular strengths include (1) applicability to the treatment of difficult patients (broad selection criteria), (2) relevance and accessibility for psychodynamically trained clinicians who want to work more effectively and more efficiently, (3) empirical scrutiny of the model, (4) a flexible framework that allows therapists to adapt it to their own unique therapeutic styles, (5) avoidance of complex meta-theoretical constructs by staying close to observable data where possible, and (6) constructs that lend themselves to an integrative perspective (Levenson, 2003).

A treatment manual describing TLDP was developed for research purposes and published in book form—*Psychotherapy in a New Key* (Strupp & Binder, 1984). A clinical casebook, *Time-Limited Dynamic Psychotherapy: A Guide to Clinical Practice* (Levenson, 1995), translates TLDP principles and strategies into pragmatically useful ways of thinking and intervening for the practitioner. In *Key Competencies in Brief Dynamic Psychotherapy*, Binder (2004) outlines basic competencies needed to conduct dynamic–interpersonal therapy in general with a strong emphasis on TLDP.

Historically, TLDP is rooted in an object relations framework. It embraces an interpersonal perspective, as exemplified by the early work of Sullivan (1953), and is consistent with the views of modern interpersonal theorists (e.g., Anchin & Kiesler, 1982; Benjamin, 1993; Greenberg & Mitchell, 1983). The relational view focuses on transactional patterns in which the therapist is embedded in the therapeutic relationship as a participant observer or observing participant; transference is not considered a distortion but, rather, the patient's plausible perceptions of the therapist's behavior and intent; and countertransference does not indicate a failure on the part of the therapist but, rather, represents his or her natural reactions to the pushes and pulls from interacting with the patient.

CONCEPTUAL FRAMEWORK

Principles

The TLDP model adheres to seven basic principles:

1. *People are innately motivated to search for and maintain human relatedness.* In attachment theory terms, the infant's orientation to stay connected to early caregivers is based on survival needs. We are hardwired to gravitate toward others (e.g., newborns are more likely to gaze at designs in the shape and structure of a face than at more abstract ones). The more we are able to establish a "secure [interpersonal] base" (Bowlby, 1973), the more likely we are to develop into independent, mature, and effective individuals.

2. *Maladaptive relationship patterns are acquired early in life, become schematized, and underlie many presenting complaints.* How one relates as an adult typically stems from relationships with early caregivers in the following manner. If caregivers (usually parents) are attuned to the needs of the child and are accessible, the child feels secure and is able to explore the environment—feeling safe and loved. If the caregivers are inconsistent, rejecting, and/or unresponsive, the child will feel insecure and could become anxious or avoidant. Bowlby (1973) held that early experiences with parental figures result in mental representations of these relationships or working models of one's interpersonal world. These experiences form the building blocks of what will become organized, encoded experiential, affective, and cognitive data (i.e., interpersonal schemas) informing one about the nature of human relatedness and what is generally necessary to sustain and maintain emotional connectedness to others. The child then filters the world through the lenses of these schemas which allows him or her to interpret the present, understand the past, and anticipate the future. Unfortunately, these schema can become a dysfunctional, self-fulfilling prophesy if early interpersonal experiences are faulty. For example, a child might be placating and deferential because his parents were authoritarian and harsh toward him. He would have an expectation that others would treat him badly if he were not compliant. The danger is not only that his submissiveness might invite the very behavior he was most afraid of (dominance by others) but also that because his "working model" of the interpersonal world was out of his awareness, he would continue to be at its mercy.

3. *Such patterns persist because they are maintained in current relationships (circular causality).* This emphasis on early childhood experiences is consistent with the basis for much of psychoanalytic thinking. However, from a TLDP framework, the individual's personality is not seen as fixed at a certain point but, rather, as continually changing as he or she interacts with others. Data from neurobiology seem confirmatory; while relationships play a crucial role in the early years, this shaping process occurs throughout life (Siegel, 1999, p. 4). Although one's dysfunctional interactive style is learned early in life, this style must be supported in the person's present adult life for the interpersonal difficulties to continue. To go back to our example—the placating and deferential behavior of the child becomes well practiced into adulthood. As an adult, his compliance allows others to take advantage of him at best and treat him harshly at worst. If he had experiences as an adult (e.g., being assertive and not being punished and being treated with respect and as if he had a voice) that ran counter to his internalized working model, from a TLDP perspective he would be expected to shift (over time) to a more robust and enlivened view of himself and his relational world.

This reasoning is consistent with a systems-oriented approach, which holds that the context of a situation and the circular processes surrounding it are critical. Pathology does not reside within an individual but, rather, is created by all the components within the (pathological) system. According to systems theory (von Bertalanffy, 1969), if we change one part of the system, the other parts must also change, because the entire system seeks a new level of stabilization.

4. *Therefore, in TLDP, clients are viewed as stuck, not sick.* Clients are seen as trapped in a rut which they helped dig, not as deficient.

5. *Maladaptive relationship patterns are likely to be reenacted in the therapeutic relationship.*[1] A fifth assumption is that the patient is likely to interact with the therapist in the same dysfunctional way that characterizes his or her interactions with significant others (i.e., transference) and may try to enlist the therapist into playing a complementary role (i.e., countertransference). From an interpersonal therapy perspective this reenactment is an ideal opportunity, because it provides the therapist with the very situation that gets the patient into difficulties in the outside world. The therapist is given the chance to observe the playing out of the maladaptive interactional pattern and to experience what it is like to try to relate to that individual. In Sullivan's (1953) terms, the therapist becomes the *participant observer* mentioned earlier. The relational–interactionist position of TLDP holds that the therapist cannot help but react to the patient—that is, the therapist inevitably will be pushed and pulled by the patient's dysfunctional style and will respond accordingly. This transactional type of reciprocity and complementarity (i.e., interpersonal countertransference) does not indicate a failure on the part of the therapist but, rather, represents his or her "role responsiveness" (Sandler, 1976) or "interpersonal empathy" (Strupp & Binder, 1984). In such reenactments, the therapist inevitably becomes "hooked" into acting out the corresponding response to the patient's inflexible, maladaptive pattern (Kiesler, 1988), or in Wachtel's (1993) terms, patients may induce therapists to act as "accomplices."

That the therapist is invited repeatedly by the patient (unconsciously) to become a partner in a well-rehearsed, maladaptive two-step has its parallels in the recursive aspect of mental development. For example, children who have experienced serious family dysfunction are thought to have disorganized internal mental structures and processes as a result; these disorganized processes impair the child's behavior with others, which causes others not to respond in empathic ways, thereby disorganizing the development of the mind still further (Lyons-Ruth & Jacobwitz, 1999). It is a case of the rich get richer and the poor get poorer.

To get oneself unhooked, it is essential that the therapist realize how he or she is fostering a replication of the dysfunctional pattern and use this information to attempt to change the nature of the interaction in a more positive way, thereby engaging the patient in a healthier mode of relating. In addition, the therapist can collaboratively invite the patient to look at what is happening between them (i.e., metacommunicate), either highlighting the dysfunctional reenactment while it is occurring or solidifying new experiential learning following a more functionally adaptive interactive process.

Because dysfunctional interactions are presumed to be sustained in the present, including the current patient–therapist relationship, the therapist can concentrate on the present to alter the patient's dysfunctional interactive style. Working in the present allows change to happen more quickly because there is no assumption that one needs to work through childhood conflicts and discover historical "truths." This emphasis on the present has tremendous implications for treating interpersonal difficulties in a brief time frame.

6. *TLDP focuses on one chief problematic relationship pattern.* While patients may have a repertoire of different interpersonal patterns depending on their states of mind and the particulars of the situation, the emphasis in TLDP is on discerning what is a patient's most pervasive and problematic style of relating (which may need to incorporate several divergent views of self and other). This is not to say that other relationship patterns may not be important. However, focusing on the most frequently troublesome type of interaction should have ramifications for other less central interpersonal schemas and is pragmatically essential when time is of the essence.

7. *The change process will continue after the therapy is terminated.* The goal in TLDP is to interrupt the client's ingrained, repetitive, dysfunctional cycle. In so doing, the intention is to promote forays into healthier behavior, which theoretically would be responded to differently (more positively) by others, thereby increasing the person's proclivity to engage in a more satisfying manner. At the end of a brief therapy, such changes have only begun to take hold. It is expected that over time, as one had more opportunity to practice such functional behaviors, the interactions with others and the resulting more positive internalized schemas would become strengthened. In other words, the therapy sessions end, but the therapy continues in the real world.

Goals

The TLDP therapist seeks to provide a *new experience* and a *new understanding* for the patient.

New Experience[2]

The first and major goal in conducting TLDP is for the patient to have a new experience. "New" is meant in the sense of being different and more functional (i.e., healthier) than the customary, maladaptive pattern to which the person has become accustomed. And "experience" emphasizes the affective–action component of change—behaving differently and emotionally appreciating behaving differently. From a TLDP perspective, behaviors are encouraged that signify a new manner of interacting (e.g., more flexibly and independently) rather than specific, content-based behaviors (e.g., being able to go to a movie alone).

The new experience actually consists of a set of experiences throughout the therapy in which the patient has a different appreciation of him- or herself, of the therapist, and of their interaction. These new experiences provide the patient with experiential learning so that old patterns may be relinquished and new patterns may evolve.

The therapist determines the types of new experiences that are particularly helpful to a particular patient based on the therapist's formulation of the case. The therapist identifies what he or she could say or do (within the therapeutic role) that would most likely subvert the patient's maladaptive interactive style. The therapist's behavior gives the patient the opportunity to disconfirm his or her interpersonal schemata. This *in vivo* learning is a critical component in the practice of TLDP. The patient has the opportunity actively to try out new behaviors in the therapy, to see how he or she feels, and to notice how the therapist responds. This information then informs the patient's interpersonal schemata of what can be expected from self and others.

These experiential forays into what for the patient has been frightening territory make for heightened affective learning. A tension is created when the familiar (though detrimental) responses to the patient's presentation are not provided. Out of this tension new learning takes place. Such an emotionally intense process is what "heats up" the therapeutic process and permits progress to be made more quickly than in therapies that depend solely on more abstract learning (usually through interpretation and clarification). As Frieda Fromm-Reichmann is credited with saying, what the patient needs is an experience, not an explanation.

There are parallels between the goal of a new experience and procedures used in some behavioral techniques (e.g., exposure therapy) where clients are exposed to feared stimuli without negative consequences. Modern cognitive theorists voice analogous perspectives (e.g., Safran & Segal, 1990) when they talk about interpersonal processes that lead to *experiential disconfirmation*. Similarities can also be found in the plan formulation method of Harold Sampson and Joseph Weiss (1986; see also Weiss, 1993; Curtis & Silberschatz, this volume) in which change occurs when therapists pass their patients' "tests."

The concept of a *corrective emotional experience* described 60 years ago is also applicable (Alexander & French, 1946). In their classic book, *Psychoanalytic Therapy: Principles and Applications*, Alexander and French challenged the then prevalent assumption concerning the therapeutic importance of exposing repressed memories and providing a genetic reconstruction. In TLDP a therapist can help provide a new experience by selectively choosing from all the helpful, mature, and respectful ways of being in a session those particular aspects that would most effectively undermine a specific patient's dysfunctional style.

With sufficient quality or quantity of these experiences, patients can develop different internalized working models of relationships. In this way TLDP promotes change by altering the basic infrastructure of the patient's transactional world, which then reverberates to influence the concept of self. This emphasis on *experiential learning* allows TLDP to benefit a wider range of patients (broader selection criteria) than many other types of psychodynamic brief therapies that emphasize understanding through interpretation.

New Understanding

The second goal of providing a new understanding focuses more specifically on cognitive changes than the first goal which emphasizes the affective–behavioral arena. The patient's new understanding usually involves an identification and comprehension of his or her dysfunctional patterns. To facilitate a new understanding, the TLDP therapist can point out repetitive patterns that have originated in experiences with past significant others, with present significant others, and in the here-and-now with the therapist. Therapists' disclosing their own reactions to the patients' behaviors can also be beneficial. Patients begin to recognize how they have similar relationship patterns with different people in their lives, and this new perspective enables them to examine their active role in perpetuating dysfunctional interactions.

Although the two TLDP goals have been presented as separate entities, in actuality the new experience and the new understanding are part of the same picture. Both perspectives are always available, but at any one time one becomes figure and the other ground. New experiences, if they are to be more than fleeting events, have elements of representations (understandings) of self and others. Similarly, new understandings, if they are to be more than mere intellectualizations, have experiential and affective components.

However, in teaching TLDP a conceptual division is made between the idea of a new experience and a new understanding for heuristic reasons; it helps the trainees attend to aspects of the change process that are helpful in formulating and intervening quickly. In addition, because psychodynamically trained therapists are so ready to intervene with an interpretation, placing the new experience in the foreground helps them grasp and focus on the "big picture"—how not to reenact a dysfunctional scenario with the patient.

The Cyclical Maladaptive Pattern

In the past, psychodynamic brief therapists used their intuition, insight, and clinical savvy to devise formulations of cases. While these methods may work wonderfully for the gifted or experienced clinician, they are impossible to teach explicitly. One remedy for this situation was the development of a procedure for deriving a dynamic, interpersonal focus—the cyclical maladaptive pattern (CMP; Schacht, Binder, & Strupp, 1984).

Briefly, the CMP outlines the idiosyncratic "vicious cycle" of maladaptive interactions a particular patient gets into when he or she relates to others. These cycles or patterns involve inflexible, self-perpetuating behaviors, self-defeating expectations, and negative self-appraisals, that lead to dysfunctional and maladaptive interactions with others (Butler & Binder, 1987; Butler, Strupp, & Binder, 1993). The CMP comprises four categories that are used to organize the interpersonal information about the patient:

1. *Acts of the self*. These include the thoughts, feelings, motives, perceptions, and behaviors of the patient of an interpersonal nature. For example, "When I meet strangers, I think they wouldn't want to have anything to do with me" (thought). "I am afraid to take the promotion" (feeling). "I wish I were the life of the party" (motive). "It seemed she was on my side" (perception). "I start crying when I get angry with my husband" (behavior). Sometimes these acts are conscious as those above, and sometimes they are outside awareness, as in the case of the woman who does not realize how jealous she is of her sister's accomplishments.

2. *Expectations of others' reactions*. This category pertains to all the statements having to do with how the patient imagines others will react to him or her in response to some interpersonal behavior (Act of the Self). "My boss will fire me if I make a mistake." "If I go to the dance, no one will ask me to dance."

3. *Acts of others toward the self*. This third grouping consists of the actual behaviors of other people, as observed (or assumed) and interpreted by the patient. "When I made a mistake at work, my boss shunned me for the rest of the day." "When I went to the dance, guys asked me to dance, but only because they felt sorry for me."

4. *Acts of the self toward the self*. In this section belong all the patient's behaviors or attitudes toward oneself—when the self is the object of the interpersonal pattern. How does the patient treat him- or herself? "When I made the mistake, I berated myself so much I had difficulty sleeping that night." "When no one asked me to dance, I told myself it's because I'm fat, ugly and unlovable."

In addition to the four categories of the CMP, the therapist should also consider his or her reactions to the patient. How are you feeling being in the room with this patient? What are you pulled to do or not do? The therapist's internal and external responses to the patient provide important sources of information for understanding the patient's lifelong dysfunctional interactive pattern. One's reactions to the patient should make sense given the patient's interpersonal pattern. Of course, each therapist has a unique personality that might contribute to the particular shading of the reaction which is elicited by the patient, but the first assumption from a TLDP perspective is that ideally the therapist's behavior is *predominantly* shaped by the patient's evoking patterns (i.e., the influence of the therapist's personal conflicts is not so paramount as to undermine the therapy).

The CMP provides an organizational framework which makes comprehensible a large mass of data and leads to fruitful hypotheses. A CMP should not be seen as an encapsulated version of the truth but, rather, as a plausible narrative, incorporating major components of a person's current and historical interactive world. It is a map of the territory—not the territory itself (Strupp & Binder, 1984). In addition, a successful TLDP formulation should provide a blueprint for the entire therapy. It describes the nature of the problem, leads to the delineation of the goals, serves as a guide for interventions, enables the therapist to anticipate reenactments within the context of the therapeutic interaction, and provides a way to assess whether the therapy is on the right track—in terms of outcome at termination as well as in-session minioutcomes. Yet the CMP is a fluid working formulation that is meant to be refined as the therapy proceeds. The focus provided by the CMP permits the therapist to intervene in ways that have the greatest likelihood of being therapeutic. Thus the therapy can be briefer *and* more effective at the same time.

INCLUSION/EXCLUSION CRITERIA AND MULTICULTURAL CONSIDERATIONS

TLDP was developed to help therapists deal with patients who have trouble forming working alliances due to their lifelong dysfunctional interpersonal difficulties. However, from a relational point of view, many symptoms (e.g., depression and anxiety) and problems in living (e.g., marital discord) stem from one's impaired relatedness to self and other; consequently a wide range of clinical issues and presentations could be successfully addressed using TLDP.

Five major selection criteria are used in determining a patient's appropriateness for TLDP (Strupp & Binder, 1984).[3] First, patients must be in *emotional discomfort* so they are motivated to endure the often challenging and painful change process and to make sacrifices of time, effort, and money as required by therapy. Most therapists have confronted the enormous (and frequently insurmountable) problem of trying to treat people who are court-referred or "dragged" into the consultation room by an exasperated family member.

Second, patients must *come for appointments and engage with the therapist*—or at least talk. Initially such an attitude may be fostered by hope or faith in a positive outcome. Later it might stem from actual experiences of the therapist as a helpful partner.

Third, patients must be *willing to consider how their relationships have contributed* to distressing symptoms, negative attitudes, and/or behavioral difficulties. The operative word here is "willing." Suitable patients do not actually have to walk in the door indicating that they have difficulties in relating to others. Rather, in the give-and-take of the therapeutic encounter, they must evidence signs of being willing to consider the possibility that they have problems relating to others.

Fourth, patients need to be *willing to examine feelings* which may hinder more successful relationships and may foster more dysfunctional ones. Also, Strupp and Binder (1984) elaborate that the patient needs to possess "sufficient capacity to emotionally distance from these feelings so that the patient and therapist can jointly examine them" (p. 57).

And fifth, patients should be capable of having a *meaningful relationship* with the therapist. Again, it is not expected that the patient initially relates in a collaborative manner. But the potential for establishing such a relationship needs to exist. Patients cannot be out of touch with reality or so impaired that they have difficulty appreciating that their therapists are separate people. It would be impossible to conduct an interpersonal therapy if the patient did not know where he or she ended and the therapist began.

The exclusionary criteria for TLDP are very similar to criteria for red-flagging patients in other brief dynamic approaches (MacKenzie, 1988). Specifically, the TLDP exclusionary criteria are:

- Patient is not able to attend to the process of a verbal give-and-take with the therapist (e.g., patient has delirium, dementia, psychosis, or diminished intellectual status).
- Patient's problems can be treated more effectively by other means (e.g., patient has a specific phobia or manic–depressive illness).
- Patient cannot tolerate the interpretative, interactive therapy process, which often heightens anxiety (e.g., patient has impulse control problems, abuses alcohol and/or substances, or has a history of repeated suicide attempts).

Because TLDP acknowledges that both therapist and client bring their own personal qualities, history, and values to the therapeutic encounter, it is potentially sensitive to the interactive factors involved in treating clients from different races, cultures, sexual orientations, and so on. However, as pointed out by LaRoche (1999), proponents of the interpersonal–relational approach could do a much better job of explicitly considering the larger context in which any therapy takes place. "It seems crucial to extend . . . [the notion] of transference to include the organizing principles and imagery crystallized out of the values, roles, beliefs, and history of the *cultural* environment " (p. 391, emphasis added). Thus, it is of paramount importance that the therapist be aware of and understand how cultural factors (in the inclusive sense of the word) may be playing a role in the patient's lifelong patterns and in interpersonal difficulties including those that might manifest between therapist and patient. From a relational point of view, the client's interpersonal style outside the therapy office is an amalgamation of one's unique problems, attachment history, sociocultural context, strengths, developmental stage, familial factors, and values, just to mention a few. All these contribute to the client's assumptive world, or working models. If a therapist did not consider these factors, important interactive dimensions could be missed or misunderstood, thereby endangering the entire therapeutic process and outcome.

As part of this understanding, the therapist should have some comprehension (based on the available clinical and empirical data) of the normative interpersonal behavior and expectations for people with similar backgrounds (cultural data). And this should be distinguished (to the extent possible) from the individual's idiosyncratic CMP. For example, in the case to be presented later, the therapist is a Caucasian man who has a medical degree. The client is an African American woman, an office administrator, and old enough to be his mother. She complains of feeling inferior and other people keeping her at arm's length. Is this to be understood as part of her idiosyncratic CMP or as part of set of experiences she shares with other women of color in our sexist and racist society. And if it is shared by others with a similar cultural background, is her manifestation of it more extreme? In this particular case, the client describes how she longs for closeness with her *female relatives* and feels different from them in her ability to achieve this intimacy. Thus, our hypothesis that these experiences have an idiosyncratic component is strengthened.

In addition, within the therapy office, the therapist must also consider how cultural factors take on an active role. Perhaps this client is saying she feels held at arm's length because she is working with a white male (a *cultural* transference–countertransference reenactment). If this is the case, her therapist could make a seriously erroneous error by inferring that this is a more global problem for her. From a TLDP perspective, it is important to be aware of the dangers of making assumptions based solely on transference–countertransference enactments. This again highlights the importance of a comprehensive and evolving formulation using the CMP categories.

The best way to judge if a CMP is more an artifact of differences between therapist and client is to gauge the therapist–patient interactions in the here-and-now of the therapy sessions in light of what the patient says about expectations of and behavior from other people (especially to the extent that they are of the same race, gender, age, or other relevant parameters). In this case, the therapist noted that the client felt her *female relatives* were not trustworthy and that she needed to protect herself from them by distancing herself. Having said this, however, the therapist must always be vigilant for cultural ignorance and bias having an untoward effect on the therapy.[4]

Regarding multicultural considerations of the short-term nature of TLDP, it has been found repeatedly that most people regardless of background prefer briefer therapies (Sue, Zane, & Young, 1994). However, until there are research data to inform us, "mental health professionals should exercise caution in using brief models with diverse populations and should adapt them to the unique cultural and social situation of the client" (Welfel, 2004, p. 347). To our knowledge there is no TLDP outcome research examining the influence of cultural variables. However, there are some intriguing (albeit limited) relevant publications. Using Asian American students, participants were randomly assigned to read either a cognitive therapy (CT) or TLDP treatment rationale for depression (Wong, Kim, Zane, Kim, & Huang, 2003). Those with low levels of white identity rated the rationale of CT as more credible than that for TLDP, while those with high white identity did not rate the two treatment rationales differently. However, further analyses reveal that these students (who were not actually clients) were only moderately involved in the task, possibly limiting generalizability to actual patient populations. On the other hand, Li (2003), in a theoretical study, makes the case for how TLDP is well suited to the needs of Chinese Americans by examining the parallels between ten TLDP values and the core principles of Confucianism, Taoism, and Buddhism. She optimistically argues that TLDP may someday become the psychotherapeutic treatment of choice for the Chinese American population.

With regard to use of TLDP with different age groups, we have seen patients from 18 to 92 in our studies and clinical practices. Noting that conflicts in current, close relationships are commonly presented complaints by older clients, Nordhus and Nielsen (1999) extended the application of TLDP to elderly adults by presenting a case illustration. "We find the cyclical maladaptive patterns format especially valuable for the therapeutic endeavour itself as well as for supervising the process" (p. 946).

Flasher (2000) also makes a case for using TLDP formulation with an age group at the opposite end of the continuum—children. She notes that while TLDP was developed for use with adults, "this interpersonally-based model is viewed as consistent with recent literature in child development and psychopathology which emphasizes the centrality of peer relationships, interpersonal schema, and social attribution biases in the development of maladaptive interpersonal behavior" (p. 239). Flasher demonstrates with a

TABLE 6.1. Steps in TLDP Formulation and Intervention

1. Let the patient tell his or her own story in his or her own words.
2. Explore the interpersonal context related to symptoms or problems.
3. Use the categories of the CMP to gather, categorize, and probe for information.
4. Listen for themes in the patient's content (about past and present relationships) and manner of interacting in session.
5. Be aware of reciprocal reactions (countertransferential pushes and pulls).
6. Be vigilant for reenactments of dysfunctional interactions in the therapeutic relationship.
7. Explore patient's reaction to the evolving relationship with the therapist.
8. Develop a CMP narrative (story) describing the patient's predominant dysfunctional interactive pattern.
9. From this CMP, outline the goals for treatment.
10. Facilitate a new experience of more adaptive relating within the therapeutic relationship and/or with others in the patient's life consistent with the CMP (Goal 1).
11. Help the patient identify and understand his or her dysfunctional pattern as it occurs with the therapist and/or others in his or her life (Goal 2).
12. Assist the patient in appreciating the once adaptive function of his or her manner of interacting.
13. Revise and refine the CMP throughout the therapy

case study that TLDP formulation can be used to individually tailor treatment for children with aggression, rejection, and other problematic interpersonal patterns.

With regard to gender bias, Levenson and Davidovitz (2000) found that male therapists devoted a significantly greater percentage of their clinical time to brief therapy than did their female counterparts and were more likely to prefer shorter-term therapies. However, little is known regarding brief therapy outcome depending on the therapist's gender.

STEPS IN CASE FORMULATION

Table 6.1 contains the steps in TLDP formulation and intervention. These "steps" should not be thought of as separate techniques applied in a linear, rigid fashion but, rather, as guidelines for the therapist to be used in a fluid and interactive manner. In the initial sessions, the therapist lets the patient tell his or her own story (Step 1) rather than relying on the traditional psychiatric interview, which structures the patient's responses into categories of information (developmental history, education, etc.). By listening to *how* the patient tells his or her story (e.g., deferentially, cautiously, OR dramatically) as well as to the content, the therapist can learn much about the patient's interpersonal style. The therapist then explores the interpersonal context of the patient's symptoms or problems (Step 2). When did the problems begin? What else was going on in the patient's life at that time, especially of an interpersonal nature? By using the four categories of the CMP and his or her own reactions (Step 3), the therapist begins to develop a picture of the patient's idiosyncratic, interpersonal world, including the patient's views of self and expectations of others' behavior. The therapist listens for themes in the emerging material by seeing commonalities in the patient's transactional patterns over person, time, and place (Step 4). As part of interacting with the patient, the therapist can be pulled into responding in a complementary fashion, recreating a dysfunctional dance with the patient. By examining the patterns of the here-and-now interaction, and by using the Expectations of Others' Reactions and the Behavior of Others components of the CMP, the therapist becomes aware of his or her countertransferential reenactments (Steps 5 and 6). The therapist can then help the patient explore his or her reactions to the relationship which is forming with the therapist (Step 7). By incorporating all the historical and present interactive thematic information, the therapist can develop a narrative description of the patient's idiosyncratic primary CMP (Step 8). From this formulation, the therapist then discerns the goals for treatment (Step 9). The first goal involves determining the nature of the new experience (Step 10). The therapist discerns what he or she could say or do (within the therapeutic role) that would most likely subvert or interrupt the cyclical dynamic nature of the patient's maladaptive interactive style. Consistent with this way of conceptualizing a new experience, Gill (1993) suggests that what is needed are *specific* mutative transference–countertransference interactions. The therapist–patient "interaction has to be about the right content—a content that we would call insight if it became explicit" (p. 115).

Traditionally in TLDP the most potent intervention capable of providing a new understanding (Step 11) is thought to be the examination of the here-and-now interactions between therapist and patient. It is chiefly through the therapist's observations about the reenactment of the cyclical maladaptive pattern in the sessions that patients begin to have an *in vivo* understanding of their behaviors and stimulus value. By ascertaining how the pattern has emerged in the therapeutic relationship, the patient has perhaps for the first time the opportunity to examine the nature of such behaviors in a safe environment.

It is usually helpful for the therapist to share his or her formulation with the patient *at whatever level the patient can comprehend it*, and to collaborate with the patient to derive a mutual understanding of the dysfunctional nature of his or her interactions. However, the degree to which a patient can join the therapist in elaborating a new life narrative is limited by such factors as his or her intellectual ability, capacity for introspection, psychological-mindedness, and the quality of the therapeutic alliance.

The therapist can help depathologize (Step 12) the patient's current behavior and symptoms by helping him or her to understand their histori-cal development. From the TLDP point of view, symptoms and dysfunc-tional behaviors are the individual's attempt to adapt to situations threaten-ing interpersonal relatedness. For example, in therapy a passive, anxious client began to understand that as a child he had to be subservient and hypervigilant in order to avoid beatings. This learning enabled him to view his present interpersonal style from a different perspective and allowed him to have some empathy for his childhood plight.

The last step (13) in the formulation process involves the continuous refinement of the CMP throughout the therapy. In a brief therapy, the ther-apist cannot wait to have all the "facts", before formulating the case and intervening. As the therapy proceeds, new content and interactional data become available that might strengthen, modify, or negate the working for-mulation.

APPLICATION TO PSYCHOTHERAPY TECHNIQUE

We consider the formulation to be essential to the understanding of the case. It is not necessarily shared with the patient but may well be depending on the patient's abilities to deal with the material. Rather than presenting intellectual generalizations to the patient, the shared understanding of what is important to work on in the therapy is a collaboratively derived process. For some patients with minimal introspection and abstraction ability, the problematic interpersonal scenario may never be stated per se. Rather, the focus may stay very close to the content of the presenting problems and concerns of the patient (e.g., wanting to be accorded more respect at work). The therapist, however, is constantly using the CMP to inform him- or her-self regarding how to facilitate a new experience of self and other in session (e.g., the patient's experiencing himself as a respected and responsible part-ner in the therapeutic process). Some patients enter therapy with a fairly good understanding of their own self-defeating and self-perpetuating inter-personal patterns (e.g., "I have decided to come into therapy at this time because I can see I am going to get fired from this job, just like all the other jobs, if I don't stop antagonizing my boss"). In these cases, the therapist and patient can jointly articulate the parameters that foster such behavior, generalize to other situations where applicable, and be vigilant to recognize its occurrence in the therapy.

The CMP is critical for guiding the therapist in the direction of the most facilitative interventions. The following examples of two patients with seemingly similar behaviors but differing CMPs will illustrate. Marjo-rie's maladaptive interpersonal pattern suggested she had deeply ingrained beliefs that she could not be appreciated unless she were the entertaining, effervescent ingenue. When she attempted to joke throughout most of the fifth session, her therapist directed her attention to the contrast between her joking and her anxiously twisting her handkerchief. (New experience: The therapist invites the possibility that he can be interested in her even if she were anxious and not cheerful.)

Susan's lifelong dysfunctional pattern, on the other hand, revealed a meek stance fostered by repeated ridicule from her alcoholic father. She also attempted to joke in the fifth session, nervously twisting her handkerchief. Susan's therapist listened with engaged interest to the jokes and did not interrupt. (New experience: The therapist can appreciate her taking center stage and not humiliate her when she is so vulnerable.) In both cases the therapist's interventions (observing nonverbal behavior; listening) were well within the psychodynamic therapist's acceptable repertoire. There was no need to do anything feigned (e.g., laugh uproariously at Susan's joke), nor was there a demand to respond with a similar therapeutic stance to both presentations.

In these cases the therapists' behavior gave the patients the opportunity to disconfirm the patients' own interpersonal schemata. With sufficient quality and/or quantity of these experiences, patients can develop different internalized working models of relationships. In this way TLDP promotes change by altering the basic infrastructure of the patient's transactional world, which then reverberates to influence the concept of self.

CASE EXAMPLE

At the time of her therapy, Mrs. Follette was a 59-year-old, African American, employed, widow with three grown daughters. She had been in individual and group therapy several times in the past. Her therapist was Dr. David, a male fourth-year psychiatry resident who was a trainee in the brief therapy program run by the first author. During his first session with Mrs. Follette, Dr. David was unsure how he could be of help to her. She presented with no clear agenda—only saying that she had some memory difficulties. She had been referred by the neurology service when they could find no evidence of an organic problem. Dr. David did some formal mental status testing but also did not find any discernible memory impairment. By the third session, Mrs. Follette said her memory was "no longer bothering me." At this point it was not clear what she wanted to accomplish in the therapy.

However, Dr. David relied on the TLDP case formulation procedures to help him begin to understand why Mrs. Follette was there and what he could do to help—to discern the "dysfunctional mental working model and corresponding maladaptive interpersonal pattern that *is hidden in plain sight*" (Binder, 2004, p. 141, emphasis added). He used the categories of the CMP to gather, classify, and probe for interpersonal information. Table

TABLE 6.2. Mrs. Follette's CMP

Acts of the self: Patient feels self-conscious in the presence of others, particularly peers in a nonworking environment. Patient maintains a "shell" around herself which allows her to keep others at "arm's length." ("I don't want to be depending on anyone. I don't care what other people think.") Although she longs for closeness and acceptance, she fears intimacy. ("It makes me nervous when other people get too close to me.") As a result, she remains somewhat isolated and alone. ("I spend most of my time alone and that suits me fine. I'm doing very well, thank you.") Patient believes she does not need other people. She repeatedly sets professional goals for herself which she eventually meets, but is then left feeling unfulfilled.

Expectations of others: Patient believes others are not dependable. ("If you depend on people, you will be disappointed every time. When you need someone, they will not be there. Other people always want you to do things for them. They really don't care about one.") She believes others are not willing to provide closeness and nurturance when needed. She expects others will be hurtful to her if she depends on them, and thinks others will treat her better the more she is independent. Patient believes others are often not honest with her. She also expects that others will perceive her as inferior.

Acts of others toward self: Patient's fears of allowing others to get close to her or to know her by revealing things about herself leads others to feel alienated and distanced. ("My aunt is just concerned with herself, and really isn't interested in what I have to say. My daughters have each other and don't need me much.") Others view the patient as being strong and independent and not interested in, or in need of their help or friendship. Some others treat the patient as if she were inferior. ("All the support I've gotten in the past has been misleading. Members of my family said I wasn't college material.")

Acts of the self toward self (introject): Patient sees herself as having an inferior mind, and therefore feels she is inadequate. ("Once I reach my goals, I feel unsatisfied with myself. My memory is failing me and that really bothers me. Maybe the way I am is because my umbilical cord was wrapped around my neck when I was born.") She considers herself to be unlovable. Patient feels guilty. She sees herself as vulnerable with a need to preserve control and appear strong. She has a heightened sense of responsibility for her own well being.

Therapist's reaction to patient: Dr. David felt superfluous and put off by her seeming self-sufficiency and apparent disinterest in his help.

6.2 contains some of Mrs. Follette's dialogue (in parentheses) from the first session organized according to the four components of the CMP.

When initially formulating the CMP, some therapists become concerned about whether they have correctly placed what the patient is saying into the right category. There are simple guidelines, such as the patient's own behavior toward others usually goes under Acts of the self, whereas behaviors directed toward the self usually go under Introject. But sometimes the meaning of a particular behavior (whether it is directed at others or toward the self) is not so obvious. Fortunately, one need not become obsessed with the correct placement because these categories are primarily designed to be of heuristic value—to help the therapist elicit, assess, and organize a large amount of incoming data; eventually all components will be combined into one narrative.

Following the TLDP steps to case formulation, Dr. David also observed how and what he was feeling and thinking in her presence. He became aware of the emotional tone and sequence of transactions with her as the sessions progressed. He took note of how her descriptions of her interactions with others displayed redundant themes which could be woven together into recurring patterns. By the end of the third session, Dr. David was able to discern a style of relating that he conjectured was quite problematical for Mrs. Follette. Based on her interactions with him, what she said about her relationships with others, and his reaction to her, he constructed a narrative version of her CMP (See Table 6.2).

Because Dr. David was able to derive a cyclical maladaptive pattern, and Mrs. Follette met the basic selection criteria for TLDP with no exclusionary criteria, she was accepted into treatment. The patient, however, could not come to therapy on a weekly basis. Every other week she had to take business training classes during the time she would ordinarily meet with Dr. David. So a revised schedule was agreed on; Mrs. Follette would come to therapy every other week. In total, she was to receive 10 sessions spread over 20 weeks.

Dr. David summarized Mrs. Follette's interpersonal narrative as follows: This is a woman who puts out signals that she does not need anything from anyone, because she fears no one will be there for her if she were vulnerable. She keeps her guard up, so as not to get harmed, but her distancing behaviors (her pseudoindependence) put others off, ensuring the very reaction she most fears.

From this initial formulation, Dr. David derived the two goals of treatment. The *new experience* was for Mrs. Follette to experience herself as letting down her guard and becoming vulnerable while interacting with a therapist who neither backed away nor intrusively made demands of her. The *new understanding* was for her to begin to appreciate how her distancing behaviors caused others to move away.

How Formulation Relates to Treatment Interventions

Dr. David could now see how Mrs. Follette's CMP had been reenacted in the early sessions with him. At the beginning of the therapy, he had felt detached and confused in the sessions. After constructing Mrs. Follette's CMP, Dr. David began to appreciate how his reaction to the patient was not a hindrance but, rather, an *in vivo* example of what needed to shift if the therapy were to be beneficial.

The first few minutes of the fifth session (which took place during the 10th week of therapy) captures the patient's interactive style. Although Dr.

David had derived his understanding of Mrs. Follette's maladaptive interactional pattern some weeks before, he found this present interchange quite consistent with his working formulation. Comparing ongoing clinical material to the CMP is one way of constantly refining the working formulation.

THERAPIST: Any thoughts?

PATIENT: Not really. No. Not any real thoughts. Things are just moving along. Do you got any thoughts? What about your thoughts? (*Laugh*) Oh, goodness!

THERAPIST: What kind of thoughts were you speaking of?

PATIENT: You mean what kind of thoughts that I was speaking of when I asked you what your thoughts were?

THERAPIST: Uh huh.

PATIENT: Oh, your thoughts about me, [Uh huh.] and what we've been doing. (*Pause*) If it is helping you.

THERAPIST: If it is helping me?

PATIENT: Yeah, right, to accomplish your goals.

THERAPIST: Hmmm. What do you see as being my goal?

PATIENT: Well, must be to become a—what—a psychiatrist or what? What? A psychiatrist?

THERAPIST: Uh huh.

PATIENT: How is that coming?

THERAPIST: It's interesting that you would view therapy as being something to help me [Yeah, it is . . .] in my goal.

PATIENT: . . . isn't it?

THERAPIST: I suppose in general everything I'm doing is leading me toward that. Ah, but I wonder if you think of our meeting as being more for me than for you? It sounded like that is what you were suggesting.

PATIENT: Hmmm. Well, I think for both, really. You know, this is a dual purpose situation. I come in here and this is to help you get, I guess your certification or whatever it is. And, ah, you're helping me, and I'm helping you—in a way.

THERAPIST: Does that, I wonder, if that leaves any room for caring?

In this exchange, Dr. David's responded (briefly) to the realities of his being in training. He confirmed the patient's perception that he was getting something for himself out of their meeting but then turned the discussion back to the larger issue of their interaction. In an attempt to introduce an affective tone into the you-scratch-my-back-I'll-scratch-yours nature of the interchange, Dr. David brought up the possibility of caring.

According to Mrs. Follette's CMP, she does not believe others will be there to provide closeness when needed. By suggesting that caring might be an important ingredient of their relationship, Dr. David was providing a mini-new experience that ran counter to Mrs. Follette's expectation of how others behave. In the middle of the same session (Session 5) termination issues are discussed. Because sessions were every other week, her treatment was half over at this point.

THERAPIST: The one thing that I'm thinking about too, is what you brought up earlier in the session about therapy's ending and, you know, where the, ah, we sort of talked about the last week of this will be the first week of June, [Uh huh.] which is June fourth. I'm wondering how you feel about that and how that's affecting . . .

PATIENT: I feel very fine about that because, ah, I don't have any burning issues . . .

It is important in a time-limited therapy for both patient and therapist to be aware of the finiteness of the therapy. Here the therapist asks the patient for her feelings about the impending ending date, to which the patient replies that she feels "fine." However, the therapist, understanding the patient's tendency to pull back during times of perceived vulnerability, explored Mrs. Follette's reaction as illustrated in the next interaction.

THERAPIST: The one thing you said once though was, ah, you wanted to make sure that you didn't start to depend on 2:30 on Thursdays. [Uh huh.] Because when that ends then you're left without, without that [Hmmm.] and that would be a very uncomfortable feeling. [Uh huh.] So it just makes me wonder, ah, that your comfortable feeling about ending June fourth, ah, is OK because the feeling that, well, I'll just make sure that I don't get too dependent on this, and make sure that I hold back to a certain degree. Then we could end June fourth and it won't matter, because I never will have allowed myself to depend on this in the first place.

PATIENT: Well, that's a form of protection, you know. If I don't protect me, who will, you know? And I'm not saying that's true, but it could be, you know, it could be.

Here the therapist did not take the patient at face value and blankly accept what she had said. Nor did he contradict her or infer that his perceptions were superior to hers. What he did was question her "comfort" in terms of other things she has previously mentioned. He reminded her that she had said she did not want to depend on their sessions. He then wondered out loud if she were feeling comfortable about ending soon because of her fears about becoming dependent.

Several times during the fifth session, Dr. David gently confronted Mrs. Follette with what she herself said in previous sessions. These interventions led the patient to justify her "holding back" as a form of "protection," so that she did not become a "babbling nut." Here again, Dr. David explored her strategy of avoiding becoming a "blithering basket case."

The patient disagreed that she had fears about becoming devastated should she get into this "old stuff" too deeply, because she had other "release valves" in her life. Again, Dr. David reminded her of what she said earlier in the therapy: "And yet you said before that that's one of the things you might do for protection is never to get involved in the first place as a way to make sure you were together when you walked out the door." In this way, Dr. David confronted Mrs. Follette's disavowal of her tendency to avoid and distance.

Dr. David used gentle confrontation several times throughout this fifth session. He stayed very close to the material Mrs. Follette was introducing and used this information in an empathic way to confront her rigid, withdrawn stance. His approach combined content and process. What he said is important in terms of her defensive pattern, but how he said it in the context of their relationship was even more significant. Dr. David was providing Mrs. Follette with a series of new experiences in which she was being heard and responded to—he was helping her wrestle with facing her fears.

Mrs. Follette then talked about how she and Dr. David need to be on the "same plane." She told him she was aware that he always had an "agenda." Midway into the session she launched into an acknowledgement of how she and Dr. David talked about the "relationship between the therapist and the client."

PATIENT: So, so we sit in here and we talk about the relationship between the therapist and the client. (*Laugh*)

THERAPIST: What do you think about that?

PATIENT: (*Laugh*) I think it's fun! I really do.

THERAPIST: Uh huh. What do you think about that? Anything come to mind? What's coming up for you . . . talking about our relationship?

PATIENT: Well, it certainly makes for a better ra . . . ah, feeling, you know, to come out here [Uh huh.] and see and talk to you, you know, because we do have that type of relationship, ah, you know, it always helps. [Uh huh.] Ah, you know, ah, you know, it help me. We won't talk about whether it helping you or not. But anyway, a dimension, ah, that, ah, that may be something else that we, I may need to throw out on the table, ah, for us to discuss.

When the patient said that talking about their relationship was fun, she said it in a very open and honest manner. At that moment she appeared to be more present and more affectively connected to Dr. David than she had been previously. Talking about the relationship within the context of that relationship is a very intimate thing to do. The very process demands trust. Continuing with the last interchange, Dr. David picked up on the patient's "hint" that there might be something else that she might need to discuss.

THERAPIST: Something particular in mind that you were . . . [Huh?] Something particular in mind that you were thinking of when you said that?

PATIENT: Uh huh, yeah, uh huh.

THERAPIST: What, what was that?

PATIENT: (*Chuckle*) It is funny, you know, ah, of all the therapy sessions I've been in, I've never brought up the fact that my step-father, ah, (*pause*) demanded, when I was about, what, 20, 21, whatever. Ah, my mother had, ah, gone to Chicago for the summer and ah, you know, we were there, and, ah, you know, and it's pretty hard to say he made me have sexual intercourse with him. But you know, it came down to that. And that didn't bother me until, oh, I guess about maybe ten years ago, and then, you know, whatever, it came back very vividly. And, ah, out of all the therapists that I've been to and talked to, I've never brought that one little aspect up. And, you know, I was really curious about that. You know, I was wondering about that, ah, why I never, you know, brought that up as an issue, that it happened. . . .

THERAPIST: (*Softly, in measured tones*) That's a pretty heavy duty [Uh huh.] thing to have gone through. [Uh huh.] This was not just a stepfather but he raised you like . . .

PATIENT: Well, right, yeah. I always looks at him as my father, right. And, ah, ah, you know, someone that you think of as your father, when they do one of those, you know, and what not, it make you very, ah, very distant, very distant.

The patient was able to tell her therapist a secret she had been keeping for 39 years. However, she told about the rape in her characteristic, intellectualized ("I was really curious"), minimizing ("that one little aspect") manner. Dr. David did not engage with the patient on this level but, rather, responded affectively in content and tone. He correctly ascertained that to engage with Mrs. Follette in a discussion about understanding the timing of her sharing her secret would be colluding with her avoidance of her need to be comforted and acknowledged and would inhibit their connecting on a more affective level. His commenting on the "heavy-duty" nature of her experience is similar to his introducing the concept of "caring" earlier. Dr. David was trying to see if Mrs. Follette could relate to him and to her own experience on a deeper emotional level. His affective reaction to hearing her secret also validated his perception that she had endured a truly traumatic incident when she was younger.

After hearing the secret, experienced therapists can imagine several different therapeutically valid ways Dr. David could have gone (e.g., referral to an incest survivor group). However, he chose to stay within the frame of the CMP and to continue focusing on Mrs. Follette's vulnerability, trust, and distance issues. The patient herself, after revealing her secret, talked about an interpersonal consequence consistent with Dr. David's conceptualization (pseudoindependence vs. intimacy). "It make you very, very distant— very distant." Dr. David maintained the focus by asking Mrs. Follette if she had felt more distant from her father since then, and then expanded this specific behavior to the broader implications of her distancing style with other people in general. This pattern recognition helps patients discover motifs in their manner of relating; "It must have made it very difficult to have anybody that you could trust, if your own father did this to you." The patient readily agreed to this interpretation.

In the closing minutes of this same session, Dr. David explored with the patient how he experienced a change in her manner of interacting with him in the session.

THERAPIST: I just want to point something out. I've commented before about that feeling of there being a shell around you—that distance. I noticed when you came in today, there was very much that feeling again [Of what?], there being a shell around you [Oh.] But that somewhere in the middle of the session it feels like that shifted. [Uh huh.] I feel a lot more openness and warmth about you [Uh huh.] now as opposed to early in the session. [Um huh.] Are you aware of that? Do you feel any difference?

PATIENT: Um . . . (*pause*). Yeah, I think I do. I think so. I've reached some, I've reached some, ah, real, ah, decisions about, you know, about myself and about where I want to go. And the fact is, I can't move on if I'm holding all these things. You know, I can't move. [Yeah.] I mean, I can't be a part of, you know, be with other people and feel comfortable [Uh huh.] as long as I'm keeping a whole lot of stuff. . . . But you know, I feel a lot looser, and alot more at ease, and a lot . . . You know, I want to let go of some of these things I've been holding. You can't hold something, what, ah, 37, 8 years and it not affect you. You have to let it go.

THERAPIST: So, in other words, you think holding some of these things inside helps to create a distance between you and other people?

PATIENT: Yeah. I guess so. I think so. Ah huh, I think so.

In this interaction, Dr. David shared the positive changes he observed in Mrs. Follette, consistent with his formulation. In brief therapy especially, one needs to make the patients aware of what they are doing right. We need to build on their strengths and make their shifts in a healthier direction obvious to them. Quite often when patients begin relating in a more positive way, they are completely unaware of it. Therapists can be quite helpful to patients in pointing out these changes. Unfortunately, often with a medical model, we become more accustomed to pointing out dysfunctions and deficits. When Dr. David introduced what Mrs. Follette was doing differently, he did so by examining its interpersonal effect on him. He said that he felt a lot more openness and warmth somewhere in the middle of the session; it was Mrs. Follette who made the connection between the openness and sharing her secret.

As the session was about to come to an end, Mrs. Follette mentioned that although she ordinarily would skip meeting the next week, she thought she might be able to get away in time to make an appointment with Dr. David the very next week. We understand this as in-session evidence that she felt more trusting and safer with Dr. David. She had taken risks in this fifth session and Dr. David had not exploited her increased vulnerability. It seemed she could now extend herself even further and let herself become more involved in her therapy with him.

By the end of therapy, both patient and therapist thought the brief therapy had been quite helpful. Mrs. Follette responded to several self-report measures to assess outcome in TLDP (Symptom Checklist-90R, Derogatis, 1983; Inventory of Interpersonal Problems, Horowitz, Rosenberg, Baer, Ureno, & Vallasenor, 1988). Her symptomatic distress level dropped to a quarter of what it was on intake. For example, at intake she indicated that a loss of sexual interest or pleasure was causing her moderate distress; at termination she reported this problem was not bothering her at all. Similarly, Mrs. Follette's interpersonal distress level dropped in half. For example, at intake she responded that trusting other people too much was causing her quite a bit of distress; by termination this had ceased being a problem. Furthermore, at termination, Mrs. Follette stated her problems were much better and Dr. David likewise thought that she had made considerable progress.

Six months after Mrs. Follette ended her brief therapy, Hanna Levenson, the director of the Brief Therapy Program, contacted her for a semistructured follow-up interview. In this interview Mrs. Follette was asked some general questions about her therapy with Dr. David. The following excerpt comes after the patient talked about what she had gained from the therapy.

INTERVIEWER: And have you been able to use what you've experienced and learned in your therapy since then? Has it made a difference?

PATIENT: Oh, yes. Oh, yes. Oh, yes. I think the amazing thing about it is that because I've come into my own, my relatives treat me differently. And I don't know if maybe instead of my being . . . Hmm. (*pause*) I don't know how to put it. But it seems as though they recognize the newness in me, and therefore things they said and did before they did not do. And maybe because they felt like, I have not become defiant or anything, but I've become my own person.

INTERVIEWER: And somehow you communicated that to them?

PATIENT: Right. Right. Without saying that. Right.

INTERVIEWER: Do you have any idea what they're picking up?

PATIENT: I have no idea. I guess it's, ah, (*pause*) I don't know. I have no idea. Maybe the video [session is being videotaped], one can see oneself. But in so much as I cannot mentally see myself, I don't know what it is that I'm now throwing out to other people that they're getting. There is a new Joan Follette. It's not the old Joan Follette. And even people that I haven't seen in a long time, there's something about me that's different and they mention it.

INTERVIEWER: They do?

PATIENT: Either you've become prettier or something. They don't know what it is. And I know what it is. Because I have decided that, that ah, I guess I have a lot more confidence in myself. And I think that's the thing that maybe's coming out and they see. (*pause*) So it's been a real growing process. In other words, I've come of age.

This interchange illustrates the chief principle whereby TLDP is thought to generalize outside the therapist's office. Ideally, a patient's experience in the brief therapy helps disconfirm his or her ingrained dysfunctional interpersonal expectations and thereby encourages him or her to try out new but shaky behaviors with other people. In this particular case, Mrs. Follette was able to be more vulnerable, trusting, and self-revealing (i.e., removed the "shell" surrounding her) in her sessions, encouraged by Dr. David's positive therapeutic stance (e.g., nonintrusiveness, empathic understanding, and gentle confrontation) and adherence to the thematic interpersonal issue. In this follow-up excerpt Mrs. Follette clearly evaluated the benefits from therapy in interpersonal terms. She gave evidence that she was trying out more available, approachable attitudes and behaviors with her relatives who began seeing her as literally more attractive. She then related how her relatives in turn "treat me differently." She was unsure ("I have no idea") exactly what she was communicating to them to get them to act differently, but she knew they saw "something about me that's different." What is critical here is not the patient's precise understanding of some abstract principle about her CMP but, rather, her ability to generalize her experiential learning with Dr. David to others in her life. Here then are the beginnings of a cyclical *adaptive* pattern. Although the brief therapy sessions had ended, Mrs. Follette continued the therapeutic work.[5]

TRAINING

Clinical Aspects of Training

For the reader who is curious to learn more about TLDP case formulation and intervention, we recommend a multifaceted approach including reading, supervision, consultation (expert or peer), and workshops with instructional videotapes. Presently two TLDP manuals are available *Psychotherapy in a New Key* (Strupp & Binder, 1984) describes the basic principles and strategies of TLDP; *Time-Limited Dynamic Psychotherapy: A Guide to Clinical Practice* (Levenson, 1995) provides a practical and pragmatic casebook approach. Instructional videotapes are also commercially available.[6] After reading further about TLDP, we advise becoming familiar with the steps in TLDP formulation and intervention outlined in Table 6.1 and reviewing the Vanderbilt Therapeutic Strategies Scale (VTSS) and accompanying manual included in the appendices of Levenson's (1995) book. Next, therapists can practice devising CMP formulations and TLDP goals for their problematic patients (e.g., those with poor therapeutic alliances). Going through this exercise even for ongoing patients in long-term therapies can be quite informative for helping therapists see more clearly where they might be unintentionally colluding with patients in some dysfunctional dynamic. For those therapists who wish to try out a TLDP therapy, we advise video- or audiotaping sessions and then reviewing these sessions using the VTSS to assess adherence and deficient areas needing further attention and/or guidance. Peer (or if possible, expert) consultation is invaluable in becoming aware of nuances in the therapeutic interchange that inform the CMP. A new learning format is now available, consisting of an interactive website where those learning TLDP can submit their formulations on three target cases and then receive an expert's version (Levenson, 2006). In addition, workshops on TLDP occur nationally and regionally through universities and professional associations.

When teaching TLDP to clinicians (whether they be neophytes to the field or experienced professionals), we have preferred to use small-group supervision focusing on video- or audiotapes of therapy hours in combination with didactic sessions, also using videotapes to illustrate teaching points (Levenson & Strupp, 1999).[7] As trainees watch the tapes of these sessions in a stop-frame approach, they are asked to say what is going on in the vignettes, to distinguish between relevant and irrelevant material, to propose interventions a therapist might use, to justify their choices, and to anticipate the moment-to-moment behavior of the patients. This learning approach is consistent with the teaching format of "anchored instruction," where knowledge to be learned is specifically tied to a particular problem using active involvement of the learner in a context that is highly similar to actual conditions (Binder, 1993, 2004; Schacht, 1991).

Each trainee videotapes a patient for an entire therapy (up to 20 sessions) and then privately reviews his or her entire videotape of that week's session and selects portions to show in the group supervision. This format allows trainees to receive peer and supervisory comments on their technique as well as to observe the process of a brief therapy with other patient–therapist dyads. In this way, trainees learn how the model must be adapted to address the particular dynamics of each case and also what is generalizable about TLDP across patients. At the beginning of therapy, trainees devise a CMP and goals for their patients. Changes are made in the formulations as clinical knowledge grows, allowing trainees to observe the reciprocal process of formulation informing the direction of the therapy, which then informs the nature of the formulation.

Levenson has delineated 10 similarities between supervision in TLDP and TLDP itself (work actively with trainee "resistance"; focus on trainees' having a new experience as well as gaining knowledge; expect trainees will continue to incorporate and integrate what they have learned after the training rotation is over) (Levenson, Butler, & Bein, 2002). The reader who is particularly interested in TLDP training is referred to the book by Levenson (1995), because it contains actual transcripts of exchanges between supervisor and trainees as they deal with clinical and didactic material.[8]

Research Studies of Training

Strupp and his research group undertook a direct investigation into the effects of training on therapist performance. These studies (Vanderbilt II) explored the effects of manualized training in TLDP for 16 experienced therapists (8 psychiatrists and 8 psychologists) and 80 patients (Strupp, 1993). The main results indicate that the training program was successful in changing therapists' interventions congruent with TLDP strategies (Henry, Strupp, Butler, Schacht, & Binder, 1993), and that these changes held even with the more difficult patients (Henry, Schacht, Strupp, Butler, & Binder,

1993a). However, a later analysis suggested that many of these therapists did not reach an acceptable level of TLDP mastery (Bein et al., 2000).

Among the more striking findings were differences in training effects due to whether the therapist was in Trainer A's or Trainer B's group. Trainer A's therapists showed greater changes in adherence to TLDP. Inspection of differences between the two trainers' styles indicated that Trainer A's approach was more directive, specific, and challenging. This finding led the investigators to suggest how to maximize training effects:

- Choose competent but relatively less experienced therapists.
- Select therapists who are less vulnerable to negative training effects (e.g., less hostile and controlling).
- Assume that even experienced therapists are novices in the approach to be learned.
- Provide close, directive, and specific feedback to therapists and focus on therapists' own thought processes.

Regarding the training of beginning therapists, Kivlighan and his colleagues found that the clients of novice TLDP therapists reported more therapeutic work and more painful feelings than those seen by control counselors (Kivlighan, 1989), and live supervision was more likely to foster TLDP skills when compared to videotaped supervision (Kivlighan, Angelone, & Swofford, 1991). Multon, Kivlighan, and Gold (1996) demonstrated that prepracticum counselor trainees were able to increase their adherence to TLDP strategies with training; furthermore, a related study (Kivlighan, Schuetz, & Kardash, 1998) found that the more trainees focused on learning as an end in itself they better they did. In another training study, Levenson and Bolter (1988) found that trainees' values and attitudes toward brief therapy became more positive after a 6-month seminar and group supervision in TLDP. Other research has supported these findings (Neff, Lambert, Lunnen, Budman, & Levenson, 1997).

In an innovative study, LaRue-Yalom (2001) sought to study the long-term outcome of training in TLDP. Participants were 90 professionals who previously (on average, 9 years ago) learned TLDP during their 6-month outpatient rotation at a large medical center. Results indicated that these professionals still used TLDP and called on aspects of their TLDP training in their present daily work. Many said they had integrated TLDP strategies into their long-term work as well.

RESEARCH SUPPORT FOR THE APPROACH

The background for TLDP comes from a program of empirical research begun in the early 1950s. Strupp (1955, 1960) found that therapists' interventions reflected their personal (positive or negative) attitude toward the patients. Later work (Strupp, 1980) revealed that patients who were hostile, negativistic, inflexible, mistrusting, or otherwise highly resistant, uniformly had poor outcomes.

Strupp reasoned that the difficult patients had characterological styles that made it very hard for them to negotiate good working relationships with their therapists. In such cases the therapists' skill in managing the interpersonal therapeutic climate was severely taxed, and they became trapped into reacting with negativity, hostility, and disrespect. Because the therapies were brief, this inability to form a therapeutic alliance quickly had deleterious effects on the entire therapy.

Henry, Schacht, and Strupp (1990) found that for poor outcome cases (no change in the patients' introjects), therapists and patients manifested more hostile communications, and amount of therapists' hostile and controlling statements were related to the number of patients' self-blaming statements. Furthermore, therapists whose pretherapy self-ratings revealed more hostility directed toward themselves were more likely to treat their patients in a disaffiliative manner. And all this occurred by the third session of therapy! A later investigation (Hilliard, Henry, & Strupp, 2000) further demonstrated that patients' and therapists' introjects have a direct effect on the therapy process, which affects outcome.

Quintana and Meara (1990) found that patients intrapsychic activity became similar to the way patients perceived their therapists treated them in short-term therapy. A study examining relational change (Travis, Binder, Bliwise, & Horne-Moyer, 2001) found that following TLDP, patients significantly shifted in their attachment styles (from insecure to secure) and increased the number of their secure attachment themes.

Johnson, Popp, Schacht, Mellow, and Strupp (1989), using a modification of the CMP, found that for a single case, relationship themes were identified that were similar to themes derived using another psychodynamic relationship model (Core Conflictual Relationship Theme method, CCRT; see Horowitz & Eells, Chapter 5, this volume). (See Henry, 1997, for more information on this CMP modification and interpersonal case formulation.)

The VA Short-Term Psychotherapy Project (the VAST Project) examined TLDP process and outcome with a personality-disordered population (Levenson & Bein, 1993). As part of that project, Overstreet (1993) found that approximately 60% of the 89 male patients achieved positive interpersonal or symptomatic outcomes following TLDP (average of 14 sessions). At termination, 71% of patients felt their problems had lessened. One-fifth of the patients moved into the normal range of scores on a measure of interpersonal problems.

A VAST Project long-term follow-up study of this population (Bein, Levenson, & Overstreet, 1994; Levenson & Bein, 1993), found that patient gains from treatment were maintained and slightly bolstered. In addition, at the time of follow-up, 80% of the patients thought their therapies had helped them deal more effectively with their problems. In a naturalistic effectiveness study of 75 patients treated with TLDP, neurotic and psychosomatic patients evidenced significant improvement at termination, as well as 6-month and 12-month follow-ups (Junkert-Tress, Schnierda, Hartkamp, Schmitz, & Tress, 2001). Those diagnosed with personality disorders also improved, but to a lesser degree.

Hartmann and Levenson's (1995) study using the VAST Project data found that TLDP case formulation is relevant in a real clinical situation. CMP case formulations written by treating therapists (after the first one or two sessions with their patients) conveyed reliable and valid data to other clinicians. Perhaps most meaningful is the finding that better outcomes were achieved the more these therapies stayed focused on topics relevant to these patients' CMPs.

ACKNOWLEDGMENTS

Portions of this chapter are reprinted from *Time-Limited Dynamic Psychotherapy: A Guide to Clinical Practice* (copyright 1995 by Hanna Levenson) with permission of Basic Books, a member of Perseus Books, LLC.

NOTES

1. Recently some clinicians and researchers have appropriately questioned the inevitability of in-session dysfunctional reenactments of the most pervasive pattern displayed with significant others (e.g., Binder, 2004; Connolly et al., 1996).
2. The goal of a new experience presented here and elsewhere in more detail (Levenson, 1995) is a modification of that originally presented by Strupp and Binder (1984).
3. Previously we endorsed the TLDP selection criteria as outlined by Strupp and Binder (1984). Now Levenson considers that TLDP may be helpful to patients even when they may not quite meet these criteria, as long as the therapist is able to discern the redundant themes involved in their interpersonal transactions.
4. Of course, one cannot overlook the fact that this client may see her relatives (i.e., people of the same race) as untrustworthy because of introjected racism from the dominant white culture. Thus, the TLDP therapist is wise to adopt the point of view that cultural parameters and interpersonal working models are inextricably intertwined.
5. Whereas all clinicians and researchers are well aware of the multiple factors that could account for such a positive self-report of treatment outcome (e.g., need to please the interviewer, avoidance of conflict, and justification of investment in the therapy), Mrs. Follette's demeanor during the interview (more eye contact,

more relaxed posture, more use of "I," fewer vague statements, etc.) were consistent with her account of the changes she had experienced in her life.

6. For instructional videotapes, contact Hanna Levenson, Levenson Institute for Training, 2323 Sacramento Street, 2nd Floor, San Francisco, CA 94115 (Liftcenter@aol.com; www.HannaLevenson.com); American Psychological Association, 750 First Street NE, Washington, DC 20002; Psychological and Educational Films, 3334 E Coast Highway #252, Corona del Mar, CA 92625.

7. See Levenson and Strupp (1999) for specific recommendations concerning training in brief dynamic psychotherapy.

8. For further discussions about training, see Levenson and Burg (2000), Levenson and Evans (2000), and Levenson and Davidovitz (2000).

REFERENCES

Alexander, F., & French, T. M. (1946). *Psychoanalytic therapy: Principles and applications*. New York: Ronald Press.

Anchin, J. C., & Kiesler, D. J. (Eds.). (1982). *Handbook of interpersonal psychotherapy*. New York: Pergamon Press.

Bein, E., Anderson, T., Strupp, H. H., Henry, W. P., Schacht, T. E., Binder, J. L., et al. (2000). The effects of training in time-limited dynamic psychotherapy: Changes in therapeutic outcome. *Psychotherapy Research, 10*, 119–132.

Bein, E., Levenson, H., & Overstreet, D. (1994, June). Outcome and follow-up data from the VAST project. In H. Levenson (Chair), *Outcome and follow-up data in brief dynamic therapy: Caveat emptor, caveat vendor*. Symposium conducted at the annual international meeting of the Society for Psychotherapy Research, York, UK.

Benjamin, L. S. (1993). *Interpersonal diagnosis and treatment of personality disorders*. New York: Guilford Press.

Binder, J. L. (1993). Is it time to improve psychotherapy training? *Clinical Psychology Review, 13*, 301–318.

Binder, J. L. (2004). *Key competencies in brief dynamic psychotherapy: Clinical practice beyond the manual*. New York:Guilford Press.

Bowlby, J. (1973). *Attachment and loss: Vol. 2. Separation, anxiety, and anger*. New York: Basic Books.

Butler, S. F., & Binder, J. L. (1987). Cyclical psychodynamics and the triangle of insight: An integration. *Psychiatry, 50*, 218–231.

Butler, S. F., Strupp, H. H., & Binder, J. L. (1993). Time-limited dynamic psychotherapy. In S. Budman, M. Hoyt, & S. Friedman (Eds.), *The first session in brief therapy*. New York: Guilford Press.

Connolly, M. B., Crits-Christoph, P., Demorest, A., Azarian, K., Muena, L., & Chittams, J. (1996). Varieties of transference patterns in psychotherapy, *Journal of Consulting and Clinical Psychology, 64*, 1213–1221.

Derogatis, L. R. (1983). *SCL-90R administration, scoring and procedures manual for the revised version*. Baltimore: Clinical Psychometric Research.

Flasher, L. V. (2000). Cyclical maladaptive patterns: Interpersonal case formulation for psychotherapy with children. *Journal of Contemporary Psychology, 30,* 239–254.

Gill, M. M. (1993). Interaction and interpretation. *Psychoanalytic Dialogues, 3,* 111–122.

Greenberg, J. R., & Mitchell, S. A. (1983). *Object relations in psychoanalytic theory.* Cambridge, MA: Harvard University Press.

Hartmann, K., & Levenson, H. (1995, June). *Case formulation in TLDP.* Presentation at the annual international meeting of the Society for Psychotherapy Research, Vancouver, Canada.

Henry, W. P. (1997). Interpersonal case formulation. In T. D. Eells (Ed.), *Handbook of psychotherapy case formulation* (pp. 223–259). New York: Guilford Press.

Henry, W. P., Schacht, T. E., & Strupp, H. H. (1990). Patient and therapist introject, interpersonal process, and differential psychotherapy outcome. *Journal of Consulting and Clinical Psychology, 58,* 768–774.

Henry, W. P., Schacht, T. E., Strupp, H. H., Butler, S. F., & Binder, J. L. (1993). Effects of training in time-limited dynamic psychotherapy: Mediators of therapists' responses to training. *Journal of Consulting and Clinical Psychology, 61,* 441–447.

Henry, W. P., Strupp, H. H., Butler, S. F., Schacht, T. E., & Binder, J. L. (1993). Effects of training in time-limited dynamic psychotherapy: Changes in therapist behavior. *Journal of Counseling and Clinical Psychology, 61,* 434–440.

Hilliard, R. B., Henry, W. P., & Strupp, H. H. (2000). An interpersonal model of psychotherapy: Linking patient and therapist developmental history, therapeutic process, and types of outcome. *Journal of Consulting and Clinical Psychology, 68,* 125–133.

Horowitz, L. M., Rosenberg, S. E., Baer, B. A., Ureno, G., & Vallasenor, V. S. (1988). Inventory of Interpersonal Problems: Psychometric properties and clinical applications. *Journal of Consulting and Clinical Psychology, 56,* 885–892.

Johnson, M. E., Popp, C., Schacht, T. E., Mellon, J., & Strupp, H. H. (1989). Converging evidence for identification of recurrent relationship themes: Comparison of two methods. *Psychiatry, 52,* 275-288.

Junkert-Tress, B., Schnierda, U., Hartkamp, N., Schmitz, N., & Tress, W. (2001). Effects of short-term dynamic psychotherapy for neurotic, somatoform, and personality disorders: A prospective 1-year follow-up study. *Psychotherapy Research, 11,* 187–200.

Kiesler, D. J. (1988). *Therapeutic metacommuniation: Therapist impact disclosure as feedback in psychotherapy.* Palo Alto, CA: Consulting Psychologists Press.

Kivlighan, D. M., Jr. (1989). Changes in counselor intentions and response modes and in client reactions and session evaluation after training. *Journal of Counseling Psychology, 36,* 471–476.

Kivlighan, D. M., Jr., Angelone, E. O., & Swofford, K. (1991). Live supervision in individual counseling: Effects of trainees, intention use and helpee's evaluation of session impact and working alliance. *Professional Psychology: Research and Practice, 22,* 489–495.

Kivlighan, D. M., Jr., Schuetz, S. A., & Kardash, C. M. (1998). Counselor trainee achievement: Goal orientation and the acquisition of time-limited dynamic psychotherapy skills. *Journal of Counseling Psychology, 45,* 189–195.

LaRoche, M. J. (1999). Culture, transference, and countertransference among Latinos. *Psychotherapy, 36,* 389–397.

La-Rue-Yalom, T. (2001). The long term outcome of training in time-limited dynamic psychotherapy. *Dissertation Abstracts International, 61*(9-B), 4991.

Levenson, H. (1995). *Time-limited dynamic psychotherapy: A guide to clinical practice.* New York:Basic Books.

Levenson, H. (2003). Time-limited dynamic psychotherapy: An integrative approach. *Journal of Psychotherapy Integration, 13,* 300–333.

Levenson, H. (2006). Time-limited dynamic psychotherapy. In A. B. Rochlen (Ed.), *Applying counseling theories: An online, case-based approach* (pp. 75–90). Upper Saddle River, NJ: Pearson.

Levenson, H., & Bein, E. (1993, June). VA Short-term psychotherapy research project: Outcome. In D. A. Shapiro (Chair), *Long-term outcome of brief dynamic psychotherapy.* Symposium conducted at the annual international meeting of the Society for Psychotherapy Research, Pittsburgh, PA.

Levenson, H., & Bolter, K. (1988, August). Short-term psychotherapy values and attitudes: Changes with training. In H. Levenson (Chair), *Issues in training and teaching brief therapy.* Symposium conducted at the convention of the American Psychological Association, Atlanta, GA.

Levenson, H., & Burg, J. (2000). Training psychologists in the era of managed care. In A. J. Kent & M. Hersen (Eds.), *A psychologist's proactive guide to managed health care* (pp. 113–140). Mahwah, NJ: Erlbaum.

Levenson, H., Butler, S. F., & Bein, E. (2002). Brief dynamic individual psychotherapy. In R. E. Hales, S. C. Yudofsky, & J. A. Talbott (Eds.), *The American Psychiatric Press textbook of psychiatry* (4th ed., pp. 1151–1176). Washington, DC: American Psychiatric Press.

Levenson, H., & Davidovitz, D. (2000). Brief therapy prevalence and training: A national survey of psychologists. *Psychotherapy, 37,* 335–340.

Levenson, H., & Evans, S. A. (2000). The current state of brief therapy training in American Psychological Association-accredited graduate and internship programs. *Professional Psychology: Research and Practice, 31,* 446–452.

Levenson, H., & Strupp, H. H. (1999). Recommendations for the future of training in brief dynamic psychotherapy. *Journal of Clinical Psychology, 55,* 385–391.

Li, W. (2004). Confucius on the couch: Time-limited dynamic psychotherapy and the Chinese American population. *Dissertation Abstracts International, 65*(1-B), 445.

Lyons-Ruth, K., & Jacobwitz, D. (1999). Attachment disorganization: Unresolved loss, relational violence, and lapses in behavioral and attentional strategies. In J. Cassidy & P. R. Shaver (Eds.), *Handbook of attachment: Theory, research and clinical applications* (pp. 520–554). New York:Guilford Press.

MacKenzie, K. R. (1988). Recent developments in brief psychotherapy. *Hospital and Community Psychiatry, 39,* 742–752.

Multon, K. D., Kivlighan, D. M., & Gold, P. B. (1996). Changes in counselor adherence over the course of training. *Journal of Counseling Psychology, 43,* 356–363.

Neff, W. L., Lambert, M. J., Lunnen, K. M., Budman, S. H., & Levenson, H. (1997). Therapists' attitudes toward short-term therapy: Changes with training. *Employee Assistance Quarterly, 11,* 67–77.

Nordhus, I. H., & Geir, H. N. (1999). Brief dynamic psychotherapy with older adults. *In Session: Psychotherapy in Practice, 55,* 935–947.

Overstreet, D. L. (1993). *Patient contribution to differential outcome in time-limited dynamic psychotherapy: An empirical analysis.* Unpublished doctoral dissertation, Wright Institute, Berkeley, CA.

Quintana, S. M., & Meara, N. M. (1990). Internalization of the therapeutic relationship in short term psychotherapy. *Journal of Counseling Psychology, 37,* 123–130.

Safran, J. D., & Segal, Z. V. (1990). *Interpersonal process in cognitive therapy.* New York: Basic Books.

Sampson, H., & Weiss, J. (1986). Testing hypotheses: The approach of the Mount Zion Psychotherapy Research Group. In L. S. Greenberg & N. M. Pinsof (Eds.), *The psychotherapeutic process: A research handbook.* New York: Guilford Press.

Sandler, J. (1976). Countertransference and role-responsiveness. *International Review of Psycho-Analysis, 3,* 43–47.

Schacht, T. E. (1991). Can psychotherapy education advance psychotherapy integration?: A view from the cognitive psychology of expertise. *Journal of Psychotherapy Integration, 1,* 305–319.

Schacht, T. E., Binder, J. L., & Strupp, H. H. (1984). The dynamic focus. In H. H. Strupp & J. L. Binder, *Psychotherapy in a new key: A guide to time-limited dynamic psychotherapy.* New York: Basic Books.

Siegel, D. J. (1999). *The developing mind: Toward a neurobiology of interpersonal experience.* New York: Guilford Press.

Strupp, H. H. (1955). Psychotherapeutic technique, professional affiliation, and experience level. *Journal of Consulting Psychology, 19,* 97–102.

Strupp, H. H. (1960). *Psychotherapists in action: Explorations of the therapist's contribution to the treatment process.* New York: Grune & Stratton.

Strupp, H. H. (1980). Success and failure in time-limited psychotherapy: Further evidence (Comparison 4). *Archives of General Psychiatry, 37,* 947–954.

Strupp, H. H. (1993). The Vanderbilt psychotherapy studies: Synopsis. *Journal of Consulting and Clinical Psychology, 61,* 431–433.

Strupp, H. H., & Binder, J. L. (1984). *Psychotherapy in a new key.* New York: Basic Books.

Sue, S., Zane, N., & Young, K. (1994). Research on psychotherapy with culturally diverse populations. In A. E. Bergin & S. L. Garfield (Eds.), *Handbook of psychotherapy and behavior change* (4th ed., pp. 783–820). New York: Wiley.

Sullivan, H. S. (1953). *The interpersonal theory of psychiatry.* New York: Norton.

Travis, L. A., Binder, J. L., Bliwise, N. G., & Horne-Moyer, H. L. (2001). Changes in clients' attachment styles over the course of time-limited dynamic psychotherapy. *Psychotherapy, 38,* 149–159.

von Bertalanffy, L. (1969). *General systems theory: Essays on its foundation and development* (rev. ed.). New York: Braziller.

Wachtel, P. L. (1993). *Therapeutic communication: Knowing what to say when.* New York: Guilford Press.

Weiss, J. (1993). *How psychotherapy works.* New York: Guilford Press.

Welfel, E. R. (2004). The ethical challenges of brief therapy. In D. P. Chapman (Ed.), *Core processes in brief psychodynamic psychotherapy* (pp. 343–359). Mahwah, NJ: Erlbaum.

Wong, E. C., Kim, B. S. K., Zane, N. W. S., Kim, I. J., & Huang, J. S. (2003). Examining culturally based variables associated with ethnicity. *Cultural Diversity and Ethnic Minority Psychology, 9,* 88–96.

Chapter 7

The Plan Formulation Method

JOHN T. CURTIS
GEORGE SILBERSCHATZ

The Plan Formulation Method (PFM) was developed as a way to opera-tionalize the process that clinicians engage in when formulating a clinical case. The evolution of the PFM was spurred by the need to develop reliable comprehensive formulations for clinical research—that is, formulations that identify not only a patient's manifest and latent problems but also the patient's stated and unstated goals for therapy, possible obstacles and resistances to achieving these goals, and how the patient is likely to work in therapy to solve the problems. Prior to the development of the Plan Diag-nosis Method (a precursor to the PFM, see Curtis & Silberschatz, 1997), comprehensive clinical formulations were not used in psychotherapy re-search because of problems obtaining adequate interjudge reliability (DeWitt, Kaltreider, Weiss, & Horowitz, 1983; Seitz, 1966).

The PFM does not constitute a new method for formulating a case. In-deed, the components of a plan formulation and the processes involved in developing it are common to most approaches to psychotherapy case for-mulation. The PFM was originally developed to study the Control–Mastery Theory of psychotherapy (Weiss, 1986, 1993) and has been used primarily in research on this theory. However, the PFM is cross-theoretical and has been employed in studies of other theories of therapy (e.g., Collins & Messer, 1998, 1991; Persons, Curtis, & Silberschatz, 1991). The PFM re-quires that clinicians review and evaluate clinical material to determine what is relevant and necessary for understanding a particular case and de-veloping a treatment plan. The PFM is unique because it allows clinicians who share a common theoretical orientation to develop a *reliable* comprehensive case formulation.

The clinical applications of the PFM are the same as those of any formulation: The PFM identifies a patient's goals, the conflicts and inhibitions that inhibit or prevent the patient from pursuing or attaining these goals, the source(s) of these conflicts and inhibitions, information that might be helpful to the patient in understanding and overcoming his or her conflicts, and behaviors or interventions on the part of the therapist that will be helpful. The PFM may differ from other approaches in one basic assumption, that an accurate formulation of an individual patient can often be developed quite early in the therapy. Indeed, for research purposes (e.g., predicting patient responses to interventions across the course of a therapy), plan formulations have been developed on as little as a single intake interview. In clinical use, the therapist is well served by trying to formulate a patient's plan as early in the therapy as possible. However, when used by a therapist, the plan formulation is not a static creation set in stone early in the therapy. Rather, it is a working hypothesis that is constantly evaluated and fine-tuned based on such factors as the patient's responses to interventions and the emergence of new history.

HISTORICAL BACKGROUND OF THE APPROACH

For over 25 years, the San Francisco Psychotherapy Research Group (formerly known as the Mount Zion Psychotherapy Research Group) has conducted studies of psychoanalyses, psychodynamic psychotherapy, and time-limited psychotherapies (for an overview of this research, see Silberschatz, 2005b). One primary focus of this enterprise has been to study the role of the analyst or therapist in the process of treatment. Specifically, the group has tried to identify what it is that a therapist does that leads to patient improvement, stagnation, or deterioration in the course of treatment. In a variety of studies, the group has tested the broad hypothesis that when a therapist responds in accord with a patient's goals for therapy, the patient will show immediate improvement in the process of the treatment and that this improvement will translate into an overall positive therapy outcome. Of course, this hypothesis is deceptively simple, for how does one identify, operationalize, and respond appropriately to a patient's goals for therapy? In clinical practice, a case formulation is usually implicitly or explicitly developed by the therapist in order to understand the meaning of an individual patient's problems, to evaluate the appropriateness of therapeutic interventions, and to measure response to treatment (see Perry, Cooper, & Michels, 1987). To keep their research as clinically relevant as possible, the San Francisco Group decided to employ individual case formulations in studies of the process and outcome of psychotherapy. However, as noted in the introduction, in order to employ clinical formulations, the research group had to address the problem of getting clinicians to agree among themselves, an issue that had bedeviled researchers for years. Joe Caston, a member of the research group who developed the Plan Diagnosis Method (Caston, 1977, 1986), the precursor to the PFM, did the groundbreaking work in this area.

The Plan Diagnosis Method was employed in studies of psychoanalyses and of time-limited psychodynamic psychotherapies to develop formulations. While the Plan Diagnosis Method proved to be very reliable (Caston, 1986; Curtis, Silberschatz, Sampson, Weiss, & Rosenberg, 1988; Rosenberg, Silberschatz, Curtis, Sampson, & Weiss, 1986), it needed to be modified to ensure the independence of judges and to tighten the procedures for developing the items on which the final formulation is developed (see Curtis et al., 1988, for a more complete description of the Plan Diagnosis Method and Curtis & Silberschatz, 1997, for a discussion of the problems with this method). A new procedure, the Plan Formulation Method (Curtis & Silberschatz, 1991, 1997; Curtis, Silberschatz, Sampson, & Weiss, 1994) was thus developed.

CONCEPTUAL FRAMEWORK

Both the PFM and the earlier Plan Diagnosis Method were developed in order to study a cognitive psychoanalytic theory of therapy (Control–Mastery Theory) developed by Joseph Weiss (Weiss, 1986, 1993; see also Silberschatz, 2005a). The Control–Mastery Theory holds that psychopathology stems largely from pathogenic beliefs that, in turn, develop from traumatic experiences usually occurring in childhood. Pathogenic beliefs suggest that the pursuit of certain goals will endanger oneself and/or someone else and thus are frightening and constricting. Consequently, an individual is highly motivated to change or disconfirm these beliefs in order to pursue his or her goals. Irrational beliefs in one's power to hurt others, excessive fears of retaliation, feelings of unworthiness, and exaggerated expectations of being overwhelmed by feelings such as anger and fear are all examples of beliefs that can act as obstructions to the pursuit or attainment of goals.

In therapy, the patient uses the relationship with the therapist to attempt to disconfirm pathogenic beliefs. The therapist's function is to help the patient understand the nature and ramifications of the pathogenic beliefs by interpretation and by allowing the patient to test these beliefs in the therapeutic relationship. The manner in which an individual will work in psychotherapy to disconfirm pathogenic beliefs, overcome problems, and achieve goals is the patient's "plan." The plan is not a rigid scheme that the patient will invariably follow; rather, it comprises general areas that the patient will want to work on and how the patient is likely to carry out this work (see Weiss, 1986, 1993, for a thorough description of the theory; also see Curtis & Silberschatz, 1986; Silberschatz & Curtis, 1986; and Silberschatz, 2005c, for further discussion of the applications of the theory to clinical phenomena). Formulations developed according to Weiss's theory have five component parts: the patient *goals* for therapy; the *obstructions* (pathogenic beliefs) that inhibit the patient from pursuing or achieving these goals; the events and experiences (*traumas*) that lead to the development of the obstructions; the *insights* that will help the patient achieve therapy goals; and the manner in which the patient will work in therapy to overcome the obstacles and achieve the goals (*tests*).

INCLUSION/EXCLUSION CRITERIA AND MULTICULTURAL CONSIDERATIONS

To formulate an individual patient's pathogenic beliefs and therapy goals, the clinician (or, in a research context, the formulating team) must consider the cultural and ethnic background of the patient (see, e.g., Bracero, 1994). One's beliefs are shaped by the meanings attributed to experience(s), and the meaning of these experiences is shaped in some measure by the family as well as by the cultural environment. For example, at a very basic level, a child who grows up with boisterous, emotionally labile parents may respond differently (and attribute different meaning) to a parent's emotional outburst than will a child whose parents are typically quiet and undemonstrative. Similarly, a child who grows up in a culture that values and promotes filial respect and intergenerational dependency may develop markedly different beliefs (and different life goals) than a child raised in a culture that promotes independence and autonomy. However, by the same token, it is important not to assume that one's cultural or ethnic background solely dictates the nature of that individual's pathogenic beliefs or his or her goals. A plan formulation is *case specific* and, to be accurate, must be developed with an appreciation of cultural and ethnic differences but without preconceptions as to what the patient's beliefs and goals are or should be. Thus it is important to understand what experiences were traumatic for the individual and why—and what beliefs developed out of these experiences.

A plan formulation can be developed for all individuals suffering from psychogenic psychopathology. For research purposes, the PFM has been applied to children (Foreman, 1989; Gibbins, 1989), adolescents, and adults of all ages (Curtis & Silberschatz, 1991), including geriatric cases (see Silberschatz & Curtis, 1991). In addition, the PFM has been employed in psychobiographical research (Conrad, 1995) and to study family therapy (Bigalke, 2004). The majority of cases we have formulated in our research program have received DSM-III-R Axis I diagnoses of dysthymia or generalized anxiety disorder, frequently accompanied by an Axis II Cluster C personality disorder (DSM-III-R; American Psychiatric Association, 1987). The cases have displayed mild to severe symptomatology, with moderate to catastrophic psychosocial stresses.

STEPS IN CASE FORMULATION

As noted previously, a plan formulation developed for clinical use may be characterized as a working hypothesis (or set of hypotheses) that is constantly being evaluated for its accuracy by the clinician. The clinician carefully monitors the patient's responses to interventions to determine whether they are in accord with what is predicted by the formulation. If not, the formulation should be modified accordingly. A formulation may also be altered or elaborated based on new data (e.g., memories and transference patterns) that emerge in the course of therapy.

In contrast, plan formulations developed for research purposes are based solely on transcripts of early therapy hours, with no additional information (e.g., concerning the subsequent treatment or outcome) included. By restricting the data from which the plan formulations are developed, these formulations can then be used, for example, to predict a patient's response to a therapist's intervention in the later hours of the therapy (e.g., Silberschatz, 1986; Silberschatz & Curtis, 1993; Silberschatz, Fretter, & Curtis, 1986). For a brief therapy, we ordinarily use an intake interview and the first 2 therapy hours of the case; for the study of a psychoanalysis, we usually employ the intake and first 10 hours of treatment. However, we have reliably formulated individual psychotherapy cases based on as little as one interview (Curtis et al., 1994; Perry, Luborsky, Silberschatz, & Papp, 1989) and a family therapy case on the first two therapy sessions (Bigalke, 2004).

For our research, we typically use three or four clinical judges. The judges are all experienced with and adhere to Weiss's Control–Mastery Theory of psychotherapy. We have used judges with widely varying degrees of clinical experience and of experience applying the theory to therapy (Curtis & Silberschatz, 1991).

The PFM involves five steps:

1. Clinical judges independently review the transcripts of the early therapy hours, and each develops a formulation for the case. Each judge then creates lists of "real" and "alternative" goals, obstructions, traumas, insights, and tests and for the case. The definitions and instructions given to the judges to complete this step follow (from the manual of the PFM):

Traumas. A trauma is the event(s) and experience(s) that lead to the development of a pathogenic belief. The following are examples of traumas and the resultant pathogenic beliefs:

- During the patient's adolescence, her mother called her a "whore" when she expressed interest in boys. Consequently, she does not enjoy sex because she believes that it is bad.
- His father was critical of his successes in school and acted hurt when his son outperformed him (e.g., beat him at chess). Consequently, the patient does not allow himself to vigorously pursue his career because he believes to do so would hurt his father.
- His mother had few friends and frequently confided in him about her disappointment with his father. Consequently, the patient has not moved away from home because he believes that his mother would feel abandoned if he left.

More than one trauma may contribute to the formation of a pathogenic belief, and more than one belief may develop out of a given trauma. For purposes of this plan formulation, you do not need to develop an exhaustive list of all the traumas that contributed to a given pathogenic belief or account for every pathogenic belief in the list of traumas you develop. Instead, identify those traumas and the resultant pathogenic beliefs that are paradigmatic of the conflicts this patient is attempting to resolve in therapy. You do not need to develop alternative (irrelevant) traumas.

When writing traumas, follow the format of describing the trauma and then noting the resultant pathogenic belief (see examples above).

Obstructions. Obstructions are the irrational pathogenic beliefs—and the associated fears, guilt, and anxieties—which hinder or prevent a person from pursuing his or her goals. Typically, these beliefs are unconscious in the early phases of therapy. These irrational beliefs act as obstructions because they suggest that certain undesirable consequences will occur if the patient pursues or attains a certain goal or goals. For example:

- The patient holds herself back from doing well in school because she feels her sister would be humiliated by her successes.
- The patient acts aloof and distant toward her peers because she believes her mother will feel abandoned if she (the patient) has friends.
- The patient stays away from people, feeling they will want nothing to do with him, because he feels that he is basically an evil, despicable person.

An obstruction is more than just a belief in that it must in some way influence the patient's thoughts, feelings, or behaviors. Thus, some negative consequence(s) must be associated with the belief for it to be an obstruction. For instance, if the first example above were written, "If the patient is successful, he will surpass a sibling," it would not be considered an obstruction as no negative consequence is associated with surpassing a sibling (in fact, this item could just be a statement of fact). Similarly, stating "the patient believes that if she is happily married she will leave her parents behind," would not qualify as a pathogenic belief without noting the consequences of the belief (e.g., "the patient stays away from men because she believes that her parents would be devastated if she married and left home").

Also keep in mind that guilt alone is not a pathogenic belief but, rather, a response to a pathogenic belief. Thus stating that "the patient avoids relationships with men because they would make her feel guilty toward her parents," or "the patient does not do well in school because he would feel guilty doing better than his brother," is not an adequate description of obstructions. In each instance, the cause or reason for the guilt needs to be elucidated. Thus, the first example, might be better written, "The patient does not do well in school because he feels that his success would humiliate his brother." The second item might read, "The patient avoids relationships with men because she believes that her parents would be devastated if she married."

A pathogenic belief may act as an obstruction in more than one area. For instance, a patient's belief that his independence will hurt a parent might lead him to inhibit himself in his interactions with his parents, restrict his social life, and/or abandon his career goals. You do not need to be exhaustive in listing all the ways in which a given belief might act as an obstruction. Rather, try to note the most important or exemplary behavior that the pathogenic belief influences. If you do note more than one way in which a pathogenic belief acts as an obstruction, please make them separate items. For example, "The patient has kept herself from dating and has not pursued her academic career because she believes that her parents need her to stay close to home to protect them," should be recast as two items, one noting how the belief has stopped her from dating and the other describing how it has affected her academic career.

When writing obstructions, follow the format of stating the effect or consequence of the pathogenic belief, followed by the pathogenic belief. That is, "[S]he does (or does not do) (*thought, feeling, behavior*) because [s]he believes that (*pathogenic belief*)."

Goals. The patient's goals for therapy represent potential behaviors, affects, attitudes, or capacities which the patient would like to achieve. These goals may be highly specific and concrete (e.g., to get married) or more general and abstract (e.g., the capacity to tolerate guilt). While at one level a patient's goal(s) for therapy can be conceptualized as overcoming a pathogenic belief(s) (e.g., to overcome her belief that getting married will destroy her mother), for the purposes of creating a plan formulation, please do not do so. Instead, list as a goal the way(s) overcoming the pathogenic belief might be manifested (e.g., to get married)—include the pathogenic belief(s) under Obstructions. Similarly, avoid writing goals that suggest the genetics of a problem (e.g., to overcome his identification with his father and be more assertive)—again, only state how the goal(s) might be manifested (e.g., to be more assertive) and leave the genetics for the Obstructions section (e.g., he believes that his father would be overwhelmed if he were more assertive than his father had been).

The patient's presenting complaints may not accurately reflect his or her goals for therapy. The patient may not be able to acknowledge his or her true desires because, for example, they are unconscious or are experienced as being too bold or ambitious. Therefore, the assessment of a patient's goals requires a dynamic formulation of the case. For instance, a patient may state a desire to get married. However, a careful reading of the early sessions may reveal a strong sense of obligation to marry. Thus, what the patient may initially want—but is unable to articulate—is the freedom to choose not to get married.

When writing goals, follow the format "To _____ " (e.g., "To feel comfortable saying 'no' to others." "To be able to look for a better job." "To feel greater self-confidence.").

Testing. One method by which a patient attempts to disconfirm pathogenic beliefs and irrational expectations is by observing the therapist's behavior in response to tests. Tests are actions by the patient that are designed to appraise the danger or safety of pursuing a particular goal(s). When testing, the patient observes the therapist's behavior to see if it confirms or disconfirms an irrational expectation or false belief. For example, a patient who feels that he will hurt others if he is forceful might test this belief by observing whether the therapist is upset when he (the patient) argues with him or acts decisive and independent. The same patient might also test by observing the therapist's reaction when he (the patient) turns passive into active—for example, by acting hurt or upset when the therapist is bold or insightful.

You will need to use your clinical judgment to infer (on the basis of the intake and first 2 therapy hours) the nature of the tests that the patient is likely to present to the therapist. Pay attention to the testing which occurs in the first 2 therapy hours as this may provide clues to how this patient will work in subsequent hours.

When writing tests, follow the format, "[S]he will do X to work on (or test) pathogenic belief Y" (e.g., "She will act indifferent to the therapist and to therapy to work on her belief that she should not make demands upon others." "He will exaggerate his occupational striving (e.g., appear 'ruthless') to see if the therapist disapproves of his legitimate professional aspirations as he felt his parents did.").

Insights. Insights are knowledge which help the patient achieve his or her goals for therapy. This knowledge pertains to the nature, origins, and manifestations of the patient's pathogenic beliefs and is generally incomplete or unavailable to the patient at the beginning of therapy. A patient might obtain insight(s) into the content of a pathogenic belief (e.g., an irrational feeling of omnipotent responsibility for the welfare of others), into the identifications and compliances spawned by pathogenic beliefs (e.g., by pining for a man, the patient is acting pathetic like, and thereby not threatening, her mother), into the historical roots of a belief (e.g., when the patient acted independent as a child, her mother acted hurt), and even into his or her goals for therapy (as in the example of the patient who wanted to feel free *not* to get married before pursuing his conscious wish to be married).

When writing the (relevant and alternative) insights for this case, follow the format, "To become aware that _____" (e.g., "to become aware that she has inhibited herself from having enjoyable sexual relationships with men because she feels guilty allowing herself greater pleasure than her mother has experienced" and "to become aware that he has inhibited his occupational progress to avoid achieving greater success than his father and to keep himself in a one-down position with his father").

All items in a plan formulation are written in a standard format to facilitate comparison between items and to help disguise which judge created which item.

As noted, the judges are instructed to include in their lists both items they believe are relevant to the case and any items they think reasonable for the case, but of lesser relevance (e.g., items of which they are unsure or items that they at one point thought were highly relevant but ultimately decided were of lesser relevance). These "alternative" items are not simply "straw men" that can be readily discounted. Indeed, these items are sometimes given high ratings by other judges.

2. The judges' lists are combined into master lists of traumas, goals, obstructions, tests, and insights. In the master lists, the authors of the items are not identified, and the items developed by any given judge are randomly distributed within the appropriate list.

3. The master lists of goals, obstructions, trauma, insights, and tests are returned to the clinical judges who independently rate the items on a 5-point Likert scale for their relevance to the case (0 = not relevant; 1 = slightly relevant; 2 = moderately relevant; 3 = highly relevant; 4 = very highly relevant).

4. Because different formulations are developed for each case, there tends to be relatively little overlap of items across cases. Consequently, reliability is measured for each of the five plan components (goals, obstructions, tests, insights, traumas) for each case by calculating an intraclass correlation for pooled judges' ratings (Shrout & Fleiss, 1979). Two figures are calculated, the estimated reliability of the average judge ($r_{(1)}$, referred to by Shrout and Fleiss as ICC 3, 1) and coefficient alpha, the estimated reliability of $\underline{K}$ judges' ratings ($r_{(K)}$, referred to by Shrout & Fleiss as ICC 3, K).

5. After determining reliability, the development of the final formulation involves a two-step process. First, items rated as being of lesser relevance to the case are dropped from the list. This is done by taking the mean of judges' ratings per item, determining the median of the mean item ratings per category (goals, obstructions, etc.), and then dropping all items within each category that fall below the median rating for that category. In our experience, this is a conservative criterion; the final items usually have received mean ratings falling at or above the "highly relevant" range. The second step entails a separate team of judges individually reviewing the final items to identify redundancies. The judges then meet and decide consensually which items are redundant and should be eliminated. The remaining items are included in the final formulation.

The plan formulation is cast in the following format: There is a description of the patient and of the patient's current life circumstances followed by a narrative of the patient's presenting complaints. Then the goals, obstructions, tests, insights, and traumas are listed for the patient. As each plan formulation is case-specific, the number of goals, obstructions, tests, insights, and traumas identified varies from case to case; there is no optimal number of these items. Depending on the nature of the formulation and how it is to be used, a paragraph summarizing the main features of the individual items may be included under each of the rubrics. (A complete manual of the PFM is available from the authors. Also see Curtis & Silberschatz, 2005, on the application of the theory to the development of case formulations).

APPLICATION TO PSYCHOTHERAPY TECHNIQUE

A basic assumption behind the development of a plan formulation is that a clinician cannot and should not proceed to treat a patient without an understanding of that individual's true goals for therapy and the conflicts that have inhibited the patient from obtaining those goals. As with all formulations, the plan formulation contains the clinician's understanding of the causes and manifestations of the patient's symptoms and conflicts. According to the Control–Mastery Theory, the causes can be discerned from the traumas that the individual has experienced (Curtis & Silberschatz, 2005; Silberschatz, 2005a; Weiss, 1986, 1993). The identification of traumas can alert the therapist to potential issues in the therapy, in particular to what Weiss describes as pathogenic beliefs. These are beliefs that suggest that the pursuit or attainment of goals will lead to danger to oneself and/or others. For instance, individuals who have experienced neglect and abandonment are likely to work on issues of basic trust and worthiness, as manifested in beliefs about their worth and/or the trustworthiness of others (Silberschatz & Curtis, 1991; Weiss, 1993). Similarly, a patient who comes from a family in which members experienced significant losses or disabilities might have survival guilt stemming from pathogenic beliefs that personal success in life would hurt others (Bush, 2005). Thus, an awareness of the traumas experienced by a patient can alert the therapist to the obstructions, or pathogenic beliefs, on which the individual will want to work in therapy. A picture of the patient's pathogenic beliefs can often clarify the patient's true goals for therapy as well as the meaning and origins of symptoms. Without a formulation, the therapist cannot determine whether the patient's stated goals represent true treatment goals or compromises (i.e., less ambitious goals) or even false goals (e.g., when patients feel guilty about their true goals and thus present with goals that may even be the opposite of their real aspirations—see Curtis & Silberschatz, 1986, 2005).

Identifying the traumas endured by a patient and the consequent pathogenic beliefs that developed can be essential to understanding the meaning of a patient's behaviors. Such an understanding enables the therapist to respond to these behaviors appropriately. A good illustration of this is when a patient is testing by turning passive into active—that is, when a patient who has been traumatized by the behaviors of others enacts similar behaviors with the therapist. For example, a patient who was repeatedly browbeaten by a parent may be critical and argumentative with the therapist as part of an effort to master this childhood trauma (see Weiss, 1993, and Silberschatz, 2005a, for a thorough explanation of testing). At such times, the patient may appear to be resisting or even sabotaging the treatment. However, a thorough understanding of the patient's pathogenic beliefs and of the manner in which these beliefs might be tested in the therapy can assist the therapist in seeing these behaviors for what they really are, the patient's active attempts to work on and master a problem by literally bringing it into the therapy. On a broader level, the case formulation can help the therapist to determine what degree of activity on the part of the therapist will be appropriate and helpful to the patient. For example, a patient who was traumatized by intrusive parents may be similarly traumatized—or, minimally, have important tests failed—by an active therapist. On the other hand, a passive, "neutral" therapist might traumatize a patient who has experienced neglect or abandonment. Finally, a formulation is necessary to evaluate the progress of the therapy. Without clear-cut goals and a sense of what must transpire for the patient to achieve them, the therapist cannot assess progress, and the therapy is likely to falter. When the therapy is not going according to the formulation, it suggests either that the therapist is not using the formulation appropriately or that the formulation is wrong and needs to be revised. Patients do not change their basic plans. They may change how they go about trying to achieve their plans—for example, they may try new testing strategies if the therapist consistently fails certain types of tests or work on different goals if the therapy does not help them progress in certain arenas (see Bugas & Silberschatz, 2005; Curtis & Silberschatz, 1986). However, these may be seen as shifts in focus, not a change in the patient's overall plan.

Should the therapist share the formulation with a patient? In a sense, the course of therapy may be seen as the unfolding and explication of a patient's plan. However, how and when this is done can be tricky. It may take time for the therapist to feel confident with a formulation, for the therapist is also, in a sense, testing the formulation in the course of the therapy. Certainly, sharing an inaccurate formulation with a patient would be problematic. Sharing an accurate formulation can also be troublesome if, for example, doing so discourages the patient's testing and/or identifies unconscious conflicts of which the patient is not yet aware or ready to consider. Thus, questions about when and how to share the formulation with a patient are best answered by considering what the formulation suggests about how the patient is likely to hear and respond to both the words and the therapist's actions (for a detailed clinical illustration, see Bloomberg-Fretter, 2005).

CASE EXAMPLE

The following case is drawn from our ongoing research on the process and outcome of time-limited psychodynamic psychotherapy (Silberschatz, Curtis, Sampson, & Weiss, 1991). The patient, "Jill," was referred to the research project by her daughter (herself, a therapist). Jill felt chronically anxious and despondent about her life circumstances, yet she felt powerless to effect any changes. Jill had no social life, outside her family, and felt lonely and frustrated.

The plan formulation for Jill presented here is not that of the therapist; rather, it was developed several years after the termination of therapy by a team of four clinicians based on written transcripts of an intake interview and the first 2 (of a total 16) therapy hours. The formulating clinicians knew nothing about the case other than what was contained in the transcripts; that is, they knew nothing about what happened in the later hours of the case or about the outcome. They were also blind as to the identity of the therapist.

Presenting Complaints

Jill is a 59-year-old widowed Caucasian female who is currently living with her widowed mother. Her children are grown and live away from home though she provides some financial assistance to her two younger children who are finishing their educations. She is employed as an executive secretary with a large corporation and also works part time selling home furnishings out of her apartment.

Jill's primary complaint on entering therapy was her inability to tolerate living with her mother who she described as excessively needy, dependent, and intrusive. She felt paralyzed about resolving the situation. She also expressed concerns about her perilous financial situation; when her husband died he left a financial "empire" that quickly collapsed, forcing her to declare bankruptcy (which included losing her home and many of her possessions) and leaving her with enduring tax problems. She expressed concerns about being overweight and about her lack of involvement with men. She felt anxious, depressed, and overwhelmed by her circumstances.

Plan Formulation

Traumas

Jill's parents were unhappily married. Jill's father was a powerful, outgoing man, while her mother was passive and lonely. Jill's mother often acted passive, helpless, and dependent and turned to Jill for nurturing and support. Jill was in fact closer to her father, and this provoked jealousy and anger in her mother. Neither parent responded to Jill's needs and wishes; instead, they followed their own agendas. Both parents were controlling and manipulative and constantly undercut Jill's accomplishments by taking credit for them or by manipulating them to their own ends. Jill was never encouraged to excel, to be independent, or to pursue her own goals.

Following are the individual traumas developed for Jill by the formulating team:

> Her mother was unhappily married, isolated, and passive. Consequently, Jill has trouble enjoying life and being assertive, because she believes her mother feels pained and humiliated by her success.
>
> Her mother was unhappily married and turned to Jill for support and comfort. Consequently, Jill felt responsible for taking care of her mother.
>
> Her mother often acted passive, helpless, and dependent. Consequently, Jill inferred that it was her job to take care of her mother's wants and needs.
>
> When Jill was a child, her mother often failed to honor Jill's feelings and needs, instead focusing on what she needed from Jill. Consequently, Jill inferred that her feelings and needs were relatively unimportant and did not deserve to be met.
>
> When she was growing up, her mother was jealous of her closeness to her father. Consequently, she became guilty over having something for herself that excluded her mother.
>
> Jill's parents constantly undercut her accomplishments by "arranging" or "fixing" things for her. Consequently, she believed she should not achieve or be competent herself.
>
> When Jill quit college, her parents let her quit and did not encourage her to go back. Consequently, she concluded she should not be independent and have a life of her own.

Goals

Jill's broad goals for therapy are to gain a sense of control over her life and the freedom to pursue her emotional and physical needs. She wants to be comfortable recognizing her abilities and her competence. At the same time, she wants to feel more comfortable being critical of others. She wants to feel less responsible for others and more entitled to pursue her own wishes and needs, even when they appear at odds with those of others.

Following are the individual goals developed for Jill by the formulating team:

> To honor her feelings and needs
> To be more assertive in taking care of her needs
> To let off steam without feeling guilty
> To be more confident in her ability to do things herself
> To feel comfortable with her competence
> To pursue enjoyable activities and interests
> To enjoy living by herself and doing things by herself

To think clearly about money and handle her finances

To feel less burdened by and responsible for others

To overcome feeling responsible for her mother's happiness

To feel less compelled to help her mother

To overcome her guilt about leaving mother behind as she enjoys her own life

To overcome her guilt about not meeting her mother's wants and needs

To get her mother to move out of her home

To be less tolerant of mistreatment by others

To avoid being manipulated by the "guilt trips" that she feels her mother lays on her

To feel less guilty about her disgust and dislike of her mother

To not feel guilty for being critical of her mother

To accept her anger at her husband

To mourn her deceased husband

Obstructions

Simply put, Jill believes that others will be hurt by her abilities and accomplishments. These beliefs appear to have developed out of her relationship with her parents. While she felt close to her father, she also felt that he expected little of her and did not truly support her independence or autonomy. Her mother was jealous of Jill's relationship with her father and acted abandoned and neglected by Jill. As a result of these experiences, Jill has inhibited herself and/or felt excessively responsible for the feelings and needs of others.

Following are the individual obstructions developed for Jill by the formulating team:

She avoids enjoying life more because she believes that others will be jealous or feel left out.

She does not have a life of her own because she thinks if she does it will hurt both her mother and father.

She is not comfortable being competent because she feels her competence humiliates her mother because of her mother's sense of inadequacy.

She acts overwhelmed and helpless in the face of her financial problems because she believes it would be disloyal to her mother to exhibit greater resourcefulness and resilience than her mother.

She does not take control of her finances because she believes, in identification with her helpless mother, that she cannot be more competent than her husband or father.

She cannot feel less burdened because she believes that if she feels better, her mother would feel worse in comparison.

She feels she must continue to take care of her mother, as her husband did, because it would be disloyal to her husband to do otherwise.

She feels guilty about not meeting her mother's wants and needs because she believes that she is being mean and/or neglecting her responsibility.

She assumes responsibility for her mother's well-being because she believes that her mother would otherwise feel abandoned and neglected.

She cannot enjoy living by herself because she believes that doing so would be disloyal to her mother, who cannot tolerate being by herself.

She takes care of her mother's wants and needs and sacrifices her own because she believes that her mother's needs would otherwise not be met.

She thinks her love for her father has hurt her mother.

Tests

In therapy, Jill will work to disconfirm her pathogenic beliefs. For example, she may test her belief that others need to see her as passive and helpless by acting bold and assertive with the therapist to see if he disapproves of and/or is threatened by this behavior. Toward the same end, she may act passive or dependent to see if the therapist needs to feel superior to her. This same behavior my also reflect a passive-into-active test. That is, Jill may act dependent or incompetent to see if the therapist feels unduly responsible for or burdened by her needs.

Following are the individual tests developed for Jill by the formulating team:

Transference tests

She will act helpless, and then see if the therapist takes over, to work on her belief that her parents needed her to be helpless.

She will act passive in taking care of her own needs to work on her belief that she should not be bold.

She will boast about her competence to see if the therapist feels threatened, as she feels her mother does.

She will act bold in relation to the therapist to see if this bothers him.

She will act dependent on the therapist for support and advice to see if the therapist enjoys being in a superior role.

She will hesitantly reveal her work successes to test her belief that being successful is disloyal to her parents.

She will demonstrate independent insight in therapy, and then undo it, to work on her belief that she should not be independent.

She will attempt to take care of her therapist's needs in order to work on her belief that others' needs are more important than her own.

She will not understand clear, accurate statements by the therapist in order to work on her belief that she should not see things clearly.

She will disagree with the therapist to test her belief that not believing what she is told would have hurt her father.

She will express anger toward the therapy (therapist) to test her belief that others are damaged by her anger.

Passive-into-active tests

She will act dependent on the therapist to see if the therapist feels responsible for her.

She will act incompetent and helpless to see if the therapist becomes overburdened, as she does with her mother.

She will complain that the therapist has neglected her needs to see if the therapist feels guilty and attempts to make it up to her.

She will accentuate the negative in her life to see if the therapist feels sorry for her and tries to rescue her.

Insights

Jill will be assisted in achieving her goals for therapy by developing insight into the genetics of her pathogenic beliefs and how these beliefs have influenced her thoughts, feelings, and actions. She will be helped by understanding how her relationships with her parents lead her to feel uncomfortable with her own competitive and independent strivings. She may discover how these experiences lead her to feel that she should protect men (e.g., her father and husband) by not challenging or disagreeing with them but, instead, behave in a dependent and passive manner toward them. Similarly, she may be helped by recognizing how her attitudes toward men reflect, in part, identifying with her passive, incompetent mother. She may see how this identification has served to protect her mother, for whom Jill feels excessive responsibility to protect and nurture. In general, Jill will be helped by understanding how she has sacrificed her appropriate desires and ambitions because of feeling omnipotent responsibility for the needs and happiness of others.

Following are the individual insights developed for Jill by the formulating team:

To become aware that she has felt guilty about her family's ill-gotten gains.

To become aware that she prevented herself from knowing about her husband's questionable business practices to protect her father (whose business practices were also questionable).

To become aware that her obliviousness to her husband's business dealings protects her mother, who was unaware of her husband's (the patient's father) business difficulties.

To become aware that she has felt guilty over having her own life, independent of mother, because she feels she is abandoning or neglecting her mother.

To become aware that she feels guilty toward her mother because of an irrational sense of omnipotence and responsibility.

To become aware that dealing with her mother more reasonably is difficult because it would mean surpassing her mother.

To become aware that her fear of being alone is an unconscious identification with her mother out of guilt over being more independent.

To become aware that she inferred that she was responsible for her mother's well-being because her mother acted passive and dependent when Jill was a child.

To become aware that she felt guilty over being closer to her father than to her mother and that she now feels that she must make up for hurting and betraying her mother in this way.

To become aware that her mother viewed life in a discouraging way and was discouraging of her ambitions, and she became discouraged out of compliance.

To become aware that her inability to control her finances stems from an identification with her mother's incompetence, due to guilt over having a better life than mother.

To become aware that her excessive feeling of responsibility for her mother represents identifying with the behavior of her husband and father.

To become aware that she feels an obligation to take care of her mother because her husband provided so well for her (Jill).

To become aware that she is often ruled by feelings of obligation and duty that are irrational and contrary to her own rights and needs.

To become aware of her unconscious guilt over having more and doing better than others because she believes they will be hurt.

To become aware that she feels guilty about being emotionally assertive with her husband, and that guilt makes it difficult for her to assert her needs.

To become aware that she unconsciously fears that she will have to pay a price for doing well and therefore holds herself back.

To become aware that her parents' difficulties allowing her to leave home and go to college caused her to feel indecisive and to lack confidence.

Several points should be emphasized concerning how the therapist should use a plan formulation. In the first place, while a plan formulation usually identifies a number of goals that a patient might want to work on in therapy; it is the patient, and not the therapist, who actually determines the focus of the treatment. As discussed in greater detail elsewhere (Curtis & Silberschatz, 1986, 1997; Silberschatz, 2005a; Weiss, 1993), a basic premise of the plan formulation and its application is that the formulation identifies the patient's plan in order to assist the therapist in helping the patient to enact that plan. In other words, it helps the therapist follow the patient, not lead the treatment.

The plan formulation also helps the therapist to understand the patient's symptoms and complaints. For example, Jill's unhappiness could be seen as a normal, expectable reaction to real-life events and their consequences (e.g., her husband's death, her financial concerns, and the burden of caring for an aging parent). However, the plan formulation makes it clear that her despair and depression are largely reactions to her identifying with her passive mother and her compliance with her overbearing father and husband. Consequently, the therapy should focus on her inhibitions about taking charge of her life and not, for example, on her grief or issues of loss.

The plan formulation also provides guidance for understanding and responding to the process of the therapy and, in particular, to the patient's tests. For instance, according to the plan formulation, Jill's protestations of being incompetent and overwhelmed can be seen as tests and as ways of trying to disconfirm her pathogenic beliefs rather than as signs of resistance. Similarly, the plan formulation can assist the therapist in assessing the true meaning of any reports by Jill of her being critical or rejecting of her mother (e.g., is she exaggerating the intensity or inappropriateness of any altercations she has with her mother due to her omnipotent feelings of responsibility for this woman and her guilt about wanting to be emancipated from this toxic relationship). (See Curtis & Silberschatz, 1986, 1997; Silberschatz, 2005a; Silberschatz & Curtis, 1986, 1991; Weiss, 1986, 1993, for more through discussions of how the plan formulation is used in psychotherapy.)

TRAINING

As noted earlier, while the PFM was developed to study the Control–Mastery Theory of psychotherapy, it has been applied by other researchers who adhere to a different theoretical stance (Collins & Messer, 1991) and to therapies conducted under widely varying theoretical orientations, both psychodynamic and nonpsychodynamic (Curtis & Silberschatz, 1991; Curtis et al., 1994; Persons et al., 1991). Thus, for purposes of training in the PFM, the first consideration is that the clinicians share and be well versed in a common theoretical position. It should be noted that this is often easier said than done. One of the interesting findings from adapting the PFM for use by other researchers is that theories and their applications are often poorly operationalized, and clinicians who think they share a common perspective may find, after applying the PFM, that they differ widely in how they understand or apply that perspective (Collins & Messer, 1991; see also Seitz, 1966). We see this as a strong point of the PFM; it does not allow for sloppy thinking. Once a group of clinicians share a common, well-operationalized theoretical perspective, the PFM can be applied with good reliability (Collins & Messer, 1988; Curtis & Silberschatz, 1991). Even relatively inexperienced clinicians have been able to develop plan formulations with reliabilities approaching those of more seasoned veterans of the procedure (Curtis & Silberschatz, 1991).

RESEARCH SUPPORT FOR THE APPROACH

We have obtained excellent reliabilities applying the PFM to long- and short-term therapies from different settings (research programs, private practice, and hospital and university clinics), treated under differing theoretical models (including psychodynamic psychotherapy, psychoanalysis, interpersonal psychotherapy, and cognitive-behavioral therapy) (Curtis & Silberschatz, 1991; Curtis et al., 1994; see also Persons et al., 1991; Silberschatz, Curtis, Persons, & Safran, 1989). Across six cases reported elsewhere (Curtis & Silberschatz, 1991), coefficient alpha averaged as follows: goals, .90; obstructions, .84; tests, .85; insights, .90.

Other investigators have used the PFM with good reliability. Collins and Messer (1988, 1991) employed the PFM and obtained good interjudge reliabilities among their judges who were generally less clinically experienced than the typical judges used by our research group. We have found no significant differences between ratings of judges who have had previous experience with the PFM and those who have not, nor have we found level of clinical experience to be a barrier to learning this method (Curtis & Silberschatz, 1991).

The validity of the PFM has been tested in studies in which formulations have been used to measure the impact of therapist interventions (Fretter, 1984; Norville, 1989; Silberschatz, 1978, 1986; Silberschatz & Curtis, 1993; Silberschatz et al., 1986; see also Silberschatz, 2005b, for an overview of this research) and patient progress in psychotherapy (Nathans, 1988; Silberschatz, Curtis, & Nathans, 1989). For instance, in several studies we have demonstrated that the "accuracy" of therapist interventions (defined as the degree of adherence of the interpretation to the individual patient's plan formulation) predicts subsequent patient progress in therapy

(Broitman, 1985; Fretter, 1984; Silberschatz, 1986; Silberschatz & Curtis, 1993; Silberschatz, Curtis, Fretter, & Kelly, 1988; Silberschatz, Curtis, & Nathans, 1989; Silberschatz et al., 1986; see also Bush & Gassner, 1986). In preliminary studies, we have also shown that a case-specific outcome measure, Plan Attainment, that rates the degree to which a patient has achieved the goals and insights and overcome the obstacles identified in his or her plan formulation correlates highly with other standardized outcome measures and is a good predictor of patient functioning at posttherapy follow-up (Nathans, 1988; Silberschatz, Curtis, & Nathans, 1989). These studies support the hypothesis that the plan formulation identifies important factors that influence the nature and maintenance of a patient's psychopathology. The clinical relevance of these findings is reflected in the fact that when therapists respond in accord with a patient's plan it leads to improvement in both the process and the outcome.

REFERENCES

American Psychiatric Association. (1987). *Diagnostic and statistical manual of mental disorders* (3rd ed., rev.). Washington, DC: Author.

Bigalke, T. (2004). *The theoretical implications of applying the Control-Mastery concept of testing to family therapy.* Unpublished doctoral dissertation, California School of Professional Psychology, San Francisco Bay Campus, Alliant International University.

Bloomberg-Fretter, P. (2005). Clinical use of the plan formulation in long-term psychotherapy. In G. Silberschatz (Ed.), *Transformative relationships* (pp. 93–109). New York: Routledge.

Bracero, W. (1994). Developing culturally sensitive psychodynamic case formulations: The effects of Asian cultural elements of psychoanalytic Control–Mastery Theory. *Psychotherapy, 31*, 525–532.

Broitman, J. (1985). *Insight, the mind's eye. An exploration of three patients' processes of becoming insightful.* Unpublished doctoral dissertation, Wright Institute Graduate School of Psychology, Berkeley, CA.

Bugas, J., & Silberschatz, G. (2005). How patients coach their therapists in psychotherapy. In G. Silberschatz (Ed.), *Transformative relationships* (pp. 153–167). New York: Routledge.

Bush, M. (2005). The role of unconscious guilt in psychopathology and in psychotherapy. In G. Silberschatz (Ed.), *Transformative relationships* (pp. 43–66). New York: Routledge.

Bush, M., & Gassner, S. (1986). The immediate effect of the analyst's termination interventions on the patient's resistance to termination. In J. Weiss, H. Sampson, & Mount Zion Psychotherapy Research Group (Eds.), *The psychoanalytic process: Theory, clinical observation, and empirical research* (pp. 299–320). New York: Guilford Press.

Caston, J. (1977). Manual on how to diagnose the plan. In J. Weiss, H. Sampson, J. Caston, & G. Silberschatz, *Research on the psychoanalytic process I: A compari-*

son of two theories about analytic neutrality (Bulletin #3, pp. 15–21). San Francisco: Psychotherapy Research Group, Department of Psychiatry, Mount Zion Hospital and Medical Center.

Caston, J. (1986). The reliability of the diagnosis of the patient's unconscious plan. In J. Weiss, H. Sampson, & Mount Zion Psychotherapy Research Group (Eds.), *The psychoanalytic process: Theory, clinical observation, and empirical research* (pp. 241–255). New York: Guilford Press.

Collins, W., & Messer, S. (1988, June). *Transporting the Plan Diagnosis Method to a different setting: Reliability, stability, and adaptability.* Paper presented at the annual conference of the Society for Psychotherapy Research, Santa Fe, NM.

Collins, W. D., & Messer, S. B. (1991). Extending the Plan Formulation Method to an Object Relations perspective: Reliability, stability, and adaptability. *Psychological Assessment, 3,* 75–81.

Conrad, B. B. (1995). *Personality and psychopathology reconsidered: A quantitative/ qualitative Control–Mastery psychobiography on Henri de Toulouse-Lautrec (1864–1901).* Unpublished doctoral dissertation, Wright Institute Graduate School of Psychology, Berkeley, CA.

Curtis, J. T., & Silberschatz, G. (1986). Clinical implications of research on brief dynamic psychotherapy. I. Formulating the patient's problems and goals. *Psychoanalytic Psychology, 3,* 13–25.

Curtis, J. T., & Silberschatz, G. (1991). *The Plan Formulation Method: A reliable procedure for case formulation.* Unpublished manuscript.

Curtis, J. T., & Silberschatz, G. (1997). The Plan Formulation Method. In T. D. Eells (Ed.), *Handbook of psychotherapy case formulation* (pp. 116–136). New York: Guilford Press.

Curtis, J. T., & Silberschatz, G. (2005). The assessment of pathogenic beliefs. In G. Silberschatz (Ed.), *Transformative relationships* (pp. 69–91). New York: Routledge.

Curtis, J. T., Silberschatz, G., Sampson, H., & Weiss, J. (1994). The Plan Formulation Method. *Psychotherapy Research, 4,* 197–207.

Curtis, J. T., Silberschatz, G., Sampson, H., Weiss, J., & Rosenberg, S. E. (1988). Developing reliable psychodynamic case formulations: An illustration of the Plan Diagnosis Method. *Psychotherapy, 25,* 256–265.

DeWitt, K. N., Kaltreider, N. B., Weiss, D. S., & Horowitz, M. J. (1983). Judging change in psychotherapy. *Archives of General Psychiatry, 40,* 1121–1128.

Foreman, S. (1989, June). *Overview of the method to study psychotherapy with children, based on the Mount Zion Method.* A paper presented at the annual conference of the Society for Psychotherapy Research, Toronto, Ontario, Canada.

Fretter, P. B. (1984). The immediate effects of transference interpretations on patients' progress in brief, psychodynamic psychotherapy (Doctoral dissertation, University of San Francisco, 1984). *Dissertation Abstracts International, 46*(6). (UMI No. 85-12,112)

Gibbins, J. (1989, June). *The plan diagnosis of a child case.* Paper presented at the annual conference of the Society for Psychotherapy Research, Toronto, Ontario, Canada.

Nathans, S. (1988). *Plan Attainment: An individualized measure for assessing outcome in psychodynamic psychotherapy.* Unpublished doctoral dissertation, California School of Professional Psychology, Berkeley.

Norville, R. L. (1989). *The relationship between accurate interpretations and brief psychotherapy outcome.* Unpublished doctoral dissertation, Pacific Graduate School of Psychology, Menlo Park, CA.

Perry, S., Cooper, A. H., & Nichols, R. (1987). The psychodynamic formulation: Its purpose, structure, and clinical application. *The American Journal of Psychiatry, 144,* 543–550.

Perry, J. C., Luborsky, L., Silberschatz, G., & Popp, C. (1989). An examination of three methods of psychodynamic formulation based on the same videotaped interview. *Psychiatry, 52,* 302–323.

Persons, J. B., Curtis, J. T., & Silberschatz, G. (1991). Psychodynamic and cognitive-behavioral formulations of a single case. *Psychotherapy, 28,* 608–617.

Rosenberg, S. E., Silberschatz, G., Curtis, J. T., Sampson, H., & Weiss, J. (1986). A method for establishing the reliability of statements from psychodynamic case formulations. *American Journal of Psychiatry, 143,* 1454–1456.

Seitz, P. F. D. (1966). The consensus problem in psychoanalytic research. In L. Gottschalk & A. H. Auerbach (Eds.), *Methods of research in psychotherapy* (pp. 209–225). New York: Appleton-Century-Crofts.

Shrout, P. E., & Fleiss, J. L. (1979). Intraclass correlations: Uses in assessing rater reliability. *Psychological Bulletin, 86,* 420–428.

Silberschatz, G. (1978). Effects of the analyst's neutrality on the patient's feelings and behavior in the psychoanalytic situation. *Dissertation Abstracts International, 39,* 3007-B. (UMI No. 78-24, 277)

Silberschatz, G. (1986). Testing pathogenic beliefs. In J. Weiss, H. Sampson, & Mount Zion Psychotherapy Research Group (Eds.), *The psychoanalytic process: Theory, clinical observation, and empirical research* (pp. 256–266). New York: Guilford Press.

Silberschatz, G. (2005a). The Control–Mastery Theory. In G. Silberschatz (Ed.), *Transformative relationships* (pp. 3–23). New York: Routledge.

Silberschatz, G. (2005b). An overview of research on Control–Mastery Theory. In G. Silberschatz (Ed.), *Transformative relationships* (pp. 189–218). New York: Routledge.

Silberschatz, G. (Ed.). (2005c). *Transformative relationships.* New York: Routledge.

Silberschatz, G., & Curtis, J. T. (1986). Clinical implications of research on brief dynamic psychotherapy. II. How the therapist helps or hinders therapeutic progress. *Psychoanalytic Psychology, 3,* 27–37.

Silberschatz, G., & Curtis, J. T. (1991). Time-limited psychodynamic therapy with older adults. In W. A. Myers (Ed.), *New techniques in the psychotherapy of older patients* (pp. 95–108). Washington, DC: American Psychiatric Press.

Silberschatz, G., & Curtis, J. T. (1993). Measuring the therapist's impact on the patient's therapeutic progress. *Journal of Consulting and Clinical Psychology, 61,* 403–411.

Silberschatz, G., Curtis, J. T., Fretter, P. B., & Kelly, T. J. (1988). Testing hypotheses of psychotherapeutic change processes. In H. Dahl, G. Kächele, & H. Thomä (Eds.), *Psychoanalytic process research strategies* (pp. 128–145). New York: Springer.

Silberschatz, G., Curtis, J. T., & Nathans, S. (1989). Using the patient's plan to assess progress in psychotherapy. *Psychotherapy, 26,* 40–46.

Silberschatz, G., Curtis, J. T., Persons, J. P., & Safran, J. (1989, June). *A comparison of psychodynamic and cognitive therapy case formulations.* Panel presented at the annual conference of the Society for Psychotherapy Research, Toronto, Ontario, Canada.

Silberschatz, G., Curtis, J. T., Sampson, H., & Weiss, J. (1991). Research on the process of change in psychotherapy: The approach of the Mount Zion Psychotherapy Research Group. In L. Beutler & M. Crago (Eds.), *Psychotherapy research: An international review of programmatic studies* (pp. 56–64). Washington, DC: American Psychological Association.

Silberschatz, G., Fretter, P. B., & Curtis, J. T. (1986). How do interpretations influence the process of psychotherapy? *Journal of Consulting and Clinical Psychology, 54,* 646–652.

Weiss, J. (1986). Part I. Theory and clinical observations. In J. Weiss, H. Sampson, & Mount Zion Psychotherapy Research Group (Eds.), *The psychoanalytic process. Theory, clinical observations, and empirical research* (pp. 3–138). New York: Guilford Press.

Weiss, J. (1993). *How psychotherapy works.* New York: Guilford Press.

Chapter 8

Case Formulation in Interpersonal Psychotherapy of Depression

JOHN C. MARKOWITZ
HOLLY A. SWARTZ

Interpersonal psychotherapy (IPT) is a simple, practical, and proven time-limited approach originally developed to treat outpatients with major depression. Its success in a series of randomized clinical trials (Weissman, Markowitz, & Klerman, 2000) has led to its expansion to treat a variety of depressive subtypes and other psychiatric syndromes. In this chapter, we focus on IPT as a treatment for major depressive disorder. Until recently IPT was practiced almost exclusively by researchers, but its research achievements have been incorporated into treatment guidelines, encouraging interest among clinicians and its spread into clinical practice. The late Gerald L. Klerman, who with Myrna M. Weissman, PhD, developed IPT, believed that process research should await proof of the efficacy of an intervention. Hence IPT research has focused on outcome more than process. Although researchers have maintained careful monitoring of IPT therapist adherence to technique (Hill, O'Grady, & Elkin, 1992; Markowitz, Spielman, Scarvalone, & Perry, 2000), most IPT studies have examined whether it efficaciously treats target diagnoses, rather than the process within sessions. Case formulation, an important aspect of the treatment process, is central to the IPT approach but has received little specific study to date.

In this chapter, we describe the elements of IPT case formulation and its function in clinical context. Case formulation in IPT is primarily a treatment tool rather than a theoretical construct (see Table 8.1). It serves both

TABLE 8.1. Features of the IPT Case Formulation

A. Simple.
B. Employs a "medical model" of psychiatric illness.
C. Based on linkage of:
    1. medical diagnosis of psychiatric illness (depression) with
    2. patient's interpersonal circumstances
D. Focuses on one of four interpersonal problem areas:
    1. Grief (complicated bereavement)
    2. Role dispute
    3. Role transition
    4. Interpersonal deficits
C. Explicitly delivered to patient.
D. Determines the focus of time-limited treatment.
E. Therapist and patient must agree on formulation for treatment to proceed.
F. Generally well accepted by patient as affectively meaningful.

to help the therapist understand the patient and to focus and advance this usually acute (12–16 session) weekly treatment.

The crux of IPT is the empirically demonstrated link between mood and interpersonal life events (Klerman, Weissman, Rounsaville, & Chevron, 1984). IPT therapists help patients to identify specific life events and interpersonal issues that appear temporally and thematically related to the onset and maintenance of their depressions, using this information to help them understand the connection between their mood and their current life situation. Patients learn that by altering their interpersonal environment, they can improve their mood and alleviate their mood disorder. The IPT case formulation is the initial means of organizing this crucial information, the focus of all further therapy sessions, and conveying it to the patient.

An IPT case formulation must be coherent, convincing to both therapist and patient, grounded in the patient's interpersonal experiences, and linked to the onset or persistence of the mood disorder. Within this framework, the case formulation encapsulates both the guiding principles of IPT and the individual patient's particular issues (i.e., those that distinguish this patient from others with similar interpersonal issues or diagnosis). That the case formulation leads logically into the treatment plan is a *sine qua non* of IPT. Indeed, case formulation drives the treatment and becomes the focus of IPT. The ability to rapidly develop and deliver such a formulation is for many therapists among the more difficult but most valuable aspects of learning a time-limited, focused psychotherapy like IPT.

HISTORICAL BACKGROUND

IPT was developed in the 1970s by the late Gerald L. Klerman, Myrna M. Weissman, and colleagues as a simple, reproducible, and testable psychotherapy for outpatients with major depression (Klerman et al., 1984). They based the therapy both on the ideas of the interpersonal school of psychoanalysis (Sullivan, 1953) and on research demonstrating the effect on mood of life events and stressors (Klerman et al., 1984). Meyer, Sullivan, Fromm-Reichmann, and other interpersonal psychotherapists of the late 1940s and 1950s had stressed the importance of environmental events as a counterbalance to the strictly intrapsychic approach that dominated psychoanalysis. Research subsequently corroborated theory in demonstrating that depressive episodes frequently arise following the loss of a loved one (i.e., bereavement-related depression), in the setting of marital strife (what IPT terms a "role dispute"), in the context of a major life change (a "role transition"), or in the absence of social supports ("interpersonal deficits") (Weissman et al., 2000). Conversely, social supports protect against depression (Klerman et al., 1984; Brown & Harris, 1978; Kendler et al., 1995).

CONCEPTUAL FRAMEWORK

IPT focuses on the intuitively reasonable concept that events in one's psychosocial environment affect one's mood, and vice versa. When painful events occur, mood worsens and depression may result in vulnerable individuals. Conversely, depressed mood compromises the ability to handle one's social role, generally leading to negative events. This simple yet powerful concept forms the core of IPT and its case formulation. IPT therapists use the connections among mood, environment, and social role to help patients understand their depression within an interpersonal context, and to teach them to handle their social role and environment so as to both solve their interpersonal problems and relieve the depressive syndrome.

IPT does not espouse a causal theory. Life events do not necessarily cause a depressive episode, which is multidetermined. Often unhappy events follow the onset of depression as the mood disorder impairs social functioning. Regardless of the etiology of a depressive episode, the human mind seeks meaning from life and willingly connects life events to their apparent consequences. The goal is to establish a connection that the patient finds credible, in order to provide a context for the depressive episode and, more important, an escape from it. Case formulation provides the vehicle for communicating this rationale to the patient.

It may help at this juncture to compare IPT and psychodynamic case formulations. Of the manualized psychotherapies for depression that have been tested in time-limited trials, IPT is among the closest to the psychodynamic psychotherapies many therapists practice. Both focus on the patient's feelings and relationships. Nonetheless, IPT case formulation differs markedly from the psychodynamic formulation described by Messer and Wolitzky (see Chapter 3, this volume). The IPT formulation concentrates on the patient's relationship to the world around him and his depressive symptoms rather than on internal processes or conflicts (Markowitz, Svartberg, & Swartz, 1998), emphasizing current rather than past interpersonal issues. The IPT therapist concedes that aspects of relationships may repeat patterns from and have roots in the past but stresses that an intervention made in the present—without addressing past conflicts—can improve the current interpersonal environment and alleviate the patient's depression.

Unlike a psychodynamic approach, IPT does not consider the patient's intrapsychic issues germane to case formulation or the thrust of treatment. Transference, dreams, and fantasies are not interpreted. Subliminally, however, knowledge of psychodynamics may inform the therapist's approach to a given patient (e.g., influencing how the therapist interacts with a histrionic, paranoid, or dependent patient). Many IPT therapists think psychodynamically but speak to the patient about—and formulate the case around—current life circumstances. Unlike a psychoanalyst, the IPT therapist is generally active and vocal in sessions. The structure and time limit of IPT require that the formulation be explicitly presented to the patient no later than the end of the third session, the culmination of the opening phase of IPT.

The IPT therapist uses a *medical model*, defining depression as a medical illness independent of the patient's personality or character. As discussed explicitly in the case formulation, this medical illness employs a stress–diathesis model: that is, depression has biological underpinnings that interact with environmental life events. The formulation offers the patient a hopeful, optimistic, empowering, and forward-looking approach by identifying a treatable illness and by encouraging the patient to seek happiness while offering strategies to achieve that goal.

As part of the case formulation, the patient is explicitly assigned the "sick role," which excuses the self-blaming depressed patient from responsibility for having gotten ill but charges him or her to work toward getting better (Parsons, 1951). This encourages the patient to separate depression from his or her sense of self, and to participate actively in IPT. It also allows the therapist to provide psychoeducation about depression, another important part of IPT formulation and treatment.

The therapist conceptualizes and presents the case formulation within the first one to three sessions. The therapeutic tasks in this beginning phase of treatment include diagnosing depression as a medical disorder, determining the nature of and changes in key relationships in the patient's "interpersonal inventory," and presenting the patient with an interpersonal case formulation that links the onset of the patient's mood disorder to one of four focal interpersonal problem areas (see Tables 8.1 and 8.2).

Although IPT uses little jargon, the IPT interpersonal problem area is labeled and explicitly included in the case formulation. In a sense, the term

TABLE 8.2. Tasks of the Opening Phase of IPT

Usually the first one to three sessions. Goals include:
1. Diagnosing the depression ("medical model")
2. Eliciting the interpersonal inventory
3. Establishing the interpersonal problem area
4. Giving the sick role
5. Developing a treatment plan
6. Making the interpersonal formulation
7. Obtaining patient's agreement to the formulation
8. Establishing the therapeutic alliance
9. Beginning psychoeducation
10. Instilling hope

becomes the case formulation. The four IPT problem areas are (1) *grief* (bereavement-related depression), (2) *role dispute*, (3) *role transition*, and (4) *interpersonal deficits*. Grief refers to depressive symptoms that extend beyond the usual severity or expectable mourning period following the death of a significant person in the patient's life. A role dispute is a disagreement with a spouse, boss, parent, friend, family member, or co-worker. Role transition encompasses major life events such as graduation, retirement, moving, changing jobs, being diagnosed with a severe illness, divorce, and so on. Conceptual "losses" (e.g., loss of a dream or an ideal) that do not involve the death of a significant other are categorized as role transitions rather than grief. The last category, interpersonal deficits, is the least well developed and worst titled and probably carries the worst prognosis. It defines a long-standing pattern of impoverished or contentious relationships. Interpersonal deficits really means the absence of life events, and hence the inapplicability of the first three options.

The case formulation explicitly assigns the patient a problem area:

> "Your move from California to New York has been very difficult for you. This *role transition* has meant coming to a strange new city while losing touch with friends and giving up a house that you loved. We'll focus on how this *role transition* is related to your depression and explore how you can make this transition more manageable for you. That should help both your life situation and your mood."

The patient must agree on the salience of the problem area proposed in the case formulation and *agree to work on it* before IPT proceeds to its second phase.

Although patients may fit into several or all of the four IPT problem areas, the need for a sharply delineated focus dictates limiting the choice to one, or at most two, problem areas, lest the treatment become diffused and lose coherence for both therapist and patient. The case formulation should be considered an organizing, simplifying fiction, a distillation of the history the patient has initially related, whose goal is to help the patient understand both what has been happening in his or her life and what will happen in treatment. As such, the narrative should be clear and concise, rather than complicated by a list of possible interpersonal foci. From a practical standpoint, if any of the first three foci exist, interpersonal deficits can be discarded. Many patients will present with both a role dispute and a role transition, but frequently treatment can subsume one within the other framework, and the therapist may choose the focus that makes the most clinical sense, or evokes the strongest affect from the patient.

How does one know the "right" formulation? Sometimes a single problem demands attention, and the course appears clear. The patient may present material leading in the direction of only one of the four problem areas. Even here, there is the danger that a covert role dispute or other interpersonal problem area may be significant, so the therapist must search for all possibilities. Even when the patient presents a complicated history characterized by multiple interpersonal problems, the therapist is obligated to select one problem area as a treatment focus. The combination of apparent face validity and "buy-in" from the patient suggests that the therapist has chosen a "good enough" focus.

IPT after the Formulation

The second phase of IPT, comprising most of the 12 to 16 sessions of a typical treatment of depression, focuses on the interpersonal problem area selected in the case formulation. Each of the four interpersonal problem areas has a particular treatment strategy. It is the coherence of these strategies, rather than particular elements of what is an avowedly eclectic approach, that make IPT a focused and distinct treatment. The IPT formulation determines the direction and mechanics of the treatment that follows.

In treating bereavement-related depression, the therapist's goal is to help the patient to mourn, then gradually to explore new activities and relationships to replace the lost one. Patients are encouraged to recount the good and bad aspects of their relationship with the deceased; to describe the things they did together or never had the chance to do; to describe details of the death and their relation to that situation. Patients are encouraged to look at mementos and picture albums, to visit the grave site, and in other ways to evoke the lost person to facilitate catharsis. Once the mourning process begins in earnest, the therapist often spends much of sessions empathically listening. As therapy proceeds, the therapist helps the patient explore new areas of interest, new activities, and new relationships.

For a role dispute, the therapist helps the patient examine the dispute and seek its resolution. Sometimes depressed patients imagine a relationship has reached an impasse, yet a simple clarification or discussion with the significant other resolves the dispute. When a serious dispute exists, the therapist helps the patient explore what he or she wants from the relationship and what options exist to negotiate those desired goals. The skills that depressed patients often need in self-assertion, expression of anger, or social risk taking can be developed in role play during sessions, with the implicit goal that the patient will attempt these behaviors during the week to come. If all the patients' efforts fail to resolve a true impasse in a role dispute, the therapist may help the patient dissolve the relationship, mourn its loss, and seek better alternatives.

A depressed patient in a role transition feels life is out of control. In formulating the case, the therapist redefines and explicitly labels this seeming chaos as a role transition involving the loss of a familiar old role and the potential assumption of a new one. The therapeutic goal is to help the patient navigate this transition as smoothly as possible and to fullest advantage. The patient is encouraged to see both the good and bad aspects of the old role and the benefits and liabilities of the new one; to mourn the loss of the past and accept the possibilities of the present and future.

Interpersonal deficits is a default category: The patient does not have complicated bereavement, a role dispute, or a role transition. Such patients tend to have little happening in their lives and few relationships. They are usually isolated and have trouble either in making or in sustaining relationships. In short, these are more difficult patients to treat with any psychotherapy, and perhaps more so in IPT because of their global deficits in the area in which IPT works (Elkin et. al., 1989). The goal is to help the patient recognize the link between mood and their social difficulties, to help the patient expand his or her social skills, and to gain social comfort. This is often akin to attempting to modify aspects of personality in a brief intervention: a more difficult but not impossible task.

By the final phase of IPT, the last few sessions, the patient has usually improved. In clinical trials, *remission rates* with IPT (typically defined as Hamilton Rating Scale for Depression [HRSD] scores = 6) generally range from 40 to 50% (Elkin et al., 1989; Markowitz, Kocsis, et al., 1998; Frank et al., 2000; O'Hara, Stuart, Gorman, & Wenzel, 2000; Mufson et al., 2004). The *response rate* to IPT alone (defined as = 50% decrease in HRSD scores) was reported as 63% in one trial (O'Hara et al., 2000). These response and remission rates are comparable to those seen in acute trials of pharmacotherapy for depression (Thase & Rush, 1997). For patients who have achieved remission, the therapist notes the approaching end to therapy, that the goals of relieving depression and solving the interpersonal problem area have been achieved, and acknowledges that it is sad to break up a good team. Sadness is addressed as a normal response to interpersonal separations and differentiated from depression. To bolster the patient's self-confidence as termination approaches, patient and therapist review the patient's accomplishments during the brief therapy—which are often considerable—in solving the interpersonal problem area and in reducing symptoms. They also review the symptoms of depression, potential for relapse, and interpersonal issues that might be likely to trigger a relapse for the patient.

Not all patients achieve full remission of depression with IPT alone, but few leave empty-handed: Most at least make progress in their interpersonal problem area. For patients with persisting symptoms, the therapist can point out that it is not the patient who has failed but the treatment, which promised to concomitantly relieve depression as the interpersonal problem was solved. It is important that such still symptomatic patients not feel guilty about their role in the therapy if they have worked at it, and that they leave IPT aware of alternative antidepressant treatment options. For instance, a sequence of IPT followed by augmentation with pharmacotherapy for nonresponders and partial responders to IPT resulted in a full remission for 79% of patients with histories of recurrent major depression (Frank et al., 2000). A recent study of another time-limited psychotherapy for depression found that among chronically depressed individuals who failed to respond to an acute course of psychotherapy, 42% subsequently responded to a course of pharmacotherapy (Schatzberg et al., 2005). The therapist can cite these encouraging results for patients, urging them to continue to look for treatment that works for them.

MULTICULTURAL CONSIDERATIONS AND INCLUSION/EXCLUSION CRITERIA

In general, IPT has not required adaptations for particular ethnic or cultural groups. The IPT therapist should always be sensitive to aspects of the patient's interpersonal environment, including cultural influences. In the only trial to specifically study ethnicity as a moderator of outcome, IPT was accepted by and yielded equal benefits to white, African American, and Hispanic patients with HIV infection and depressive symptoms, whereas a poorer outcome was found for the handful of African American subjects treated with cognitive-behavioral therapy (CBT) (Markowitz, Spielman, Sullivan, & Fishman, 2000). Grote et al. (2004b) demonstrated that IPT can be adapted to meet the needs of low-income, antepartum, depressed women from a public obstetrical clinic by utilizing a pretreatment ethnographic interview to understand the cultural context of the patient's depression and by systematically facilitating access to social services as these needs became apparent. Pilot work with this mostly African American group of women suggests that flexibility in scheduling and increased attention to basic needs (e.g., adequate food and housing) help to make IPT relevant to this population (Grote et al., 2004a). Mufson et al. (2004), who treated depressed adolescents with IPT in a predominantly Latino section of New York City, trained bilingual therapists and translated instruments into Spanish so that both Anglo and Latino subjects could participate in the project.

IPT seems to require few adaptations to work with patients of different cultural backgrounds. As IPT requires that the therapist take a detailed history of the patient's interpersonal relationships and functioning, therapists can easily use this framework to find out what constitutes "normal" and "abnormal" expectations in the patient's culture. For instance, an authoritarian father's interactions with an obsequious child may sound initially like a covert role dispute, but probing the patient's cultural background may lead the therapist to conclude that this represents a culturally acceptable standard within the patient's milieu. It is sometimes helpful to inquire whether the patient has concerns about working with a therapist of a different cultural background and to invite the patient to indicate when the therapist seems to misunderstand aspects of the patient's interpersonal life due to such differences.

Developed in the United States, IPT has been used with little cultural adjustment in North America, much of Europe, Puerto Rico, and Brazil. In the only controlled psychotherapy trial ever conducted in Africa to date, an IPT-based group intervention produced dramatic improvements for depressed, HIV-infected villagers in Uganda compared to treatment as usual (Bolton et al., 2003). This version of IPT used local conceptualizations of depression and incorporated social customs. For example, whereas in standard IPT, patients are encouraged to communicate directly about their dissatisfactions within the context of interpersonal relationships, Ugandan women do not directly confront men. Instead, a woman who was dissatisfied with her husband's behavior was encouraged to assert her displeasure more obliquely but culturally syntonically: by pointedly cooking him a bad meal. This was readily understood as uxorial disapproval (Verdeli et al., 2003). In Ugandan society, social roles of men and women are distinct, which required that the researchers conducting this trial form unisex groups for therapy within the villages and that therapists be of the same gender as their patients. Yet this study underscored that basic interpersonal issues related to depression were similar across widely varying cultures.

Inclusion and exclusion criteria for IPT depend on the syndrome under treatment. IPT has been used successfully to treat acute major depressive disorder; various subpopulations of depressed patients including adolescent, geriatric, HIV-positive, and postpartum patients (Weissman et al., 2000); other psychiatric syndromes such as bulimia (Fairburn, Jones, Peveler, Hope, & O'Connor, 1993; Weissman et al., 2000); and less successfully, substance abuse (Rounsaville, Glazer, Wilber, Weissman, & Kleber, 1983; Carroll, Rounsaville, & Gawin, 1991). For each of these studies, a syndromal diagnosis based on contemporary diagnostic criteria was an inclusion criterion and (except in the substance abuse studies) IPT proved superior to a control condition in randomized controlled trial. Further, less validated applications of IPT include treatment of depressed pregnant women (Spinelli & Endicott, 2003), social phobia (Lipsitz, Markowitz, Cherry, & Fyer, 1999), dysthymic disorder (Markowitz et al., 2005) and adjunctive therapy for lithium-treated patients with bipolar disorder (Frank et al., 2005). Hence the modal IPT patient suffers from a significant mood disorder or other Axis I diagnosis.

IPT has been most frequently used to treat moderately depressed outpatients. Concurrent pharmacotherapy does not exclude a patient from IPT (unless so specified by research protocol); indeed, its emphasis on a medical model makes IPT easily compatible with antidepressant medication. A "mega analysis" of patients treated with psychotherapy (IPT or CBT) ($n = 243$) alone or IPT plus antidepressant pharmacotherapy ($n = 243$) found that combination treatment offered no incremental advantage for mildly depressed patients but had significantly greater efficacy for severely depressed patients (Thase et al., 1997). Depressed women treated with combined IPT and pharmacotherapy from the outset had significantly lower remission rates than depressed women treated first with IPT alone, with pharmacotherapy then added for IPT nonresponders only (66% v. 79%, $p = .02$) (Frank et al., 2000).

Combined psychotherapy and pharmacotherapy for depression never fares worse than monotherapy, even if the combination is not always superior. In a 12-week study of another psychotherapy, investigators assigned 681 individuals with chronic depression to pharmacotherapy alone (nefazodone), psychotherapy alone (cognitive-behavioral analysis system of psychotherapy), or their combination. In this chronic patient population, response rates were significantly higher in individuals assigned to combination treatment relative to either treatment as monotherapy (Keller et al., 2000). Anecdotally, many individuals seem to benefit from the combination of pharmacotherapeutic symptom relief and psychotherapeutic support, skill building, and change in outlook.

Typical exclusion criteria for IPT research studies include psychosis, severe suicidal or homicidal risk, and—save in studies addressing these disorders—active substance abuse. These criteria reasonably apply to nonresearch patients. Another group that may fare poorly in IPT is individuals with severe interpersonal deficits. Reexamination of data from a large study comparing IPT with CBT suggested that patients with severe interpersonal deficits do better in a cognitive-behavioral treatment than IPT (Sotsky et al., 1991). This counterintuitive finding suggests that patients may need, *a priori*, a modicum of interpersonal skills or a focal interpersonal crisis in order to benefit maximally from IPT.

As IPT spreads from clinical trials into general practice, its primary focus will likely remain on specific diagnostic indications—a boast few other psychotherapies can make. As noted, targeting a specific, medicalized diagnosis is part of the treatment formula. Yet the principles of IPT are in essence universally applicable: Almost all people can find a relationship between their mood and interpersonal situation. How diagnostically diluted IPT may become in clinical practice remains to be seen.

STEPS IN CASE FORMULATION

IPT case formulation usually requires between one and three sessions of a 12–16-week treatment. Its length depends on the complexity of the patient's presenting history and the proficiency of the therapist. To formulate the case, the therapist needs to (1) diagnose depression as a medical illness; (2) evaluate interpersonal relationships, taking an *interpersonal inventory*; (3) establish a focal *interpersonal problem area*; and (4) make initial therapeutic interventions.

Diagnosing Depression

The therapist takes a formal psychiatric approach, diagnosing psychopathology based on current diagnostic criteria (i.e., DSM-IV-TR; American Psychiatric Association, 2000). Therapists rely on a standard psychiatric interview to carefully review the duration and severity of symptoms. Because diagnosing depression is vital to the case formulation, the therapist must accurately assess all relevant criteria.

Therapists frequently use measures such as the HRSD (Hamilton, 1960) to ensure a thorough review of symptoms and to educate the patient about them. Using a standardized instrument emphasizes that the patient is not (as he or she often feels) idiosyncratically lazy, willful, bad, or mysteriously overwhelmed but suffers from a common, discrete, understandable, and treatable disorder that is not the patient's fault. Assessment measures should be repeated regularly to demonstrate the patient's progress in therapy. The therapist must collect enough data in the initial interview to be able to incorporate into the case formulation a statement about the nature, onset, and severity of a patient's illness. In the context of diagnosing a depressive episode, the patient is also assigned the sick role.

Evaluating Interpersonal Relationships
(Taking the *Interpersonal Inventory*)

In the initial interviews, the therapist also develops the "interpersonal inventory," a catalogue of important relationships in the patient's life. This is not a formal instrument but refers to a thorough anamnesis, in which the therapist inquires about the important people in the patient's life, and particularly his or her current life: relationships with spouse, children, parents, boss, friends, and others. The therapist attempts to establish a temporal relationship between the onset of the depression and changes in the patient's interpersonal relationships, using both open- and closed-ended questions.

It is important to explore omissions in the interpersonal inventory as well as relationships the patient more easily discusses. For instance, if a patient describes in detail relationships with friends and bosses but skips romantic interests and family, the therapist should probe these areas. The therapist cares not only about the relationships themselves but their patterns, qualities, level of intimacy, and nonreciprocal wishes and intentions that the patient and significant others may have. How does the patient assert needs and confront people? The therapist must elicit enough detail to understand these relationships. For instance, if a patient said, "The most important person in my life is my wife and we get along wonderfully," the therapist would inquire, "Tell me more about the two of you." If an open-ended question failed to yield the degree of detail required, the therapist would follow with more structured questions, such as:

> "How long have you been married?"
> "Does your wife know how badly you've been feeling?"
> "Is she someone you can easily tell your feelings? (If not, whom do you tell?)"
> "What exactly have you said to her? How do you divide household responsibilities?"
> "How are your finances?"
> "What about your sexual relationship?"
> "Do you argue a lot? How do those disagreements start? How do they end?"
> "Has anything changed between the two of you in the past few months?"

The therapist's stance is inquiring, empathic, and respectful.

Although the past importantly determines these patterns and their chronicity, the therapist focuses on current relationships and on recent changes in relationships that may provide the interpersonal focus in the middle phase of IPT. The therapist asks about the patient's childhood relationships with family members and friends but does not explore these past relationships in the same depth as current significant relationships. Information about the patient's psychosocial development is useful background material, but it is not incorporated into the case formulation except in passing. For example, a case formulation might include the following statement about the patient's past relationship with her father. Notice, however, that the patient's attention is drawn to the present:

> "Your difficulties with your husband sound similar to problems you had with your father, with your camp counselor, and with a number of boy-

friends in the past. You seem to put up with what the men in your life want, and then silently resent it. That seems to be part of your role dispute with your husband, and to be contributing to your depression. There may be other ways of handling these situations: you are in a position to expect, to insist on, better treatment from your husband. Does that make sense to you? . . . Let's talk about how you might be able to improve the way you handle things with your husband."

Establishing an *Interpersonal Problem Area*

Having completed an interpersonal inventory, the therapist must decide into which of the four IPT problem areas the patient's problem falls (viz., grief, role dispute, role transition, or interpersonal deficits). At Cornell, therapists use a checklist called the Interpersonal Problem Area Rating Scale (IPARS; Markowitz, 1998). The IPARS merely ensures that the therapist has considered all relevant possibilities in choosing among the four interpersonal problem areas. Therapists learning IPT may find the IPARS a useful reminder of the range of possible formulations for this therapy. Audio- or videotaping treatment sessions may also help therapists to review material as they seek to construct interpersonal problem areas for patients.

In choosing a problem area, the therapist should focus on salient interpersonal events in the patient's life that are temporally proximate to the onset (or exacerbation) of the disorder. Such events usually emerge from the history. Occasionally the history and interpersonal inventory are bare. Such a patient has an impoverished social life with few meaningful relationships, none of which may have changed. Such patients often have schizoid or other personality disorders, which makes treatment more difficult but not impossible. These patients fall into the default category of "interpersonal deficits." The therapist typically describes the problem to the patient as "a difficulty in making or sustaining relationships." The goal of therapy then becomes finding a better, more comfortable social adjustment. Alternatively, these patients may suffer from dysthymic disorder, whose chronicity leads to a paucity of interpersonal relationships and events (Markowitz, 1998).

The elements of a patient's situation will vary, and it is important to subsume the patient's specific issues under a general problem area. By labeling the problem (much as one labels the depression), the patient begins to impose meaning and order on an experience that has felt random and out of control. This immediately reduces anxiety and gives patient and therapist a common language in which to discuss issues as the treatment unfolds.

Making Initial Therapeutic Interventions

From the start the therapist offers hope, an alternative optimistic viewpoint to the patient's depressed outlook, the conviction that depression is a treatable disorder. Many patients experience an initial symptomatic improvement just from beginning therapy in this newly hopeful atmosphere. This provides momentum for the treatment. (Of course, if the therapist then fails to deliver the goods, these initial gains may evanesce.) A sympathetic, understanding listener, a setting, a ritual, and an explanation for the patient's woes constitute part of the nonspecific armamentarium of most psychotherapies (Frank, 1971) and explicit ingredients of IPT. Provision of a simple, clear, intuitively reasonable case formulation, grounded in the patient's recent interpersonal life experience and carrying affective meaning, probably has a therapeutic benefit over and above its functions as an explanation and technical frame for the treatment.

Selecting Appropriate Treatment

Before presenting the case formulation, the therapist must decide whether IPT is an appropriate option for the patient. Does the patient have a disorder for which IPT has demonstrated efficacy (e.g., major depressive disorder)? Does the patient seem interested in treatment and able to engage with the therapist? Would the patient be better suited to another treatment modality, such as CBT or pharmacotherapy?

Presenting therapeutic options to the patient should follow from and complete the case formulation. Differential therapeutics should indeed determine *which* kind of case formulation the therapist gives the patient. If it were apparent that IPT was not the treatment of choice, the therapist should abandon the IPT case formulation and instead present a psychotherapeutic or psychopharmacological alternative.

Making the Interpersonal Formulation

Although further sessions flesh out the interpersonal problem area, the first one to three sessions should provide its solid skeleton. Once comfortable with a case formulation, and having decided that IPT is an appropriate option, the therapist presents it to the patient directly. In IPT, the formulation is stated explicitly and marks the end of the opening phase of treatment.

The patient must agree with this formulation before IPT can proceed into its middle phase. This agreement is more than symbolic acquiescence. It underscores the patient's expectedly active role in the treatment, and it affirms the therapeutic alliance. Perhaps most important, agreement signals that patient and therapist share an understanding of the patient's situation and can try to jointly address it. Without such agreement, therapy might trail off vaguely and inconclusively rather than focusing on the area of greatest affective valence to the patient.

Should the patient disagree with the therapist's formulation—which happens rarely, in our experience—therapist and patient would further explore the patient's interpersonal environment and situation. Based on this added information, the therapist might then propose a new formulation for the patient to consider.

> A depressed woman, who had refused to speak to her mother for the preceding 6 months because of a perceived slight, was initially presented with a case formulation that linked her depressive symptoms to a role dispute with her mother. The therapist suggested that the mother had previously provided important support for the patient, and that their "feud" had significantly contributed to the patient's despair and isolation. The patient contested this view, arguing that she and her mother had had frequent difficulties, that her mother often absented herself from her life for long stretches of time, and that she experienced this episode "like all the other times." On the other hand, she felt that a change in her relationship with a coworker, which had deteriorated over the same period of time, was more meaningful because "it affects me every day." Seemingly to prove this to the therapist, the patient contacted the mother between sessions and made plans to see her—but denied any connection to her depression because this did not alleviate her symptoms.
>
> The therapist collected further information about the patient's work difficulties, learning that work had functioned as a refuge for the patient from her difficult family situation but now had become fraught with conflict. The formulation was reframed as a role dispute with the patient's coworker. Although the therapist felt the dispute with the mother was also important, the patient's affective investment in her struggle with her coworker was impressive. Feeling that either role dispute could serve as a treatment focus, the therapist selected the one that meant most to the patient, who accepted the reformulation and proceeded with IPT.

APPLICATION TO PSYCHOTHERAPY TECHNIQUE

Case Formulation in the Initial Phase of Treatment

In the beginning phase (sessions 1–3), the IPT therapist explains the time limit, the goal of treating the interpersonal problem area and mood disorder (rather than personality traits or other aims), the sick role, and the therapist's expectations of the patient in the treatment. These expectations are that the patient become expert in the nature and treatment of depression, learn the connection between mood and interpersonal issues, and use this knowledge to confront his or her interpersonal problem area.

Case Formulation in the Middle and End Phases of Treatment

In the middle and end phases of therapy (sessions 4–12 or 16), the case formulation receives frequent mention. It is useful to repeat at least a compressed version of the formulation for two reasons: It corrects the tendency of depressed patients to lapse into self-blame, and it maintains thematic continuity and the focus of treatment. During sessions, the therapist repeatedly raises the interpersonal problem area at the core of the formulation: the depressive illness and "complicated bereavement," "your role dispute with your husband," "the role transition you're going through." Such terms reify as external the problems and issues that the depressed patient has previously internalized and blamed him- or herself for. The approach to patients with interpersonal deficits differs somewhat. Because saying a patient has "interpersonal deficits" may sound critical and is probably unhelpful, the therapist refers instead to "your discomfort in getting close to people" or "your social isolation" rather than using the formal label of the problem area.

The IPT therapist spends the bulk of each session addressing issues raised in the case formulation. Each session begins with the question, "How have you been since we last met?" in order to immediately focus the patient on contemporary interpersonal issues. Should the patient deviate from the focus (recall a dream, discuss an unrelated problem, etc.), the therapist listens empathically but then guides the patient back to the original focus by invoking the case formulation. The therapist might say:

> "It sounds like your children have been really difficult for you to manage this week. Because depression often makes people feel frustrated and overwhelmed, it's not surprising that child care may be difficult for you right now. But let's get back to what has been happening with your husband. As we discussed before, that role dispute seems connected to your depression; if you can work through that problem, your depression will lift and you will probably find it easier to cope with your children."

Alternatively, the therapist might seize on the issue of parental division of child-care responsibilities to lead back into the marital role dispute.

Therapists only abandon the case formulation under unusual circumstances. For instance, if the patient suddenly developed new, life-threatening symptoms such as active suicidal ideation or frank psychosis, the case formulation would be abandoned in order to attend to patient safety. If the patient experienced an unexpected important life event in midtreatment (the death of an important person, significant changes in socioeconomic status, etc.), it would be reasonable to suspend the initial treatment focus in order to attend to the patient's pressing needs. One would hope to return to the focus as soon as possible but, alternatively, could consider renegotiating the interpersonal focus or abandoning the IPT treatment approach.

The brevity of treatment leaves little room for error in formulating IPT cases. The therapist must use the initial treatment sessions to aggressively pursue all potential interpersonal problem areas and to determine a treatment focus prior to embarking on the middle phase of treatment. It is unlikely for a diligent therapist to discover, midway through treatment, that he or she has seriously misjudged the salience of a chosen problem area. If a covert, imposing interpersonal problem area should arise in the middle phase, however, the therapist would have to renegotiate the treatment contract to address it.

Other Applications of IPT Case Formulation

To put depression (or other psychiatric disorders) in an interpersonal and social context may also be a useful technique for non-IPT therapists. Depressed patients tend to look inward and to blame themselves as weak, lazy, impotent, flawed, and bad, forgetting the usually intuitive connection that events affect our moods, and vice versa. Patients receiving antidepressant medication, for example, might be relieved to be reminded of the effect environmental stressors have on their lives, and to hear that medication may soon give them greater energy and initiative to deal with these stressors.

CASE EXAMPLES

Case Example 1

The first case is an example of the "formula" used to share the case formulation with the patient during the beginning phase of treatment. The tone of voice should be serious, empathic, yet relaxed and conversational:

> "You have an illness called major depression, as we discussed when we did the Hamilton Depression Rating Scale. Again, it's not your fault, not something to blame yourself for, but we do need to treat it. Your job over the next weeks will be to be a patient with the medical illness called depression. You should focus on your treatment and not worry too much if you don't yet feel like your usual self. The good news is that depression is very treatable, and I expect that you'll be feeling much better in a matter of a few weeks.
>
> "From what you've told me, I think your depression has something to do with what's been going on in your life: namely, [the role transition you've been going through in your career/things haven't been the same since your husband died, and you've had trouble really grieving his death/the role dispute you're having with your wife/what hasn't been going on in your life: the difficulties you have in making or keeping relationships]. If you solve that problem, not only will you be better off for having solved it, but your depression should also clear up. Does that make sense to you?
>
> "There are a number of proven ways to treat depression. One is

with interpersonal psychotherapy, which is a brief antidepressant treatment that focuses on the connection between your mood disorder and what's going on in your life. Understanding that connection and using that understanding should allow you to choose the best options to deal with your situation and help you to feel better. If you're willing, and this makes sense to you, what I'd suggest is that we spend the next 12 weeks working on this. IPT has been carefully tested in research studies and shown to effectively treat the kind of depression you have. So we have a good chance of doing *two things* in the next 12 weeks: of helping you solve your [interpersonal problem: e.g., role dispute] and, at the same time, getting you out of this horrible episode of depressive illness."

Case Example 2

This case is an example of a role dispute. It illustrates the processes necessary to elucidate a case formulation from clinical material. It also shows how long-standing behavioral patterns are acknowledged but not directly addressed in IPT.

Ms. A, a 31-year-old recently married Catholic businesswoman, presented with her first episode of major depression, which had endured for 11 months. She had begun to feel pressured by her husband of one year, to whom she had been engaged for 3 years prior to wedding. Mr. A, although "for equal rights for women," had begun subtly, and then forcefully, to encourage her to leave work in order to have children. She loved her husband and welcomed eventual motherhood but had long defined herself through her work, had recently been promoted, and was reluctant to give up her job. Around this time Ms. A noted the onset of sleep disturbance, loss of energy, appetite, and libido. She felt guilty about her unexpressed but conscious anger toward her husband, feeling that if they were having such troubles so early in marriage, their future was doomed. She began seeing a psychotherapist but dropped out after 8 months, feeling that she was making no progress. What precipitated her second search for treatment was a late menstrual period that made her fear she was pregnant.

Ms. A reported an HRSD score of 28 (i.e., significantly elevated) and easily met DSM-IV criteria for major depression. She reported no history of substance abuse, dysthymia, or other psychiatric disorder. Her mother had been treated for depression. When her father had died 3 years previously, she had been able to grieve, feeling sad but not depressed. The elder of two sisters, Ms. A described a reasonably happy childhood with overly strict and demanding, but loving, parents. Her role in the house had been to achieve high grades and school honors for her parents' approval and to serve at times as surrogate mother to her sibling. She had had two significant sexual relationships, lasting several years each, prior to meeting her husband. Appreciated at her job for her hard work, she described good re-lations with her boss and coworkers. Ms. A described herself as generally being an "up person" who made the best of things, handled disappoint-ments stoically, and did not like to get angry. She and her husband had had few disagreements before the issue of her job arose, as she generally de-ferred to his wishes. He, although increasingly worried by her deteriorating state, seemed not to grasp the importance of her work to her, nor the effects of his own wishes: Her worsening depression was to him just another rea-son for her to stop working.

At this point the reader may want to stop and take stock. Which inter-personal problem areas appear likely prospects as a focus for therapy? There is little suggestion here of complicated bereavement, given Ms. A's re-ported ability to grieve and the lack of temporal connection between her fa-ther's death—a significant interpersonal stressor—and the onset of her mood disorder. Nor is there evidence of a role dispute in her workplace. At home, however, we find an obvious role dispute with her husband, which Ms. A seems bewildered about how to handle. Her marriage and job pro-motion might each constitute role transitions (as would pregnancy): In-deed, they appear to pull from opposing directions on her sense of identity and life trajectory. Her good relationships and marriage argue against inter-personal deficits; given the presence of alternative problem areas, we would in any case avoid using that focus. Hence the choice lies between a role dis-pute and a role transition.

Ms. A's therapist decided to frame the formulation as a role dispute, feeling that the struggle with her husband was more central than the role transitions. *(A role transition focusing on the marriage would have differed mainly in semantics.)* She said:

> "We've diagnosed the problem as a major depression; although you feel guilty about your situation, that's just a symptom of your illness, called depression. It's not your fault. Your Hamilton score is quite high: 28. But don't worry, within a few weeks we'll try to have you down below 7, in the normal range. And, you know, your depression seems to have started with your husband's pressure on you to stop the work that's been, and still is, so important to you. You don't seem to know how to handle that situation, and I think that's contributing to your depres-sion. We call this a role dispute.
>
> "There are several effective treatments for depression, including antidepressant medication, which you've said you don't want. We can talk about the reasons for and against medicine. Another approach is called interpersonal psychotherapy, or IPT. IPT works by helping you understand the connection between what's going on in your life and how that might affect your mood; once you understand that, you can figure out how to handle your life situations. As you solve those inter-

personal issues—for you, the role dispute with your husband—you're very likely to feel better. IPT has been tested in research studies and found to be a highly effective treatment for depression like yours. It works in a matter of weeks, too: we should be able to treat your depression meeting weekly for 12 weeks. Does that sound OK to you?"

It did. Although she at that point saw little prospect of extricating herself from the "mess" of her life, Ms. A was relieved by the formulation and agreed to IPT. She returned the next week feeling considerably better, happy to discover that she was not pregnant. Therapy focused on learning to assert her needs to her husband, first role playing with her therapist, and on seeing anger as a normal, useful response to her social environment that could be expressed without guilt.

After 4 weeks the Hamilton score had fallen to 9, by 8 weeks to 4, and at termination it was 3. Ms. A used the weeks of therapy to open a more balanced dialogue with her husband, who began to recognize the importance of his wife's work role, was delighted by her symptomatic improvement (if somewhat taken aback by her new assertiveness), and agreed to postpone parenthood for a couple of years.

The therapist acknowledged that many of Ms. A's patterns were longstanding but focused sessions on her current relationships outside the office rather than on her childhood. In midtherapy Ms. A reported that she had had a long and helpful talk with her mother about women's rights and the role of the wife in marriage. They agreed that Ms. A would do well not to repeat her mother's too submissive stance. In the final sessions Ms. A dealt with the issues of termination smoothly. Six months and 12 months later, the therapist received letters from Ms. A reporting continuing euthymia. Several years later, she received a baby announcement in a letter explaining that Mr. and Ms. A had now happily agreed on parenthood. Ms. A, who had received another promotion, planned to continue working part time after her maternity leave.

Case Example 3

This case presents a patient with complicated bereavement.

Ms. B, a 26-year-old pregnant, single, African American woman, was referred to the mental health clinic by her obstetrician, who was concerned about Ms. B's attitude toward her pregnancy. Ms. B had missed several prenatal visits and refused to get prenatal blood tests as requested by the obstetrician.

On presenting to the mental health clinic, Ms. B was initially wary of her therapist, who was white and considerably older than she. Ms. B answered questions with "yes" or "no," reluctant to elaborate. Concerned that Ms. B would not return for follow-up if issues of engagement were not addressed, the therapist set her formal depression assessment aside and began talking with Ms. B about how she felt coming to a mental health clinic. Ms. B conceded that it felt like another burden and believed it would not be worth the roundtrip bus fare to sessions. The therapist ventured that perhaps Ms. B was wondering how "some old, white lady" would be able to understand her situation, much less help her with it. Ms. B's curiosity was piqued by the therapist's willingness to discuss age and race so openly. Ms. B smiled and said that she was indeed worried about that: "Sometimes white folks think what's normal for us is abnormal." The therapist asked if Ms. B would be willing to educate her about Ms. B's world and tell her if she "didn't get it." Ms. B said she would, especially if the therapist promised to "not look at me funny" when she revealed her story.

Rather than beginning with a formal depression assessment such as the HRSD, the therapist invited the patient to tell her story. Ms. B revealed a poignant history of early neglect, shuttled from home to home as a child because her crack-using mother was unable to care for her; a 5-year period of heavy drug and alcohol use in late adolescence; and a series of unsatisfactory relationships with men during adolescence and adulthood. Nonetheless, Ms. B had received her GED and had worked at the same receptionist job for 5 years. Although Ms. B related this part of the history matter-of-factly, she became tearful in reporting that 2 years before, another pregnancy had ended with a stillbirth at 8 months' gestation. She had been uncertain of the paternity of this first baby because she had become pregnant during a period of promiscuity associated with drug use. She tried unconvincingly to say she didn't "care" about this loss and had been glad to return to work without having to worry about supporting a fatherless child.

The therapist, sensitive to potential rifts in the therapeutic relationship, was empathic but gently suggested that the prior pregnancy might be influencing her feelings about her current pregnancy. Although Ms. B initially denied this possibility, she soon admitted fearing that her current pregnancy would also result in stillbirth because she had smoked marijuana a few times during the pregnancy and believed prior drug use had caused the last stillbirth.

Over the first two sessions, the therapist gave Ms. B positive feedback about her willingness to express her thoughts and feelings, complimenting her on her willingness to disclose her fears and beliefs. The therapist also gradually elicited a history of depressive symptoms, learning that Ms. B's mood had dropped and her sleep became erratic 5 months before, when she learned she was pregnant. Using the Edinburgh Postnatal Depression Scale (EPDS; an instrument designed to assess depressive symptoms during pregnancy) (Cox, Holden, & Sagovsky, 1987), the therapist determined that Ms. B had a moderately elevated score of 14 and would benefit from treatment.

The interpersonal inventory made it apparent that Ms. B was isolated. She had no contact with her family of origin. Her baby's father was married to another woman and unaware of Ms. B's pregnancy. She had a few friends from work but did not socialize outside the office. Many of her friends from adolescence continued to abuse drugs and alcohol, and she had had little contact with them since achieving sobriety following her first pregnancy. Her only source of support was her church. She attended every Sunday and participated in a Bible study group once a week. Her pastor had visited her house a few times after her first pregnancy, but she reported having felt numb at the time and rebuffed most offers of help and support.

At this point, the therapist considered two possible problem areas: a role transition (pregnancy) and grief for the lost baby. Because there were other options, the therapist did not consider interpersonal deficits. It would have been plausible to frame this case as a role transition from "not pregnant" to "pregnant," but she chose to frame the problem as unresolved grief because the patient admitted that she often thought about the dead baby and prayed to ask forgiveness for her sins which, she believed, had led to the baby's death. The therapist formulated the case for the patient as follows:

> "You noticed that your mood changed soon after you learned you were pregnant. Although you were initially excited about having a baby, you soon began to worry that this baby would die also. You haven't been sleeping well and haven't been gaining as much weight as you should. These are both symptoms of depression. You've also avoided appointments with your OB because you feel hopeless about having a healthy baby. Hopelessness is another symptom of depression. It seems to me that your depression is linked to unresolved feelings about your first pregnancy. Although part of you feels the baby wasn't a "real person," another part of you was strongly affected by losing your first child. Losing a child is a terrible experience. You were able to push these feelings away for 2 years and not think about the baby, but now that you are pregnant, those feelings—unwanted as they are—have become a big part of your life. I suggest that we focus on your feelings about the loss of your first baby and how they're affecting your current pregnancy. Your mood should improve as we unravel the links between your two pregnancies and help you understand and express your feelings about the baby who died."

Note that in this case formulation, the therapist deliberately used emotionally loaded phrases such as "your first child" and "the baby who died." She watched the patient's response to these phrases to make sure that the patient could tolerate the affectively charged material. The patient became tearful but not unduly distraught or disturbingly detached during the formulation. This gave the therapist reason to believe that she was on the right track with the case formulation. Had the patient indicated an inability to handle this kind of emotional processing, the therapist might have decided to reframe the case as a role transition, which would have allowed the patient to address the grief issues obliquely while focusing on more neutral issues around the current pregnancy.

During the treatment, the therapist urged Ms. B to review the experience of the first pregnancy, her expectations about the first baby, her drug use, and the delivery. It became clear the Ms. B had never asked her doctors about the reason for the stillbirth: She admitted that they might have told her at the delivery but remembered little about that day. At the therapist's urging, Ms. B asked her current OB to discuss the medical reasons for the stillbirth. When her OB reviewed the chart, it seems that the baby died because the umbilical cord was wrapped around the neck—not because of drug use. The OB reassured Ms. B that this is an unfortunate but rare outcome that was unlikely to recur. She advised Ms. B to stop using marijuana during pregnancy but reassured her that all tests to date were normal, and that there were no indications of fetal malformations on a recent sonogram.

Relieved of guilt for the stillbirth, Ms. B began the grieving process for her lost baby. She related that the baby had been a girl and that she had picked out a name for her. She stopped referring to the lost baby in generic terms, using instead her chosen name of Tamika. Although her EPDS score initially worsened to 20 during the difficult grieving process, it dropped down to 4 (normal range) as therapy progressed. Ms. B allowed herself to think about the new baby and began to plan for the birth. She attended prenatal appointments regularly. In preparation for the demands of the postpartum period, the therapist encouraged Ms. B to build her social network and persuaded her to accept offers of help from her church.

Ms. B's final IPT appointment took place 3 weeks after the uncomplicated birth of a healthy baby girl. Ms. B proudly introduced her baby to the therapist and reported that she was doing well despite the demands of caring for a newborn by herself. In addition to congratulating Ms. B on both her baby and her hard work in IPT, the therapist reviewed the risk of new depression during the postpartum period, urging Ms. B to call the clinic if she noticed the reemergence of depressive symptoms. Ms. B agreed to follow up as needed.

Case Example 4

This case describes a patient with interpersonal deficits. As is typical for such patients, IPT produced significant gains, including new awareness of and changes in interpersonal behaviors, but underlying personality style was not altered in 16 weeks. The patient required referral for additional treatment at the end of the course of IPT.

Ms. C, a 42-year-old divorced paralegal, was referred by her internist after workup for a series of medical complaints was unrevealing. Ms. C reported feeling sad and hopeless for many months. Her multiple somatic concerns included recurrent headaches, stomach pains, backaches, and bloating. She was satisfied with her internist's thorough workup, but stated, "I still don't feel right." Her HRSD score was 16, reflecting a high level of somatic complaints.

There were no clear recent stressors. Ms. C had worked in the same legal offices for 12 years. She was proud of her work and known at the office as someone who could "always come through in a pinch." Despite her reputation and obvious pleasure in her work, Ms. C had little contact with coworkers. She generally worked alone in a cubicle and spent her lunches at a local restaurant reading novels. Ms. C lived alone. She was estranged from her family, who lived far away. She had one friend, Ms. D, with whom she spoke daily by telephone but saw rarely. She enjoyed reading and sewing. An avid folk dancer, she attended group dancing sessions twice a week. She interacted with group members there but did not form relationships outside the scheduled activities.

Ms. C had no current romantic relationships but had been married briefly in her early 30s. She had met a man at a folk dancing weekend and become intimately involved. They spent several nights together over a 2-month period before Ms. C realized she was pregnant. Against the man's wishes, Ms. C terminated the pregnancy. Paradoxically, she felt so guilty about the abortion that she later agreed to marry him when pressed. The marriage ended less than a year later.

The therapist had now reviewed all interpersonal arenas and found a paucity of relationships. Ms. C nevertheless met criteria for major depressive disorder and wanted help. The therapist was left with the interpersonal deficits category *by default and agreed to treat the patient. The data about the marriage, which emerged as a surprise given her socially isolated presentation, show the importance of taking a careful history and seeking levels of higher functioning. The therapist offered the following formulation:*

> "Your many physical problems may be related to a mood disorder. According to this Hamilton score and my clinical impression, you have a major depressive disorder, which will often cause or worsen the physical problems that you describe. Depression also makes it hard for you to feel motivated to go out and spend time with people. You have talked about how much you enjoy socializing during folk dancing but find that you interact very little with people at other times. You've said that you'd like to see more of Ms. D and perhaps get involved in another romantic relationship. I feel that your depression is related to your diffi-

culty meeting and being with people. We could think about ways for you to develop more satisfying interpersonal relationships and at the same time help to relieve your depressive symptoms. Does that make sense?"

Ms. C was surprisingly enthusiastic about this formulation and agreed to treatment. Initially, the therapist asked Ms. C to consider changes she would like to make in her one existing relationship. Ms. C thought she would enjoy spending more time with Ms. D in person, rather than over the phone, but feared Ms. D would "not be interested." The therapist encouraged her to think about options for raising this possibility with Ms. D. Encouraged by role play in therapy sessions, Ms. C decided to risk asking Ms. D to go to a movie. To her astonishment, not only did Ms. C enjoy the outing but Ms. D asked her to dinner the following week.

Pleased by this success, Ms. C began to consider widening her social contacts. Although she stated she would like to spend time with more people, she lacked the social skills necessary to initiate contact. Taking a social skills training approach, the therapist suggested that she consider striking up a conversation with a fellow folkdancer, Ms. E, whom she wanted to get to know. They again role played to test the situation in a "safe" environment before Ms. C tried it out of the office.

As this example illustrates, the therapist must be quite active with these patients, encouraging them to take interpersonal risks and to deviate from their routine. Because these patients lack interpersonal skills, direct suggestion, role play, and communication analysis become particularly important interventions. It is important not to push such socially anxious patients too far too fast but to build slowly on initial successes.

Ms. C successfully engaged Ms. E in conversation at the next folk dance session and was surprised when Ms. E asked her to join her and two male companions for a drink afterward. Reflexively, Ms. C declined the invitation. Reviewing the events in therapy, Ms. C admitted that she was frightened of repeating the events that led to her marriage and felt that a drink with men would inevitably lead to "sex and complications." The therapist encouraged her to find a more neutral activity. Ms. C finally agreed to suggest to Ms. E that they go out for frozen yogurt—rather than a drink—after the next class.

With much coaxing and practice, Ms. C began to spend time regularly with Ms. D and Ms. E. At the end of 16 sessions, she was socializing every week but still far from her stated goal of a romantic relationship. Her physical symptoms had relented somewhat and her mood was much brighter. Her Hamilton score of 10 was somewhat improved but remained in the mildly depressed range.

The therapist congratulated Ms. C on the strides that she had made in therapy and told her that because she had made progress already, she was a good candidate for ongoing psychotherapy to continue to work on her goals. She referred her for continuing supportive psychotherapy with another clinician. (Continuation IPT would have been another reasonable option.)

TRAINING

IPT training is available to therapists of all mental health disciplines. Prerequisites are several years' experience as a psychotherapist and clinical experience with the disorder to be treated (e.g., major depression). To obtain specific IPT training, interested therapists should read the IPT manual (Weissman et al., 2000) and ideally attend a training workshop. Because of growing demand for time-limited, diagnostically specific therapies of demonstrated potency like IPT, more workshops are being held for experienced therapists, and psychiatric residents are learning IPT in a number of training programs (Markowitz, 1995, 2001). Training sessions are often posted on the website of the International Society for Interpersonal Psychotherapy (ISIPT) (www.interpersonalpsychotherapy.org).

Review of the manual (Weissman et al., 2000) and a training workshop will usually suffice for experienced clinicians to gain a general appreciation of IPT technique, which they can then try to apply to their practices. To master the technique, however, therapists should videotape or audiotape three training cases and closely review them, session by session, with a trained IPT supervisor. Serial measurement of symptoms is also important. Successfully completing three supervised cases gives a therapist informal certification in IPT. At present there are no specific clinical credentials for therapists with IPT expertise, although the ISIPT is exploring how IPT therapist groups in different countries are addressing this issue.

RESEARCH SUPPORT FOR IPT

In developing IPT, Klerman and Weissman placed outcome ahead of process research. They felt that process research held limited interest if the treatment could not be proven to have efficacy. Now that the efficacy of IPT has been demonstrated (Weissman et al., 2000; Elkin et al., 1989; Frank et al., 1990), process research appears indicated. To date little has been done, however.[1]

A few preliminary data support the reliability of IPT case formulations. Three IPT research psychotherapists listened to 18 audiotapes of initial IPT treatment sessions with dysthymic patients using the IPARS to test agreement on choosing interpersonal problem areas. Kappas for the presence or absence of each of the four IPT problem areas were 0.87 for complicated bereavement, 0.58 for role dispute, 1.0 for role transition, and 0.48 for interpersonal deficits. Kappa for agreement on which of the available problem areas would provide the best clinical focus was 0.82 (Markowitz, Leon, et al., 2000). These findings suggest that IPT therapists tend to agree in determining focal problem areas based on intake histories.

Another preliminary study indicates that IPT treatments actually focus on the interpersonal problem area chosen in the case formulation and that patients and therapists perceive gains in resolving these problems. Investigators assessed small samples of patients with either dysthymic disorder or posttraumatic stress disorder (PTSD) using the Interpersonal Psychotherapy Outcome Scale (IPOS), a crude 5-point measure of whether the focal problem area changed during therapy. Patients ($n = 24$) and therapists ($n = 7$) in a time-limited IPT outcome study of dysthymic disorder, and patients ($n = 10$) in an open trial for PTSD, completed the IPOS at treatment termination. All responding dysthymic subjects ($n = 24$) and therapists ($n = 21$) reported interpersonal gains: dysthymic patients scored 4.39 ($SD = 0.52$) out of 5, therapists 4.27 ($SD = 0.53$). PTSD patients rated 4.77 ($SD = 0.34$). Patient and therapist IPOS ratings showed trend correlations with symptomatic improvement (Markowitz, Bleiberg, Christos, & Levitan, 2006). This initial testing of the IPOS supports the theorized link between resolving interpersonal crises and clinical improvement in IPT, which provides indirect support for the clinical value of the IPT case formulation.

Research at the University of Pittsburgh also provides indirect evidence for reliability and validity of case formulation in IPT. Frank and colleagues found that patients in a 3-year study using monthly, maintenance IPT had better outcomes when their maintenance sessions focused on a clear interpersonal theme. Patients whose sessions had high interpersonal specificity survived a mean 2 years before developing depression, whereas those with a low interpersonal focus gained only 5 months of protection before relapse. In fact, however, this study allowed maintenance therapy sessions to focus on *any* interpersonal theme, which hence may have diverged from the original, acute case formulation (Frank, Kupfer, Wagner, McEachran, & Cornes, 1991).

CONCLUSION

Case formulation is a relatively unstudied but important facet of the initial phase of IPT. Now that the efficacy of IPT has been demonstrated for several mood and nonaffective disorders, research on the ingredients of IPT, including case formulation, deserves greater attention. Readers of this chapter who are not trained in IPT may nonetheless experiment with using the principles inherent in formulating IPT cases in the evaluation and treatment of patients with depression and other psychiatric disorders.

NOTE

1. One nice exception shows that more difficult, "help-rejecting" patients drive
   therapists out of a pure IPT paradigm, whereas initial symptom severity does
   not affect therapist performance (Foley, O'Malley, Rounsaville, Prusoff, &
   Weissman, 1987). Foley et al. do not, however, directly address case formulation.

REFERENCES

American Psychiatric Association. (2000). *Diagnostic and statistical manual of mental disorders* (4th ed., text rev.). Washington, DC: Author.

Bolton, P., Bass, J., Neugebauer, R., Verdeli, H., Clougherty, K. F., Wickramaratne, P., et al. (2003). Group interpersonal psychotherapy for depression in rural Uganda: A randomized controlled trial. *Journal of the American Medical Association, 289,* 3117–3124.

Brown, G. W., & Harris, T. (1978). *Social origins of depression: A study of psychiatric disorder in women.* New York: Free Press.

Carroll, K. M., Rounsaville, B. J., & Gawin, F. H. (1991). A comparative trial of psychotherapies for ambulatory cocaine abusers: Relapse prevention and interpersonal psychotherapy. *American Journal of Drug and Alcohol Abuse, 17*(3), 229–247.

Cox, J. L., Holden, J. M., & Sagovsky, R. (1987). Detection of postnatal depression: Development of the 10-item Edinburgh Postnatal Depression Scale. *British Journal of Psychiatry, 150,* 782–786.

Elkin, I., Shea, M. T., Watkins, J. T., Imber, S. D., Sotsky, S. M., Collins, J. F., et al. (1989). National Institute of Mental Health treatment of depression collaborative research program: General effectiveness of treatments. *Archives of General Psychiatry, 46,* 971–982.

Fairburn, C. G., Jones, R., Peveler, R. C., Hope, R. A., & O'Connor, M. (1993). Psychotherapy and bulimia nervosa: Longer-term effects of interpersonal psychotherapy, behavior therapy, and cognitive behavior therapy. *Archives of General Psychiatry, 50,* 419–428.

Foley, S. A., O'Malley, S., Rounsaville, B., Prusoff, B. A., & Weissman, M. M. (1987). The relationship of patient difficulty to therapist performance in interpersonal psychotherapy of depression. *Journal of Affective Disorders, 12,* 207–217.

Frank, E., Grochocinski, V. J., Spanier, C. A., Buysse, D. J., Cherry, C. R., Houck, P. R., et al. (2000). Interpersonal psychotherapy and antidepressant medication: Evaluation of a sequential treatment strategy in women and with recurrent major depression. *Journal of Clinical Psychiatry, 61*(1), 51–57.

Frank, E., Kupfer, D. J., Perel, J. M., Cornes, C., Jarrett, D. B., Mallinger, A. G., et al. (1990). Three-year outcomes for maintenance therapies in recurrent depression. *Archives of General Psychiatry 47,* 1093–1099.

Frank, E., Kupfer, D. J., Thase, M. G., Mallinger, A. G., Swartz, H. A., Fagiolini, A. M., et al. (2005). Two-year outcomes for interpersonal and social rhythm therapy in individuals with bipolar I disorder. *Archives of General Psychiatry, 62,* 996–1004.

Frank, E., Kupfer, D. J., Wagner, E. F., McEachran, A. B., & Cornes, C. (1991). Efficacy of interpersonal psychotherapy as a maintenance treatment of recurrent depression. *Archives of General Psychiatry, 48,* 1053–1059.

Frank, J. (1971). Therapeutic factors in psychotherapy. *American Journal of Psychotherapy, 25,* 350–361.

Grote, N. K., Bledsoe, S. E., Swartz, H. A., & Frank, E. (2004a). Culturally relevant psychotherapy for perinatal depression in low-income Ob/Gyn patients. *Clinical Social Work, 32*(3), 327–347.

Grote, N. K., Bledsoe, S. E., Swartz, H. A., & Frank, E. (2004b). Feasibility of providing culturally relevant, brief interpersonal psychotherapy for antenatal depression in an obstetrics clinic. *Research on Social Work Practice, 14*(6), 397–407.

Hamilton, M. (1960). A rating scale for depression. *Journal of Neurology, Neurosurgery, and Psychiatry, 25,* 56–62.

Hill, C. E., O'Grady, K. E., & Elkin, I. (1992). Applying the collaborative study psychotherapy rating scale to rate therapist adherence in cognitive-behavior therapy, interpersonal therapy, and clinical management. *Journal of Consulting and Clinical Psychology, 60,* 73–79.

Keller, M. B., McCullough, J. P., Klein, D. N., Arnow, B., Dunner, D. L., Gelenberg, A. J., et al. (2000). A comparison of nefazodone, the cognitive behavioral-analysis system of psychotherapy, and their combination for the treatment of chronic depression. *New England Journal of Medicine, 342,* 1462–1470.

Kendler, K. S., Kessler, R. C., Waters, E. E., et al. (1995). Stressful life events, genetic liability, and onset of an episode of major depression in women. *American Journal of Psychiatry, 152,* 833–842.

Klerman, G. L., Weissman, M. M., Rounsaville, B. J., & Chevron, E. S. (1984). *Interpersonal psychotherapy of depression.* New York: Basic Books.

Lipsitz, J. D., Markowitz, J. C., Cherry, S., & Fyer, A. J. (1999). Open trial of interpersonal psychotherapy for the treatment of social phobia. *American Journal of Psychiatry, 156,* 1814–1816.

Markowitz, J. C. (1995). Teaching interpersonal psychotherapy to psychiatric residents. *Academic Psychiatry, 19,* 167–173.

Markowitz, J. C. (1998). *Interpersonal psychotherapy for dysthymic disorder.* Washington, DC: American Psychiatric Press.

Markowitz, J. C. (2001). Learning the new psychotherapies. In M. M. Weissman (Ed.), *Treatment of depression: Bridging the 21st century* (pp. 281–300). Washington, DC: American Psychiatric Press.

Markowitz, J. C., Bleiberg, K. L., Christos, P., & Levitan, E. (2006). Solving interpersonal problems correlates with symptom improvement in interpersonal psychotherapy: Preliminary findings. *Journal of Nervous and Mental Disease, 194,* 15–20.

Markowitz, J. C., Kocsis, J. H., Bleiberg, K. L., Christos, P. J., & Sacks, M. H. (2005). A comparative trial of psychotherapy and pharmacotherapy for "pure" dysthymic patients. *Journal of Affective Disorders, 89,* 167–175.

Markowitz, J. C., Kocsis, J. H., Fishman, B., Spielman, L. A., Jacobsberg, L. B., Frances, A. J., et al. (1998). Treatment of depressive symptoms in human immunodeficiency virus-positive patients. *Archives of General Psychiatry, 55,* 452–457.

Markowitz, J. C., Leon, A. C., Miller, N. L., Cherry, S., Clougherty, K. F., &

Villalobos, L. (2000). Rater agreement on interpersonal psychotherapy problem areas. *Journal of Psychotherapy Practice and Research, 9*, 131–135.

Markowitz, J. C., Spielman, L. A., Scarvalone, P. A., & Perry, S. W. (2000). Psychotherapy adherence of therapists treating HIV-positive patients with depressive symptoms. *Journal of Psychotherapy Practice and Research, 9*, 75–80.

Markowitz, J. C., Spielman, L. A., Sullivan, M., & Fishman, B. (2000). An exploratory study of ethnicity and psychotherapy outcome among HIV-positive patients with depressive symptoms. *Journal of Psychotherapy Practice and Research, 9*, 226–231.

Markowitz, J. C., Svartberg, M., & Swartz, H. A. (1998). Is IPT time-limited psychodynamic psychotherapy? *Journal of Psychotherapy Practice and Research, 7*, 185–195.

Mufson, L., Dorta, K. P., Wickramaratne, P., Nomura, Y., Olfson, M., & Weissman, M. M. (2004). A randomized effectiveness trial of interpersonal for depressed adolescents. *Archives of General Psychiatry, 61*(6), 577–584.

O'Hara, M. W., Stuart, S., Gorman, L. L., & Wenzel, A. (2000). Efficacy of interpersonal psychotherapy for postpartum depression. *Archives of General Psychiatry, 57*(11), 1039–1045.

Parsons, T. (1951). Illness and the role of the physician: A sociological perspective. *American Journal of Orthopsychiatry, 21*, 452–460.

Rounsaville, B. J., Glazer, W., Wilber, C. H., Weissman, M. M., & Kleber, H. D. (1983). Short-term interpersonal psychotherapy in methadone-maintained opiate addicts. *Archives of General Psychiatry, 40*, 629–636.

Schatzberg, A. F., Rush, A. J., Arnow, B. A., Banks, P. L. C., Blalock, J. A., Borian, F. E., et al. (2005). Chronic depression: Medication (nefazodone) or psychotherapy (CBASP) is effective when the other is not. *Archives of General Psychiatry, 62*(5), 513–520.

Sotsky, S. M., Glass, D. R., Shea, M. T., Pilkonis, P. A., Collins J. F., Elkin, I., et al. (1991). Patient predictors of response to psychotherapy and pharmacotherapy: findings in the NIMH treatment of depression collaborative research program. *American Journal of Psychiatry, 148*, 997–1008.

Spinelli, M. G., & Endicott, J. (2003). Controlled clinical trial of interpersonal C psychotherapy versus parenting education program for depressed pregnant women. *American Journal of Psychiatry, 154*, 1028–1030.

Sullivan, H. S. (1953). *The interpersonal theory of psychiatry.* New York: Norton.

Thase, M. E., Greenhouse, J. B., Frank, E., Reynolds, C. F. III, Pilkonis, P. A., Hurley, K., et al. (1997). Treatment of major depression with psychotherapy or psychotherapy-pharmacotherapy combinations. *Archives of General Psychiatry, 54*(11), 1009–1015.

Thase, M. E., & Rush, A. J. (1997). When at first you don't succeed: Seguential strategies for antidepressant nonresponders. *Journal of Clinical Psychiatry, 58*(Suppl. 13), 23–29.

Verdeli, H., Clougherty, K., Bolton, P., Speelman, L., Ndogoni, L., Bass, J., et al. (2003). Adapting group interpersonal psychotherapy (IPT-G) for a developing country: Experience in Uganda. *World Psychiatry, 2*, 114–120.

Weissman, M. M., Markowitz, J. C., & Klerman, G. L. (2000). *Comprehensive guide to interpersonal psychotherapy.* New York: Basic Books.

Chapter 9

Plan Analysis

FRANZ CASPAR

Plan Analysis is a method developed to serve as a basis for clinical case conceptualizations and therapy planning. Clinically relevant information about an individual's behavior and experience is gathered through careful observation and synthesized into a meaningful whole. The instrumental perspective and the extent to which it is taken throughout the analysis is a specialty of the approach that stands behind its clinical usefulness and its clarity.

The fundamental questions that guide Plan Analysis are as follows: For what reason does a person behave in a particular way? Or, specifically, which conscious or nonconscious purpose could underlie a particular aspect of an individual's behavior or experience? The focus of Plan Analysis is thus on means–ends or instrumental relations. A patient's instrumental strategies are represented in drawn Plan structures, a visual aid used in practice and research to get an overview of the patient's functioning and thus as a basis for developing case conceptualizations (Figure 9.1).

Plans (based on the definition by Miller, Galanter, & Pribram, 1960) and in some contrast to the colloquial meaning (which is reflected by their capitalized writing of "Plan"), are often not conscious. They are not viewed as real entities in a patient's functioning but rather as constructs in the observers' view. In contrast to the meaning of "plan" in the Mount Zion "Plan Diagnosis" concept (Curtis & Silberschatz, Chapter 7, this volume; Weiss & Sampson, 1986), in the Plan Analysis concept, patients are seen as having many Plans that are independent, complement each other, or are in conflict with each other. In addition, Plans are not only related to what a patient wants in therapy: The whole of a patient's interpersonal and intrapsychic strategies are viewed as a hierarchical structure of Plans. Other

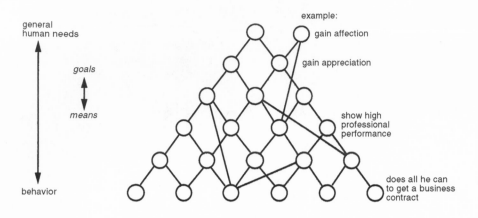

FIGURE 9.1. Schematic Plan structure. Goals or purposes (superordinate elements) are higher in the vertical dimension than the means that serve them (subordinate elements). The lines relate Plans that are in a direct instrumental relation with each other. Elements at the level of behaviors are formulated in the indicative form; Plans in the imperative form.

aspects beyond instrumental strategies, such as cognitions and emotions, are also incorporated in Plan Analysis, but they are approached from and organized by the instrumental structure of Plans. In contrast with other clinical approaches that one-sidedly emphasize either behavioral or motivational aspects, Plan Analysis integrates both into a balanced concept.

Plan Analysis does not claim to be a comprehensive psychological theory. It is rather a pragmatic theoretical approach combined with a concrete methodology. Plan Analysis can be viewed as a set of heuristic rules ready to be used in a more or less complete way. These features—theoretical parsimony and flexible use—along with the inclusion of several aspects each of which are in the foreground of one or the other traditional form of therapy make Plan Analysis an instrument that can be used by therapists with various backgrounds. It is especially useful for therapists emphasizing explicit functional analysis (such as cognitive-behavioral therapists), be it related to interpersonal or intrapsychic functioning, and to the growing group of therapists with an integrative stance, as most of these therapist like to combine concepts as well as techniques on an individual level, and a flexible case conceptualization model which is independent of therapeutic orientations can provide useful guidance in analysis as well as therapy planning. Since the first edition of the Eells case conceptualization reader, the need has rather increased, as in spite of huge progress with empirically supported disorder specific treatments, practitioners feel nevertheless left alone with all the patients who do not fit into one of the diagnostic categories (Beutler et al., 2003), or come with complicating features.

As long as the repertory of possible interventions was limited, case conceptualizations may have been of limited use: It did not make all that much of a difference in the therapeutic procedure. The great range of possible interventions the increasingly integrative therapists can use nowadays needs direction, which they can gain from flexible case conceptualizations. Plan Analysis is perfectly in line with approaches oriented toward principles rather than disorder-specific techniques (Castonguay & Beutler, 2005), although it is also reasonable to use the latter as a part of a more complex therapy. The approach is dedicated to optimizing therapy rather than providing "okay standard" therapy (Beutler et al., 2003), and rather than using quantitative information (like the approach of prescriptive therapy by Beutler & Harwood, 2000), it uses mainly qualitative information to develop a functional understanding of the individual patient. These concepts share the basic orientation and complement each other.

HISTORICAL BACKGROUND OF THE APPROACH

The Plan Analysis approach in its original form (designated "*vertical* behavior analysis" because of the hierarchical analysis of means and goals) was developed around 1976 by Klaus Grawe and Hartmut Dziewas as an aid to better understanding the interactional behavior of patients in behavioral group therapy. Traditional functional behavior analyses (designated "horizontal" because of the characteristic *chains* of stimulus, reaction, consequence, etc.) were too exclusively concentrated on the patient's problems, and they were an insufficient basis for dealing with difficult therapeutic relationships. Therefore, they were increasingly perceived as reductionistic and thus inadequate for the theoretical and clinical understanding of patients' behavior and experience.

Vertical behavior analysis was, however, originally not a comprehensive approach to problem analysis. It explicitly left many questions open, in terms of both theory and practical application. In 1980, Grawe elaborated the relationship between his Plan approach and the information-processing approach. The systematic analysis of emotions, of the patients' problems, and of other parts of the patients' functioning were then elaborated by Caspar (1984). An awareness of the lack of an adequate notion of how *changes* within and outside therapy could be explained and predicted stimulated the development of Klaus Grawe's (1986) *schema theory*. Schema theory is more comprehensive than Plan Analysis in that it includes a theory of change and a model for a heuristic understanding of psychotherapy (see Grawe, Donati, & Bernauer, 1994; Grawe, 2004). Grawe pursued the approach of ever enlarging his approach by including stepwise more concepts (Grawe, 2004) while the Plan Analysis approach was more "conservative" in limiting itself to a minimum of concepts and assumptions immediately needed for an approach of case conceptualizations. For many years, the Plan approach was viewed as a model that was already very powerful in helping therapists understand the phenomena with which they were confronted in therapy, and that would ideally once become so powerful that in most cases it would not need to be supplemented by any other approaches. In the meantime, we emphasize that Plan Analysis should not try to account for everything but, rather, limit itself to the theoretical assumptions and practical heuristics essential to its specific purpose. It should have a clearly defined function for therapists: that is, to deliver a current picture of a patient from a certain perspective, specifically, an instrumental one. Other tasks and perspectives (e.g., the functioning of larger systems) must be brought in by other approaches. Concepts going beyond Plan Analysis were formulated and published in related but separate publications (Caspar, Rothenfluh, & Segal, 1992; Caspar, 1998, 2003; Caspar & Berger, 2006, Caspar, Koch, & Schneider, 2004). The payoff of resistance to the temptation of increasing the approach's power by adding more and more elements is robustness and compatibility with other, complementary approaches and, above all, those therapists have learned before meeting Plan Analysis.

Plan Analysis has roots in, has similarities to, and is compatible with a great number of concepts in the fields of psychotherapy, basic and social psychology, and related domains. The accordance with the state of development of an empirically oriented psychology and the use of its concepts is indeed an identifying characteristic of Plan Analysis, which is worth mentioning here, although space limitations do not allow to make more than a few links explicit in the text that follows.[1] The older Plan Analysis concept is also very compatible with more recent concepts, such as the regulation model by Carver and Scheier (2002; Berger, 2005), which conveys a new understanding of what Plans are all about.

CONCEPTUAL FRAMEWORK

The Therapy Procedure as a Creative Construction Process

Certain rules concerning technique are very general and their application does not differ greatly from patient to patient. Examples are the classical rules of Rogerian therapy. However, the vast majority of intervention techniques available to therapists from the different schools of therapy can only be applied in an efficient manner if they are selected and custom-tailored for a specific patient in a specific situation. The view that a therapist has a repertoire of techniques ready to be applied that can, for example, be described in manuals, is common. Of course, this "application" view includes the concept of adapting the procedure to every individual patient (with some tension resulting between the claims of proceeding in a standardized and in an individually adapted way). We believe that it is more realistic and ultimately more useful to conceptualize the therapeutic procedure not as an application of techniques but rather as a process of continuously constructing anew an individualized procedure to do justice simultaneously to as many relevant factors as possible. Such factors or premises are, as mentioned previously, the individual case conceptualization, general knowledge about disorders and change, knowledge of therapeutic techniques used as prototypes of therapeutic procedure rather than following manuals literally, and professional and private preconditions on the therapist's side. Some of these factors remain stable over time, and thus the procedure with different patients may look similar on the surface. In addition—just as in everyday life—much of the construction process runs in an automated way. Therefore, we may not experience or observe the therapeutic procedure as necessarily always constructing something anew. From a truth point of view, however, a construction perspective is more appropriate than an application view, as can easily be demonstrated by microanalysis of therapists' information processing. In addition, from a pragmatic point of view a construction perspective makes the construction process more accessible to reflection and optimization. One concern must always be that in the "individualized" procedure personal needs of therapists could play a greater role than the needs of the patient in a way which is disadvantageous for the latter. A diligent case conceptualization contributes to maximizing the extent to which the actual needs of a concrete patient and situation are met, and quality controls should monitor process and outcome independent of the therapist's view.

The Elements of Plan Analysis

Plans

Every Plan consists of both a goal or motivational component and the means to reach this goal, or, in other words, an operations component. Plans are structured in a hierarchical fashion. One Plan can instrumentally serve another Plan, that is, the former is hierarchically subordinated to the latter. The criterion is—although the two criteria overlap—not abstraction (as in Horowitz et al., 2006) but instrumentality. A superordinate Plan determines the goal component of a subordinate Plan, which in turn serves as the means for the superordinate Plan. Human behavior can be understood as the attempt to fulfill one's most important basic needs in a given, but also changeable, environment. The hierarchical structure of Plans is equivalent to the sum of conscious and nonconscious, interpersonal, and intrapsychic strategies an individual has developed throughout his or her life to this end (Gasiet, 1981). While it is assumed that in principle, all individuals have the same basic needs, the weight of Plans varies from person to person and situation to situation.

The regulation of behavior is largely not conscious. Not conscious we mean in a neutral, everyday language sense rather than in a psycho-analytical sense of the unconscious. Given the limited capacity for conscious information processing, it would be impossible to consider the large number of premises or constraints relevant in most situations without nonconscious control. Especially the regulation of nonverbal behavior is largely nonconscious. The automated parts of social behavior are seldom incorporated in the self-concept, or, more specifically, in subjective explanations an individual gives for his or her behavior, especially for problematic aspects. In an approach that seeks to do justice to the person as a whole and to support his or her further development, access to the less conscious parts of behavior regulation is especially important: A professional therapist should, of course, not only deal with a patient's self-concept but also with what Grawe (1986) designates the actually "regulating self." Concretely speaking, this involves above all observing and interpreting nonverbal as well as verbal behavior in a systematic fashion and relating emotions to the Plan structure.

It is typical for Plan structures that each superordinate element (goal) of some importance has several subordinate elements (means), given that suitable means never have a perfect and guaranteed effect (especially in the interpersonal domain). Therefore, one usually combines several means or strategies simultaneously or sequentially; depending on only one strategy to achieve an important goal leads to fragile functioning and is one factor contributing to psychopathology (see below). It is also typical for Plan structures that means serve multiple goals. Usually behaviors or Subplans are not developed to serve one Plan at a time but to do justice to as many Plans and other constraints as possible. This principle, represented by multiple lines going from one Subplan to several superordinate Plans, is designated "multiple determination." The degree to which a person succeeds creatively integrating several Plans in one behavior or subordinate strategy is one factor determining mental health.

It is practical and helps develop an overview of the entire functioning if elements such as emotions and cognitions are also viewed and integrated from an instrumental perspective. For example, the idea (cognition) "I need to be perfect," which would be a typical element of cognitive case conceptualizations (Persons, 1989; Persons & Tompkins, Chapter 10, this volume) can be embedded in a person's functioning in many ways. It may represent a desperate wish of finally getting others' attention and appreciation, because as a perfect being one simply deserves this, it may represent resistance of a depressed patient against trying out less than perfect solutions which could lead to new disappointment, and so forth. Whether and how the idea "I need to be perfect" should be treated depends, of course, on a valid view of the deeper meaning of the idea.

Emotions

Emotions are an important aspect in an individual's functioning, and in psychotherapy it is of particular importance to develop a sound understanding of why emotions arise in particular situations. Plan Analysis incorporates a pragmatic approach that is in line with several psychological approaches conceptualizing emotion as their central target and, of course, in much greater detail. There are theories differentiating between feelings, emotions, and affects according to the criterion of consciousness. In contrast, Plan Analysis views the extent to which an emotion is conscious on a continuum from conscious to nonconscious. At a closer look, usually some *parts* or *aspects* of an emotion are rather conscious, others not conscious. One may, for example, be aware of the trigger of a particular emotion, but not of the emotion itself, or vice versa. Thus we do not systematically distinguish between categories of emotion. In our context it is also not fruitful to differentiate between so-called basic emotions and derived emotions but, rather, to maintain a broad understanding of what an emotion is. This perspective is supported by similar positions in general psychology (e.g., Ortony, Clore, & Foss, 1987) and clinical psychology (Greenberg & Safran, 1987), and by our experience in analyzing concrete situations. In the Plan Analysis conceptualization of emotions there is equal room for "basic" emotions, such as "sad" or "happy," "cognitive" emotions such as "upset," "action-oriented" emotions such as "vigorous," and "physiological" emotions such as "dizzy."

In the analysis of individual cases, emotions are approached in terms of their relations to instrumental Plans, of which a *direct* instrumental function of an emotion is only one possibility. Four aspects are considered: (1) which Plans are blocked or threatened (when negative emotions arise), (2) which additional Plans determine the nature of the emotion that actually develops, (3) which Plans serve to overcome and deal with emotions, and finally, (4) for which Plans the emotion itself has possibly an instrumental function.

Blocked/Favored Plans. We assume that negative emotions, such as fear, anger, shame, and sadness, usually arise when important Plans are threatened or blocked (in essence, "threatened" and "blocked" stand for the same concept, but usually one or the other term is more appropriate depending on the concreteness of the threat and other factors). As long as a person is able to act according to his or her most important Plans, there is no significant arousal. A person becomes (negatively) aroused when Plans are blocked or threatened, or (positively) when new opportunities arise to pursue important Plans (favored Plans). Central aspects of an individual's self-concept and view of the world play an important role in the individual's functioning and thus can be viewed from an instrumental perspective. Therefore, having experiences incompatible with one's previous experience and self-concept also represents a form of threatening or blockage. If a threat causes strong emotions one may assume that important Plans are involved and that alternatives within the existing structure that could be readily applied are lacking and cannot be developed easily. This approach is in line with the concepts by Mandler (1979) and Lazarus and his colleagues (Lazarus, 1966; Lazarus, Kanner, & Folkman, 1972).

For example, to be sick before an exam brings about stronger emotional reactions depending on whether a success in the exam stands for important Plans (to finally finish one's studies, get a well-paid job, satisfy one's father's expectations, etc.) or whether alternatives are available (exam at a later date, alternatives to finishing studies in this particular field, etc.).

The threat or blockage may consist in a restriction in one's ability to act due to a change in the environment, a loss of individual abilities (due to aging, illness, or as a result of strong emotions), or the loss of important persons or objects. A threat can also stem from an individual's Plan structure itself, for example, when Plans conflict with each other. More concretely, this means that a behavior serving one Plan has negative side effects on another Plan. All actions, after all, have positive and negative side effects beyond the primarily intended effect. A threat may be linked to a concrete situation, or it may be diffuse and of a long-term nature. An example of the latter would be when a basic need is neglected over a long period of time due to the lifestyle a person has chosen. The notion of conflicts as resulting from side effects on other Plans is clinically extremely powerful, as it brings conflicts "out of the clouds" of the abstract down to a very concrete level: looking into a drawn (partial) Plan structure, therapist and patient can trace directly which side effect of which Subplan has negative consequences for which other Plan, why this strategy is used in spite of the side effects (third Plans excluding more adaptive alternatives?), what more adaptive alternatives could be developed in therapy, and so on.

A threat need not exist objectively. It is the *subjective experience* of threat which matters. Thus a single situational cue, which was impressed on an individual, can trigger a sense of threat in a situation that objectively speaking is not threatening at all (classical conditioning). Or, an interpretation may be distorted (as emphasized by cognitive approaches). The appraisal of threat need not be conscious. In many cases, a Plan Analysis can help the therapist and patient understand which specific Plans were threatened, resulting in emotional reactions the patient could not previously understand.

In making these assumptions, our concept does not follow the therapeutic approaches that assume emotions are "postcognitive," that is, that emotions are caused by a series of cognitive operations in a narrow sense. In particular, by emphasizing analogous (in particular nonverbal) communication, the Plan Analysis approach is highly compatible with the approach represented by Zajonc (1980) and more recently Damasio (1995) in which emotional reactions can be much faster than cognitive appraisal. With the assumption that the blocked Plans are usually Plans of an interpersonal nature, the Plan Analysis approach is in agreement with Averill's (1980) theory of emotion given its emphasis on the social dimension. Plan Analysis allows us to trace in detail, how complex emotions develop in the individual patient in a given context over time, be it over years or splits of a second (Scherer, 2001).

Positive emotions develop in a converse manner to negative emotions (i.e., when situations or perceptions arise that are favorable for important Plans). Positive emotions are given less attention here than negative ones, not because such emotions or psychological well-being in general are less important but, rather, because Plan Analysis is a method for developing an understanding of the current state of *patients*, and in this context a detailed understanding of negative emotions is of particular importance.

There are two reasons why the concept of threat or blockage is of special significance in understanding emotions within the context of therapy. First, patients come to therapy when they have come into an impasse, that is, when they are confronted with a blockage or many blockages. Such situations—with some typical exceptions—are accompanied by strong negative emotions, and in therapy one wants to understand these emotions and relate them to the concrete blocking situation. In addition, the extent of inconsistencies due to conflicts between Plans and a reality that is not in line with a person's Plans is directly related to psychopathological states (Grosse Holtforth & Grawe, 2003; Grawe, 2004). Second, the therapy situation is characterized as a situation in which the therapist repeatedly gives impulses that are disturbing for the patient because he or she cannot (and is not supposed to) integrate them easily without adapting his or her structures. This incompatibility between the therapist's interventions and the patient's existing structures has been extensively discussed under the theme of "resistance" (Caspar & Grawe, 1981). Based on Piaget's (1977) assimilation–accommodation concept, Grawe (1986) views this focused disturbing function as a major change factor in therapy. In line with this perspective, some negative emotions arising during therapy are viewed as unavoidable.

Plans Shaping the Emotion. The aspect of threatening or blocking captures, however, only one factor in the development of negative and positive emotions. Which particular emotion arises in response to a threatening or blocking situation may depend on further Plans. For example, if the character of the situation would suggest aggressive emotions (e.g., a patient's mother-in-law restricts the patient's rights in a domineering manner), such emotions may be prevented by aggression-avoiding Plans. This increases the likelihood of other negative emotions, such as anxiety. There may even be a complete lack of conscious emotion, with tensions being expressed in psychosomatic symptoms. At times the type of threat already suggests a specific emotional reaction. Usually, however, a certain range of emotional reactions is possible. Here one sees the tremendous—often culture-specific—influence of previous experience in handling emotions.

Coping Plans. Another aspect of the relation between Plans and emotions is the obvious tendency to avoid negative emotions and seek positive ones. Most human activities could be understood from this perspective. If a negative emotion actually exists or is anticipated, usually a person activates more or less adaptive Plans in order to remove or prevent it. These coping strategies may aim at the source of the disturbance; that is, the person may try to remove the source of the threat. These would be the most thorough strategies. Examples are completing work that has caused sleepless nights, looking for new friends when one is depressed due to a loss, or if the threat has arisen internally due to conflicts between Plans, trying to develop an understanding of one's conflicts through therapy. Frequently skills and abilities must be acquired and anxieties must be decreased in therapy before adequate coping activities become possible.

Unfortunately, it is not always possible to remove the disturbance at its source. For example, the threat of losing one's job during an economic depression, terminal illness, or technical and natural disasters cannot simply be averted by the individual. In such cases, palliative coping behavior aimed at dealing with the negative emotions themselves may be necessary. Depending on the situation, it may be more efficient to face the emotion directly or to limit one's awareness of the emotion, up to and including the extreme of complete repression.

Coping and avoidance strategies can be a large part of human activity. If this is the case (as often with severely troubled patients) most coping plans are not oriented toward concrete threats and emotions related to them but, rather, toward protecting "sore spots." It is plausible that these avoidance strategies originally developed from concrete situations in which Plans were threatened and blocked. Early sore spots are probably related to the threat of losing one's primary caregivers or at least of losing their love and attention and the ensuing threats of shame and embarrassment. In the adult, however, these sore spots, and the avoidance strategies related to them, have become independent from the conditions under which they developed and manifest themselves in determining behavior directly.

Positive emotions are not avoided but rather sought out, or so one would think. Although this is true in general, if one examines the matter more carefully one realizes that for almost everyone, certain situations, which in general would elicit positive emotions at best elicit ambivalent emotions. A generalized fear of being dragged along by positive emotions may be present: Doing well in exams means doing better than others, which may be taboo; completing professional training may lead to insecurity about the future; an increase in the importance of a relationship may activate anxieties surrounding the possible loss of the partner or of one's own autonomy. Weiss and Sampson (1986; Curtis & Silberschatz, Chapter 7, this volume) have elaborated the idea of guilt and fear developing from positive developments in a way that is highly compatible with Plan Analysis—which is, by the way, just one example of how concepts of different origin can be referred to and used when using Plan Analysis.

Plans for Which the Emotion Has an Instrumental Function. Finally emotions themselves, or facts related to emotions, may have an instrumental function within the Plan structure of an individual. To begin with, they may have the general function of supporting behavior. It is, for example, difficult to withdraw from a source of conflict if one is full of energy. This is much easier if one is powerless, anxious, or depressed. It is difficult to approach other people if one is not in an appropriate mood or able to bring oneself into such a mood. An illustration of this are socially anxious patients who can only assert themselves when they succeed in entering a state of rage beforehand. This example shows once more how inseparably linked intrapsychic and interactional functions are. In this case we see how rage energizes and removes doubts (intrapsychic) and at the same time enhances expressive behavior likely to impress others (interactional).

Many examples could be given of how anxious emotions support and justify avoidance behavior, depressive emotions support and justify depressive withdrawal, rage supports and justifies aggressive behavior, and so forth. This direct instrumental function of emotions is so common that it is only given explicit consideration in a Plan Analysis when it helps to explain a specific observation.

Another frequently observed function of emotions is the *interactional* impact they may have when they are expressed. The attention agoraphobics often get as a result of their anxiety is a classic example of the instrumental reinforcement of a particular disorder. A depressed mood can have a similar impact, depending on the interactional system. Showing hostile nervousness can cause another person to back off and maintain greater distance after having come too close. An example of a concrete *intrapsychic* function is the paralyzing effect of anxiety or depressive states, justifying the avoidance of a conflict tat seems unsolvable (divorce from a suicidal partner, coming out of an aging homosexual teacher in a conservative rural community, etc.). Generally, elaborate coping strategies are developed when emotions are or would be strong and lasting, and instrumental functions have particularly to be considered when an emotion lasts in spite of obvious negative effects.

These are the most important aspects of the relation between emotions and Plans. Readers especially familiar with one emotion theory or another can take the basic ideas presented here as a point of departure. Obviously, such readers will be able to consider different aspects in a much more sophisticated way than would be possible without the specific knowledge they have. In spite of some limitations in the Plan Analysis conceptualization of emotion, we should emphasize that in our experience, considering the aspects presented earlier, it is usually possible to understand the emotions relevant in therapy adequately. Beyond this general experience, a specific argument in favor of our approach is the emphasis in Plan Analysis on a careful analysis of instrumental and reactive *nonverbal behavior*, and its relation to motivation. This is of special importance given that emotions are often only expressed nonverbally in subtle ways. The analysis of emotion has been given much space in this chapter because (1) understanding and dealing with emotions is a cornerstone in every psychotherapy, and (2) the issue exemplifies how Plan Analysis in spite of its emphasis on instrumental relations is not limited to the analysis of overt instrumental behavior.

Disorders

In the view of Plan Analysis, disorders may have a *direct instrumental function*. That is, they have been developed and/or are maintained by an intrapsychic or interpersonal advantage they have in the functioning of a person. Of course, such an advantage is usually not conscious, and often it is hidden by the obvious disadvantages and a patient's subjective suffering. For example, one patient's painful and frightening panic attacks hypothetically served the purpose of distracting from unbearable grief related to neglect by his mother. Initially successful symptom-oriented therapy ran against diffuse resistance of a generally very cooperative patient, but panic disappeared after a phase of opening up to and treating grief.

An individual analysis of Plans lays out the whole of a person's instrumental strategies and helps find points at which instrumental hypotheses make sense without prematurely pressing the patient into a single hypothesis. Common examples, which are, of course, known to therapists of various orientations, are agoraphobias obliging a partner to stay home, psychosomatic disorders providing an acceptable reason to withdraw from an overdemanding job, compulsive behavior reducing diffuse anxiety, and so on. Whereas such hypotheses can easily be applied to a patient without preceding Plan Analysis, questions such as "under what conditions will a patient be able to give up using this problem as part of a strategy" require more diligent analysis, and often we are actually surprised by a disorder not having the "common" instrumental function. Caspar (1987, 2000), for example, describes a case in which agoraphobic anxiety and depression does not serve to bind a partner but, rather, to paralyze the powerful patient's strong but subjectively extremely threatening wish for a divorce from her violent husband.

In sum, disorders can sometimes but not generally be viewed as having an instrumental function, which often develops later in a pathogenic process. If they do not have an instrumental function, it does not mean that they are independent of an individual's instrumental strategies. Often they are *side effects* of instrumental strategies. For example, when people withdraw from subjectively threatening situations, this represents typical avoidance, which characterizes anxiety disorders often more than actual feelings of anxiety in the present, and often avoidance and withdrawal also lead to a loss of active behaviors and positive experiences, which is typical for depressive disorders. The depression may or may not have an instrumental function in itself; mainly, it must be seen as a consequence of the avoidance and withdrawal which seem to have an instrumental function. Even if strategies one-sidedly determining an individual's life do not serve only obvious avoidance goals (e.g., when a person works excessively), there is a high risk of neglecting important needs and overstraining oneself, with all kinds of well-known consequences.

The more situations activate a person's Plans serving to protect sore spots and the less flexible the Plan structure is in the sense of enclosing only few alternatives, the more the few available Plans are also used when they have strong negative side effects, and the higher the probability that not many situations and domains remain in which the person can have positive experiences. Plans are often executed in the sense of poor "more-of-the-same" strategies, not because they are effective but, rather, because they are not, in the absence of more effective alternatives: If an individual has sound strategies to reach a goal, they can be eased once the effect is there. It is the inability to reach a positive stable state that causes the individual to continue with the available strategies despite the fact that they are ineffective and full of side effects.

Although there may be very rigid and poorly developed structures for which it is hard to imagine an environment in which they would function free of troubles, the interactionistic view of Plan Analysis suggests always viewing problems as an interaction of individual structures and situations that need to be mastered (though situations usually do not occur independent of an individual's Plan structures, the development as well as the interpretation of a situation strongly depends on the structure!). There may be structures enabling an individual to master a broad range of difficult situations or tasks coming up in a lifespan, but there is no such a thing as a "perfect structure." This is illustrated by posttraumatic stress disorders: Although some individuals seem to be superior to others in overcoming even extreme traumata, there are probably traumatic impacts that would be too severe for any individual.

It is therefore the task of a therapist not to superimpose simplistic concepts of pathogenesis to individuals but to trace how it was possible that a disorder has developed with the given structural and situational preconditions and their interaction. We do not strive for an impressively *complex* analysis but for a *useful* basis for producing ideas of what could be done therapeutically and for guessing what individual effects (including resistance) can be expected from any one intervention.

Although the Plan analysis of disorders is typically very individualized and takes a great deal of individual data into account, existing etiological and therapeutic concepts from various origins can and should be used to the advantage of the patient, as exemplified with "prototypical" Plan Structures for depression, anxiety, and psychosomatic disorders in Caspar (1995). For example, the understanding of a patient's depression can be furthered by Lewinsohn's (1974) loss of reinforcement theory, Seligman's (1975) learned helplessness approach, Beck, Rush, Shaw, and Emery's (1979) concept of dysfunctional thinking, Klerman, Weissman, Rounsaville, and Chevron's (1984) interpersonal approach, psychodynamic concepts of avoiding overt aggression, and systemic concepts. Typically it depends on the individual case how much any one concept can contribute, and usually it is by combining concepts, often complemented by ideas developed for a specific patient, that a sufficiently comprehensive view is gained.

Overall, the disorder concept of Plan Analysis is very open and individual. The primary reason for a disorder may be in the past, it may be in the present, it may be intrapsychic or interpersonal. Typically, in Plan Analysis one does not one-sidedly focus on *"the"* cause but considers different causal factors operating at different points. It is normally the interaction of these factors that brings about and maintains a problem. The price for this (supposedly more veridical) view is that normally it yields more complex case conceptualizations. The payoff is that usually it also yields several points at which therapeutic change can be brought about: It gives a therapist—specifically one whose repertoire is not limited by the restrictions of one specific school of therapy—a broader range of possibilities in comparison to most approaches of which we are aware (Grawe, Caspar, & Ambühl, 1990; Grawe, 2004; see also below).

This section on the conceptual framework of Plan Analysis should not be concluded without mentioning the vision of "second-generation theories" by Grawe (Grawe, Donati, & Bernauer, 1994). Grawe designates theories of psychopathology and therapy that are available today as "first-generation theories": They have been developed based on a limited range of empirical observations which are usually selected for their consistency with a particular theory. In contrast, second-generation theories should be in line with all empirical findings relevant to the domain for which validity of the theory is claimed. For example, a theory of anxiety therapy should include concepts explaining why anxiety is often diminished by exposure, but it would be incomplete without referring to the fact that anxiety can also be treated without exposure (as proven, for example, by client-centered therapy). The goal is thus to strive for a comprehensive "general psychotherapy" (Grawe, 2004) without disadvantageous *a priori* limitations.

INCLUSION/EXCLUSION CRITERIA
AND MULTICULTURAL CONSIDERATIONS

Plan Analysis is a flexible approach leaving much space for concentration or emphasis on the aspects which are of particular interest to the user, including cultural aspects. With the inclusion of verbal and nonverbal channels of communication, whatever expresses something relevant (e.g., clothing, status symbols, and subtle nonverbal cues) can be included in the analysis. The concept gives much weight to the environment in which a Plan structure develops: Desired effects as well as undesired effects of behaviors depend on the cultural environment. It also determines which assumptions about oneself and others are correct and adaptive, which emotions are acceptable, which resources a person has, what behaviors are conspicuous or not, and so on. A therapist who is familiar with a (sub)culture can more easily recognize what is special for a particular patient and needs attention. Information on cultural aspects can be made explicit in the structure itself ("avoid conflicts with father's cultural norms"), in additional "frames," which can be used like footnotes, or in the written case conceptualization. Halcour (1997) has used the method to compare problem solving in different cultures, Schütz (1992) to analyze politicians' self-presentation in the American and the German cultures.

Plan Analysis, as stated previously, has originally been developed to understand the patterns of interactional behavior of patients in group therapy. With later developments it became an approach that is generally suited to support an understanding of instrumental aspects of human functioning, whether intrapsychic or interpersonal, related or unrelated to the problems that brought a patient into therapy, or related to psychotherapeutic or other relationships. Although the instrumental structure is emphasized, other elements, such as preconditions ("the world is always on the edge, and I must harmonize to avoid the catastrophy") and consequences of instrumental functions, or other parts of patterns (such as states of mind; Horowitz, 1979; Horowitz & Eells, Chapter 5, this volume), are included in the analysis, and often their role becomes clearer when embedded in a functional analysis. Although the emphasis is on the present structure, there can—depending on the case—be greater emphasis on trying to understand how the structure originally developed, and to what extent the preconditions under which this development took place have changed, opening up new possibilities for the future (see below).

Unless there are severe incompatibilities with a few fundamental assumptions (e.g., that behavior can occur without conscious control, or that behaviors with some kind of advantage in the survival have a higher probability of surviving and generalizing), the general Plan Analysis approach can easily be combined with other existing concepts specialized for a specific type of disorder or group of clients. At this point it seems fair to state that the approach has its potential wherever interpersonal and intrapsychic conscious and not conscious strategies need to be understood, given that the instrumental aspect is always a central if not the most central key to an understanding of such strategies.

Instrumental strategies play a role for the (relatively) healthy person (e.g., in the self-therapy of a therapy trainee), for those who have traditionally been designated "neurotically disturbed" patients, but also for psychotic patients or people with a state strongly determined by an obviously physical handicap, be it in the genes, the brain or other parts of the body (e.g., after an accident). A problem is never a complete explanation for a patient's state, but there are always complicating or alleviating interpersonal factors, more or less appropriate coping strategies, and so on, that determine to a large extent whether a patient has reached the best possible adaptation or is in an impasse that makes him or her look for therapeutic support. The biological basis of healthy as well as pathological functioning can never be seen in isolation, and influences always go several ways (Caspar, 2003; Caspar et al., 2004).

Some disorders that are presently among the more difficult ones for psychotherapy, such as personality disorders, clearly have a strong interpersonal component, and there is a great potential for the use of Plan Analysis in this domain. Therapists of patients with DSM Axis I disorders and comorbid, "ego-syntonic" personality disorders need to deal with challenges for the therapeutic relationship originating in personality disorders or accentuations, and this is home ground for Plan Analysis and its concept of complementarity. Cognitive concepts like the schema approach by Young (1994) are easily compatible with Plan Analysis, which can use preformulated schema contents of particular personality disorders to complement the more individualized, inductive approach of Plan Analysis. Finally, one does not need to be sick in the sense of the classical psychiatric disorders to take advantage of a Plan Analytical reflection of one's instrumental functioning in its adaptive as well as maladaptive aspects. Therefore, the approach is also very useful in the own therapy of therapists in training and in nonclinical contexts.

Until recently, Plan Analysis has been broadly used in the therapy of anxiety, depression, and psychosomatic disorders, and to some extent in obsessive–compulsive disorders and addictions. Colleagues have used it in other domains, such as work with children (Schonauer, 1992; Klemenz, 1999). The analysis of cultural differences (Halcour, 1997) or self-presentation of politicians (Schütz, 1992) has already been mentioned. In an experimental study, Schmitt, Kammerer, and Holtmann (2003) have shown that the use of Plan Analysis in the training of medical doctors improves their ability to get along with patients on a relationship level. Because the approach is so general and compatible with more specific approaches, it is hard to see a limitation for its use. If there are limitations, they come from a utility perspective—that is, whether it is actually necessary to do a detailed individual analysis of every new case of agoraphobia, for example. It is true that many insights can be transferred from "the typical" agoraphobic to a new agoraphobic patient. But it is also true that if one takes a closer look, a "standard" agoraphobic often has some surprising peculiarities that are crucial for successful therapy, in particular if therapy is not limited to alleviating the main complaint but also to making a patient happier and more resistant to relapses.

With limited resources, comprehensive individual analyses may be reserved for a select group of different patients. It is, however, often not easy to know in advance when a comprehensive analysis pays and when it does not. With respect to this question of maximizing usefulness, another advantage of Plan Analysis is relevant, namely, the possibility of flexibly adapting the level of resolution to specific domains in a patient's functioning (see below), and developing a concept of the *problems* within the same framework as the concept of the *therapeutic relationship*. Plan Analysis is not a method that is either applied or not but, rather, a set of heuristic rules of which a larger or more narrow selection can be applied to a patient or a part of his or her total functioning. Thus, even in settings in which a comprehensive case conceptualization would be a luxury (e.g., in a psychiatric emergency unit), some heuristic rules from Plan Analysis can be used (e.g., in establishing a good alliance).

Exclusion criteria are related rather to therapists than to patients. Although good Plan Analyses require sound clinical intuition in many parts of the procedure, the method also requires (besides intuition) some rational-analytic thinking. Even when combined with a great deal of creativity, some therapists are not keen on disciplined reasoning, and a few seem to be unable to handle complexity mentally. An additional difficulty for therapists who like simple truths, as provided by dogmatic schools of psychotherapy, seems to be in accepting a constructivist perspective. On the other hand, therapists who are tired of dogmatic or simplistic approaches find rich and rewarding possibilities of working toward an individualized understanding of their patients, even of difficult aspects of their functioning.

STEPS IN CASE FORMULATION

General Comments

The richness of available technical advice for flexibly and individually inferring Plans and developing Plan Analysis case conceptualizations is a distinguished property of the approach. The technique of inferring Plans has been developed in much more detail than could possibly be described here (Caspar, 1995). Nevertheless, the most important principles can be briefly summarized.

The procedure varies depending on the purpose of the analysis. Whereas the research procedure is necessarily somewhat more systematic (see Caspar, 1995), the procedure in everyday practice can, within certain limits, be flexibly adapted to suit individual needs and preferences. Plan Analysis is a heuristic approach by nature. A step-by-step description in an algorithmic sense would make a first application easier; it would, however, be counter to the nature of the approach. The advantages of a heuristic approach become obvious very quickly. Experiences from past analyses can be used in subsequent ones, and psychotherapists become increasingly efficient. We emphasize that Plan Analyses should always be very individual. The use of standard elements (as they are used in other approaches) is discouraged because from our point of view the risk of jeopardizing individual fit und thus usefulness in favor of speed and easy comparability is too great (Caspar, 1988). That analysis does not need to start from scratch but may build on existing concepts, such as schemas typical for particular disorders (e.g., Young, 1997), or prototypical Plans, has been mentioned earlier.

Because the graphical representation of instrumental Plan structures are such a characteristic part of Plan Analysis it may be necessary to emphasize that such a structure is only an intermediate step: The crucial product is a case conceptualization which is based on an analysis of Plans but could, if need be, be completely formulated without explicitly referring to the Plan construct. The typical elements of such a case conceptualization are described later along with a case example.

Information Used in the Process of Inferring Plans

In Plan Analysis, all kinds of information can and should be used. The following sources are normally the most important ones:

- Observations inside or outside therapy
- Patients' reports about their behavior and about events inside and outside therapy
- Patients' introspective reports about their experiences and thoughts, including fantasies and daydreams
- Effects of the patients' behavior on interaction partners (therapist and observers, group members in group therapy, and interaction partners outside therapy), including thoughts, emotions, and behavior tendencies stimulated in them
- Questionnaires
- Reports by relatives, friends, nurses, members of a therapy group, etc.

It is typical of Plan Analysis to give much weight to directly observable information, and particularly to instrumental and reactive *nonverbal behavior*. Clearly, a comprehensive yet practically manageable case conceptualization needs to concentrate on the conspicuous, that is, on information that can be expected to be informative for the individual case.

As stated previously, it is assumed that only parts of an individual's functioning are conscious. The range of the searchlight making parts of one's own functioning conscious is limited by nature, and its range is further restricted by a tendency to protect "sore spots." Therefore, introspective reports often provide significant information, but many aspects of a patient's functioning are not accessible to him- or herself. Information provided by the patient is never directly used but always needs to be evaluated: Can it be used directly as true information (patient says: "I believe I am attractive to this woman because I am reliable," analysis: "show yourself as reliable" serves the plan "make yourself attractive") or does the statement need to be interpreted further (e.g., with respect to its function in the therapeutic alliance: "let the therapist know you are reliable," or with respect to the self-concept: "sticks to his view of being reliable" serves the Plan "maintain the self-concept of being an attractive person")?

Basics of Inferring Plans

Normally a Plan hypothesis develops based on several observations. For example, "the misbehavior of this child could serve the Plan of getting the mother's attention: It is more frequent when she is busy with other things, and the child gets upset when the Plan is blocked by continued attention to competing tasks."

Helpful questions in the process of inferring Plans are:

- What emotions and impressions does the patient trigger in me and in others?
- How does the patient want me and others to be? What does the patient want me or others to do?
- What image of him- or herself does the patient try to convey to me and others?
- What image of him- or herself does the patient try to attain or maintain for him- or herself?
- What behavior of mine or others in this situation would not feel right or would be difficult for me or others to do or accomplish. What behavior of mine or others does the patient try to prevent?

The answers to all these questions are, of course, only hypothetical. As a next step one should look for confirming, disconfirming, or differentiating information. Related to the aforementioned example, one could ask:

"Does the child also show the same misbehavior with other people, always with the mother, or only in certain types of situations?"

In practice, there are four general ways to infer Plans:

- From one behavior one infers a Plan directly and subsequently examines whether other observed behaviors confirm this hypothesis, or one searches for such confirming (or differentiating) behavior.
- One looks for a common denominator in several behaviors, infers a Plan, and then looks for further substantiating behaviors.
- One infers a Plan from the patient's impact on an interaction partner, looks for the means by which the patient causes this impact, and then seeks further substantiating behavior.
- Plans are inferred from the traces they leave in a patient's reactions (e.g., in emotions when a Plan is blocked).
- Plans are inferred from the top down, in contrast to the bottom-up procedure in the other four ways of inferring Plans. One asks oneself, for example, "How does this patient satisfy his or her need for such and such?" This search direction complements the common bottom-up search and is especially useful for finding *deficit* domains in a patient's Plan structure.

It is important to include aspects that represent strengths and resources of a patient, and to pay attention to how the individual structure is interlocked with the functioning of a patient's environment. For the former it is helpful that the concept of Plan Analysis in no way suggests an a priori emphasis on the problematic parts. Plan Analysis is an especially good means of showing how problematic parts can be viewed as related to generally well-functioning parts, and how even problematic parts enclose positive elements that can be used and furthered. As far as the functioning of an individual in his or her environment is concerned, the compatibility of the approach with systemic approaches due to the shared instrumental view is a special advantage.

Formulation

Plans should be formulated as individually characterizing as possible. Often idiosyncratic terms used by the patient him- or herself can help to develop a very distinctive structure. We recommend formulating the label of behaviors in the indicative form (e.g., "tells others about his initiative for the homeless"), and Plans in the form of an imperative directed toward oneself (e.g., "gain other people's appreciation"). The former indicates that at present one does not intend to break down the respective behavior into components (Subplans), the latter helps avoid involuntarily including noninstrumental elements. For example, "anxiety" in this form would not be a proper element of a Plan structure; it should be formulated in such a way that its position in the structure becomes more obvious (e.g., "maintain anxiety"—serving the Plan of keeping the husband at home—or "cope with anxiety"—with the means of excessive drinking). The imperative form is not meant to suggest conscious awareness for the respective part of one's functioning.

The Process of Inferring Plans

The process of inferring Plans extends over the whole course of therapy, never really completed. Interventions are always based on a provisional understanding. Nevertheless, the first few minutes in therapy are often very informative because patients try to shape the interactional situation in line with their dominant interactional needs, in the sense of Argyle's (1969) interactional problem solving. Following (or with increasing routine, even during) a well-conducted intake interview, it is usually possible to infer the Plans that are most important for custom-tailoring the therapeutic relationship. This part of therapy planning has the greatest priority in the beginning of a therapy, and it is pivotal because many therapies that stall in the initial phase do so as a result of a poor therapeutic relationship.

As stated earlier, the level of resolution can be flexibly adapted in different parts of the patient's functioning. For example, if "perfectionism" is conspicuous but not considered very important, it may be represented in only one Plan without consuming further space and attention, whereas it may be addressed extensively when considered important. Often an issue is first represented in a simple way and differentiated in more detail later on when its importance becomes obvious, or if the range of validity of a Plan needs to be specified.

Concepts from various sources (from common sense to traditional learning theories, psychodynamic ideas, etc.) can be used as a source of ideas of how the individual elements of an individual's functioning may be interrelated. In any case, theoretical concepts should be used in such a way that a given idea makes immediate sense in the individual case conceptualization. For example, Willis's (1982) "collusion" concept can be useful, but the psychoanalytic concepts have to hold for the individual patient using common sense.

The process of analyzing Plans may appear predominantly rational-analytic, especially when describing explicit practical rules. It is indeed desirable for obvious reasons that as great a part of the process as possible should be rational and explicit. On the other hand, when one endeavors to process raw information and fit it together in such a way that a meaningful model of an individual patient develops as a basis for a therapy which goes beyond the surface, it must be acknowledged that intuitive processes unavoidably come in. They play an especially important role in the steps of "framing" the raw information, creatively speculating about possible instrumental functions, and judging whether an elaborated case conceptualization actually captures what is the essence of a case from an intuitive point of view. Rational-analytic and intuitive processing should be combined in such a way that they complement and control each other.

Of course, the search and collection of data and the inference of Plans are normally not neutral from the outset. They are determined by the therapist's schemas or hypotheses and many other factors limiting or enhancing access to and processing of information. However, if one follows the rules of always supplying several concrete pieces of evidence for each hypothesis, of remaining curious concerning the unexpected, and of paying attention to possible biases and honestly engaging in openness, severe distortions can usually be avoided; early explicit hypotheses tend to help reveal rather than hide what is not in line with them. Plan Analysis, as all comparable approaches, always moves between the Scylla of being overinterpretive and inappropriately projecting concepts onto a patient and the Charybdis of not taking clinically important factors into account, based on a reluctance to engage in deeper interpretations. There is no way of minimizing the risk of one type of erring without increasing the risk of the other. By following the foregoing rules and by always being aware of the risk of erring, and of the degree to which one has chosen to be interpretive in a concrete analysis, errors can be kept within an acceptable range. In a research context, interjudge agreement has repeatedly been checked and turned out to be satisfactory to good. If it turns out in the course of therapy that predictions based on the case conceptualization (among others about the effects of interventions derived from the case conceptualization) are correct (or not), such observations cannot validate or invalidate a conceptualization in a strict sense but are a contribution to correcting at least obvious errors.

APPLICATION TO PSYCHOTHERAPY TECHNIQUE

Plan Analysis is supposed to provide a picture of the present functioning of a patient, including some insight into how a structure has developed and what the potential for the future is. For example, it can be worked out that the state of helplessness and dependence, in which a particular structure has been developed, no longer exists objectively. In other cases threats that prevented the development of important parts of a healthy structure no longer exist, and so on. Based on such a case conceptualization, the therapist determines what parts need to change in order to increase the chances for solving the obvious problems and eventually leading to a more satisfactory life overall. For example, one could emphasize the need of furthering insight into some aspects of one's own functioning to increase the degree of freedom from old patterns; one could emphasize the need for acquiring skills to make it more probable that a difficult situation will be mastered; or one could emphasize the need to work through particular emotions to minimize the need of avoiding such emotions in the future.

Normally several prototypical procedures of various origin promise to lead to the same main effect. For example, emotions can be stimulated and worked through by Gestalt two-chair techniques, by client-centered working out the emotional content of what a patient reports, or by behavioral exposure and subsequent discussion of the experiences. Obviously, all possible procedures have positive and negative side effects determining to a large extent the overall effect of therapy. For example, one of the procedures may, in addition to dealing with an emotion, further insight; another may enhance self-efficacy expectations; another may instead stress the therapeutic alliance, the other improve it, and so on. A Plan Analysis case conceptualization should answer the question regarding what—negative side effects (e.g. resistance) or positive (e.g., a good alliance as a consequence of patients feeling understood in central parts of their person or being supported by the therapist)—can be expected. The less a therapist is restricted a priori by exclusive preferences for one school of therapy the higher the chance of actually achieving the desired *main* effect with an optimal balance of *side effects*. We favor a sober, school-independent, strictly functional view of therapy methods, which should be used as prototypes in a process of constructing an individually optimized procedure (see above).

Plan Analysis case conceptualizations serve several purposes: They serve as a basis for a general planning of a therapy in the sense just described (i.e., to determine desirable change and to predict main and side effects of interventions). Such planning is done partly outside the therapy session and partly during it.

In addition, case conceptualizations are (often in a simplified form) present in a therapist's mind whenever he or she sees a patient or thinks about him or her, serving as a basis for quick interpretations, predictions, and decisions. For example, a patient may bring up a completely unexpected topic, and a therapist needs to decide very quickly whether it is better pursuing what was originally planned for the session (e.g., because the new topic is interpreted as an indicator of resistance), completely switching to the new topic, or utilizing the new material for the old goal. It seems to be typical for therapists using the Plan concept that they are flexible in a strategic sense (Thommen, Ammann, & von Cranach, 1988). They stick to important therapeutic plans, yet they do it in a flexible way as far as the means are concerned, and they are able to take advantage of the possibilities offered by a concrete situation. In most therapies there are parts in which a therapist plays a very active, structuring role, and there are parts in which processes are developing well without much overt therapist action, and the therapist only monitors them on a high level of mental presence, always ready to intervene when needed.

A case conceptualization is always used for the analysis of the patient's problem(s) as well as the requirements and possibilities in the therapeutic relationship. Problem and therapeutic relationships can be interlocked in many ways. Whatever specific relations may exist, a good relationship is the basis for freeing the resources a patient needs to work on the problems— with the need of good dosage of closeness with patients to whom a good relationship is threatening. Ideally, a therapist develops ideas about a patient's most important interpersonal Plans in the back of his or her mind parallel to the conversation in the first encounter. Thus a therapist can begin immediately to offer a complementary therapeutic relationship. Although some elements of a therapeutic relationship are favorable for most patients, such as empathy and unconditional acceptance, a complementary relationship offer in our sense is usually much more specific. It does justice to the fact that interactional needs vary between different patients and may be very difficult to meet for patients with problems and conflicting needs in the interactional domain. The more precise and custom-tailored a therapist can act, the more he or she can reach with limited resources.

Although it is certainly good if therapist and patient are well matched from the outset, it is not always possible to find an ideal combination for external reasons, nor is it always possible to recognize and predict all the interactional needs a patient will have during the course of therapy. Finally, there are patients who do not match any therapist, unless the latter adapts a great deal to the patient's requirements. The therapist's adaptability is more powerful than patient–therapist matching (Beutler & Clarkin, 1990).

In many therapeutic relationships which are interactionally less complicated, an intuitive understanding is sufficient to prevent severe mistakes and to allow a solid therapeutic bond to develop. Friendly–submissive patients are in general easier than cold and hostile patients (Caspar, Grossmann, Unmüssig, & Schramm, 2005). Elaborated analyses reveal more precise points where the therapist can intervene. The more flexible therapists are in their procedure, the lower the risk of stressing the relationship unnecessarily. In addition, a comprehensive case conceptualization should include the information needed to construct an individualized complementary relationship offer. Complementary therapist behavior does not simply mean *reacting* in the way a patient seems to suggest by problematic behavior. Learning theory might even lead one to expect that such contingent behavior would have a reinforcing effect, and this is not without validity. From a Plan Analysis point of view, however, a therapist should not react on the behavioral level but actively develop a strategy that is complementary on the level of superordinate Plans, which themselves are unproblematic.

For example, a patient may spend a lot of time in therapy complaining, guided by hypothetical superordinate Plans such as "show the therapist how badly off you are," which serves a Plan of causing the therapist to treat the patient carefully, or a Plan of causing the therapist to take the problems seriously and to fully engage in therapy. With such a patient, the therapist should not react contingently (in a learning theory sense: immediately following in time) with reluctant pity. Depending on the individual analysis, the better strategy would be to actively show that one is fully engaged in therapy, that one has understood how bad things are, that one will not be overdemanding, and so on. The process of developing a complementary strategy starting with an analysis of patient behavior is illustrated in Figure 9.2. The concept is explained in greater detail in Caspar et al. (2005).

If complementary behavior in this sense can be realized, patients can give up their problematic strategies because they have already got what they want. It is crucial not to go too high in the hierarchy, as things become too abstract and general as one approaches general human needs, but high enough to leave problematic strategies/means behind and arrive at unproblematic motives which as such do not restrict the therapist. The therapist actively appeases and even oversatiates these motives wherever possible, but not immediately following problematic patient behavior, as this could reinforce the behavior. Although long-standing problematic behavior is often very persistent, frequently a patient's behavior changes dramatically when the therapist finds and does precisely the right thing. Time and attention that were absorbed by the patients' attempts to bring the therapist into the desired interactional position are now suddenly freed for real work on the problem(s). This does not exclude confronting patients with some aspects of their functioning by behaving in a noncomplementary way, but this

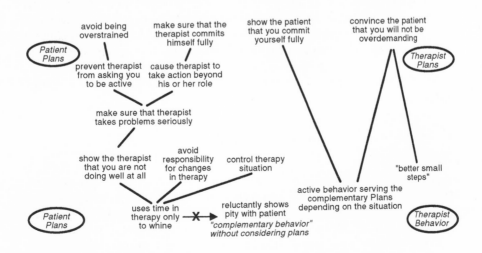

FIGURE 9.2. Complementary therapist behavior. Explanation in the text.

should be an intervention in the foreground, with a safe background of a generally complementary relationship.

A final issue in using Plan Analysis in therapy is communication with patients about "their Plans." Plan Analysis primarily gives *the therapist* a means of developing a clear view of a patient. As increasing insight is an important goal in most therapies, therapists will usually communicate with their patients at least about parts of their view, but rather in terms of an essence or a derived insight, not necessarily in terms of Plans. If parts of a Plan structure are discussed explicitly, the discussion should be restricted to a limited number of Plans and relations. Everything else would be too demanding for most patients, and patients who do well with complex kinds of analysis are often the ones who's tendency to rationalize the therapist does not wish to further.

CASE EXAMPLE

The case example follows a real case. While it remains a typical example, some elements have been changed to protect the patient's rights and to add some aspects illustrating the approach. It was not selected for demonstrating how crucial aspects can be discovered *exclusively* by Plan Analysis. The analysis corresponds to the typical state after three or four sessions. Its complexity is below what would be typical for a research case conceptualization, and at the lower end of what would be needed to derive a sensible therapy planning. To readers with some experience structures look much less complicated, but here readers to whom such structures are new should not be scared away. The structure in Figure 9.3 certainly looks complicated to them but the first impression is deceiving, and the text that guides through the structure should make it intelligible and digestible. Similarities of the addressed topics to other approaches included in this book are obvious, as discussed in detail in Caspar (1995). *Explanations that would not normally be included in a case conceptualization are printed in italics.*

1. The Patient's Present Life Situation (Summary without Deeper Analysis)

Mr. W, a single man of 37 years, works in an administrative position. He likes his work, in which he is and feels very competent, and he earns more than he needs for his modest lifestyle. Originally he had no higher education, but with an amazing investment of energy he has done additional training as an adult in parallel to his work. He is relatively small, a little overweight, not ugly but certainly physically not very attractive. He dresses inconspicuously, and in his nonverbal behavior, he does not attract a lot of

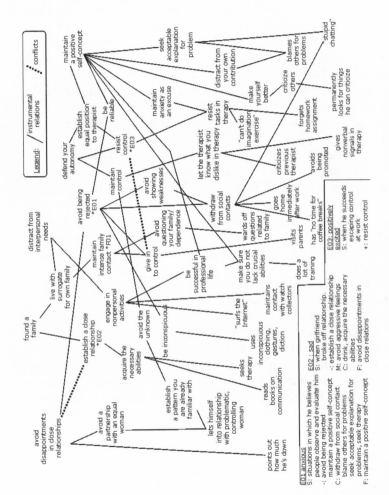

FIGURE 9.3. Drawn Plan structure of the case illustration. Abbreviations in the structure (*F01, *E01 . . . *E03) point to additional, not instrumentally related information (F = "general" frame with unspecified information; open to whatever additional information has to be stored explicitly; E = emotion frame with information related to emotions following the concept explained above: S = Situation, M = Plans shaping the emotion (*manifestation*), C = coping Plans, F = Plans for which the emotion has an instrumental function). Further explanation in the text.

277

attention. In his leisure time he attends various courses, most of them related to his work, and collects and repairs old watches.

He is still heavily entangled with his parents. They live in a village in the neighborhood and he visits them several times a week, often for dinner. In addition, his mother calls several times a week, which he experiences as controlling. He brought his parents to the second interview (we usually invite at least one person close to the patient), and indeed they seemed very interested in him in the helpless controlling manner he had already described, but not very understanding of the psychological dimension of his problems. In their view he was well off; they expected that one day he would have a family, but there was no hurry. The therapist was addressed like a physician able to help in some way but actually not important because there was no real problem. The parents were rather silent and did not interact with each other. The mother controlled the patient by little, often nonverbal cues.

The patient does not have many experiences with women due to his shy nature, but recently had a closer relationship with a woman who had mental problems and was dependent yet exploiting and controlling to an extent that he finally finished the relationship.

Mr. W's difficulties are in the domain of private contacts; he suffers from social phobia. He is anxious and avoidant mainly with women, but also with men (e.g., at work when the issue of a conversation is not professional or related to his watches). However, he has managed to get into a position where, at work, he does not suffer too much from his impairment. The reasons to seek therapy are that he still feels involved with his past relationship and that he feels he would have difficulties establishing a stable and intense relationship with a woman, although his ideal would be to have a good family including children. He has seen another therapist for four sessions for the same reason but ended the therapy because in his view the therapist simultaneously imposed too many of his own concepts on him and pressured him to do things yet did not support him enough when he needed it.

Mr. W has no significant medical, financial, or other problems.

2. Biography (Summary without Deeper Analysis)

The patient grew up in a village near a larger city. He describes his parents as good parents, who, however, never showed a lot of affection or personal interest in him. It sounds as if they were reliable but rather unromantic partners to each other. He is the only child.

He passed school without problems but also without a lot of excitement. He did not have intense contacts with girls or boys, and it sounds as if he has lived in a world of (passive) sports and building aircraft models.

When he was about 3 years old, his parents founded a little factory for underwear, which consumed all their energy and time. They gave it up when he was 15 due to difficult economic conditions. As the patient believes, they also lacked the ability required to convince banks to provide the loans needed to survive a difficult period. The episode ended without significant gain or loss. Now his father works as an employee in the same field, and both parents have excessive time to look after the patient.

Originally his parents came from farmer families. Apart from a mysterious early death of his mothers' mother nothing conspicuous is known about the family, and the patient seems not very interested in this topic.

(Normally, a section with results from an assessment battery answered by the patient himself and a person close to him would follow here, but it is omitted to save some space and because it is not specific to the Plan Analysis approach.)

3. The Patient's Most Important Positive Plans and Resources

The description given here refers to the drawn structure in Figure 9.3. Positive Plans, in contrast to avoidance Plans, are Plans serving positive needs of a person. Often superordinate avoidance Plans also contain subordinate positive Plans, and vice versa; the distinction is thus not a distinctive classification but serves to give the description some structure. Whenever the text says that the patient "has" a Plan, this is to be understood as a hypothesis in a constructivist sense. The description of Plans in topics 3 and 4 is more detailed than in most cases; most often only the most important Plans would be highlighted for readers already familiar with the concept.

There are several positive Plans worth mentioning: The patient wants to start a family, which includes establishing a close relationship (representing a goal in itself). This Plan is not supported by a sufficient repertoire of strategies, which is the primary reason for the patient to seek therapy. His remaining in close contact with his parents can, in part, be viewed as replacing an own family. The Plan of establishing a close relationship was important enough to make him engage in a relationship in which he could have recognized the problems much earlier. He took into account negative side effects as at least subjectively he had few alternatives. *(In a more detailed Plan Structure, one would, for example, instrumentally relate the distortions in his perception of this woman to the dominant Plan of establishing a close relationship.)*

The Plan of maintaining a positive self-concept *(which everybody has in some way but which is emphasized for him because several conspicuous Subplans can be related to this Plan)* determines a broad range of behavior. Positive parts of this Plan, which also have a value in themselves, are as follows: his striving for professional success, which includes ongoing education, and his leisure activities. His being very reliable is an important resource, along with an obvious strong will and intellectual abilities that were not fully used because his parents did not care much about education, nor were they good models; his striving for autonomy and for an equal position with the therapist are at the same time positive and avoidance Plans (see below). In spite of his need to maintain control and lacking routine in more personal communication, he has good skills in conversations related to nonpersonal topics.

4. The Patient's Most Important Avoidance Plans

The patient is characterized by a long list of avoidance Plans. Very relevant is a Plan of avoiding rejection, which includes avoidance strategies that are typical for social phobics, such as not exposing himself to situations in which weaknesses could be revealed, and general withdrawal from situations in which a nonpersonal topic giving structure is lacking. He thus pretends to have no time for conversation after work, for coffee breaks and "stupid chatting," and avoids being promoted into a position where social skills would be required to a higher degree. These avoidance Plans have also led to a lack of skills and experience related to such situations, which increases the risk of failure and thus the tendency to avoid. He avoids drawing attention to himself, among other things by inconspicuous dressing and inconspicuous gestures and diction. A specific Subplan of avoiding rejection is his giving in to being controlled by his parents. His maintaining intense contacts with his old family, and the engagement in nonpersonal contacts, have, apart from a positive function, also a function in distracting from unfulfilled interpersonal needs with which he would be fully confronted otherwise. He protects the relationship with his parents and at the same time his self-concept, with which dependence would be incompatible, by avoiding a debate about the relationship.

Another, related Plan is the avoidance of disappointments in close relationships. Because he desperately wants a close relationship and because he has no experience in constructively coping with disappointment, he sees the need to avoid further disappointment absolutely. His pointing out how much he is down after the last negative experience and also his social anxiety may have the function of preventing him from engaging in a new relationship.

His making sure that he does not lack crucial abilities certainly has a positive function as mentioned previously, but also serves to avoid repeating his parents' negative experiences with the lack of abilities in their business.

Plans serving the maintenance of autonomy and control can historically be understood as resulting from the need to defend himself from his parents' attempts to control him (e.g., by their own interests). He maintains control in an active way, among others by verbally and nonverbally indicating what he expects the therapist to do or not to do. He also shows signs of passive resistance (e.g., by not being able to let himself go in imagination exercises—which would require giving up some control—and by forgetting homework assignments).

His problems are a threat to his self-esteem. He therefore blames others and circumstances for failures and seeks acceptable situational and somatic explanations. Not focusing on his own contribution may also be interpreted as an attempt at maintaining his anxiety, which is embarrassing, yet protects him from letting himself into potentially even more embarrassing situations. Another subordinate Plan is to make himself (relatively) better by criticizing others; at times he appears to be actively monitoring his environment in an endeavor to find something he can criticize. This was also a dominant impression reported by his previous therapist.

In sum, his avoidance Plans make it difficult for him to use situations that would allow him to have positive experiences in line with his positive Plans.

5. Conflicts between Plans

Mr. W's structure is characterized by a number of conflicts between Plans, resulting in ambivalent behaviors and problematic compromises.

A central conflict is between establishing a close relationship and avoiding disappointments/being rejected. His avoidance Plans made it difficult to develop abilities and seek situations that would increase the chances of finding a good relationship. The fact that he has been engaged in a relationship with a dependent, unequal (seemingly riskless) woman can be viewed as a compromise between the two Plans. Surfing the Internet (which was less common at the time) can be seen as a compromise between engaging in and avoiding contact.

Achievement Plans are also in conflict with withdrawal and avoidance Plans. The compromise is to involve himself in nonpersonal activities in which personal contacts are limited.

His control Plans are in conflict with his Plan of maintaining intense family contact and the Plan of improving his situation by therapy, because they are related to accepting strong control by his mother and potentially giving at least some control to the therapist. His compromises are to avoid awareness of his dependence of his parents and occasional weak attempts at escaping the control, and in therapy persistent attempts at controlling the therapist.

6. The Patient's Self-Concept

(This includes the most important means of maintaining it for her- or himself, and means of conveying it to others. Also included is information about which parts of his or her functioning the patient is apparently unaware.)

The patient sees himself as a reliable, competent person with good qualities as a potential family man. It is important for him to have an equal position to the therapist. Probably he is, based on neglect by his parents, secretly afraid that he might not be lovable, and therefore tries to repress or justify weaknesses. The degree to which his behavior and experience is determined by avoidance Plans and dependency from his parents is not represented in his awareness.

7. The Most Important Stressors and the Most Important Positive Situations for the Patient: Strong Positive and Negative Emotions

The most stressful situations are clearly those in which he would expose himself to scrutiny and rejection, in particular by women. Usually he can avoid them; if not, he experiences anxiety. The loss of his close relationship, even if it was not a good one, was very painful to him. When he experiences the conflict between escaping from the control of his parents and being rejected for such attempts, he feels stressed and annoyed, although he is not as much aware of his dependency as observers are.

Positive are success experiences in his job and leisure activities (e.g., receiving compliments for his watch collection and skill in repairing them). He also experiences positive excitement when he can escape control at his workplace and plays games to have such experiences.

(Some of the experienced emotions are explicitly mentioned and related to the Plan structure [Figure 9.3] by the types of relations described in the text earlier. Establishing such explicit relations often gives additional information and is a test to what degree the patient has already been understood.)

8. Relation between the Problems and the Plan Structure: Where Did the Patient (Partially) Succeed in Solving Problems?

Social phobia is the result of his Plans of avoiding rejection and maintaining a positive self-concept is being threatened by exposure and achievement situations, and by conflictual positive Plans. The resulting concrete avoidance occupies him and restricts positive experiences. In particular, in contact with women he has not yet developed skills and experience, which leads to a vicious circle. Plans of avoiding rejection by his parents keep him in an environment that additionally inhibits a development appropriate for his age. It is positive that the patient has succeeded in acquiring good training and a good position. The work and hobby-related contacts and the contact with his parents prevent complete isolation, but the latter is obviously a dead end.

9. The Patient's View of His or Her Problems and Why the Patient Got into an Impasse

In general, the patient has a view of his problems that corresponds to topic 8, with the exception of a tendency of blaming others, of using his being down and his anxiety as excuses against change, and of denying his dependence on his parents. The impasse developed as a consequence of lacking encouragement from his parents or others, which prevented him from developing skills and experiences appropriate for his age and necessary to achieve a situation corresponding to his wishes. A vicious circle developed with avoidance and increasing lack of self-efficacy expectation.

10. The Therapeutic Relationship

The patient's strong Plans of maintaining control along with his wish that the therapist should structure the situation and take responsibility, and the permanent search for things the patient can criticize, are certainly handicapping. The fear of rejection and of threats to his positive self-concept also need to be considered. The fear of disappointments in close relationships may lead the patient to test the therapist before he lets himself into a closer relationship with the therapist.

In line with the concept of a complementary relationship, the therapist should actively encourage the patient to maintain control and always ask for permission when he needs to restrict the patient's control. He should actively and positively enhance the patient's self-esteem and emphasize his equal position (e.g., by addressing the patient's abilities whenever he can, mentioning the patient's expertise in his work, and openly but assertively admitting insecurity when it occurs). The general strategy is to make the patient's problematic control and defense strategies superfluous as far as possible and instead to prevent their use rather than react contingently to them in time.

11. General Outline of What in Therapy Could Help the Patient to Develop in a Desirable Direction

The therapeutic relationship is a major concern in this therapy and should be developed as described earlier.

In line with what the patient expects from therapy, social phobia and his ability to achieve and maintain a close relationship should be treated with high priority. Goals to be achieved are a reduction in dysfunctional thoughts ("to be rejected would kill me," "one is either loved or rejected completely," etc.), working through emotions related to scrutiny and rejection (including experiences he had in the past), building up concrete skills needed in interpersonal interaction (above all with women), and skills needed for coping with failures and anxiety. It is crucial that the patient has positive experiences with previously avoided situations to enhance his self-efficacy expectation. Much could be gained if he would satisfy part of his interpersonal needs in other relationships so that not everything would be loaded on that one close relationship he wants so badly.

Means to reach these goals would, for example, be the following:

- Debating his assumptions and interpretations (as in cognitive therapy)
- Activating previously avoided emotions—for example, using Gestalt therapy techniques (although one would need to pay a lot of attention not to threaten his need for control)—and, above all, by well-prepared exposure
- Enhancing his skills by role playing and assignments for his real world, plus building up self-instructions in the sense of Meichenbaum (1974)
- Concrete discussions and assignments related to establishing several personal relationships
- Including his parents occasionally in an attempt to gain their support for the processes their son needs to go through, or at least try to neutralize possible undermining from their part

The procedure would partly be planned and partly would take advantage of chances provided by situations occurring in the patient's life and of fluctuations in Plan activations and motivations in the patient's life.

TRAINING

Plan Analysis should be seen as a set of heuristic concepts, rules, and strategies. Although developing good Plan Analysis case conceptualizations requires having at one's disposal most of this set, the use of Plan Analysis is not an all-or-nothing issue. Some of the elements required for Plan Analysis (such as diligently observing nonverbal behavior; heuristic etiological concepts of the development of depressive states, etc.) are generally useful in psychotherapy practice and not specific to Plan Analysis. The extent to which a therapist or trainee has such elements available determines largely what is left to be trained and on what level of proficiency the approach can be used after the training. Based on generally useful concepts and skills, some additional, special elements need to be conveyed to most therapists interested in Plan Analysis.

A basic body of conceptual and technical knowledge can be acquired by reading. There is literature describing the handling of many details and proposing exercises that can be done by individuals or small groups without a human trainer (Caspar, 1995). The ideal is, of course, when, based on previous reading, practical skills can be trained in direct contact, for example, by role playing and then analyzing actual patients in therapy with workshop participants. Trainees not only learn a technique but also learn a lot about themselves in comparing themselves and their conclusions with others: They see blind spots in their perception, tendencies of overinterpreting, or the opposite, missing clinically important points by being too reluctant with interpretations, and so forth.

Because the first few analyses include many necessary discussions and clarifications, they are much more time-consuming than later analyses, but they represent necessary learning steps in becoming an expert. Whereas one may need a day or more for a first comprehensive case conceptualization, an expert in his or her regular practice needs an hour or even less to work out the crucial points for a case of average difficulty. In our experience, students generally familiar with psychotherapy need about two guided weeks to develop the proficiency needed to produce reliable, comprehensive research analyses, but for most therapists a 2- or 3-day workshop, ideally with some time to practice on their own, enables them to develop reasonably good and clinically useful case conceptualizations.

RESEARCH SUPPORT FOR THE APPROACH

Interrater Agreement

It is obvious that attempts at determining the "reliability" of complex Plan structures and case conceptualizations in the same way as it would be done for quantitative values from, for example, personality scales, or themes (e.g. Luborsky & Barrett, Chapter 4, this volume) would be inappropriate. We have argued in greater detail elsewhere (Caspar, 1995) that simple coefficients of agreement hide rather than reveal the factors determining the actual accuracy of case conceptualizations. Comparisons reported by Caspar (1995) and continued ever since (see, e.g., Caspar et al., 2005) show that on average, the clinically significant agreement is reasonably good but varies just as is the case for similar approaches, depending on, among others, the homogeneity of the analyzers' background, and properties of patients. Although we can be satisfied with reliability, we would at the same time emphasize the usefulness in clinical and research practice, which is harder to quantify but is an important criterion.

Contents of Plan Structures and Effects of Using Plan Analysis

Several studies have worked out typical Plan structures: for example, in comparing structures of patients with social phobia to structures of patients with psychosomatic disorders, or by searching typical Plans for patients with depression, borderline personality disorder, and schizophrenia and people with extraordinary experiences. In a series of studies, Plan Analysis has been used to analyze resistance of patients and has turned out to be useful in understanding and predicting resistance phenomena. The relation of complementarity in the relationship and outcome and the probability of complementarity depending on patient variables has also been investigated (Caspar et al., 2005).

Effects of using Plan Analysis case conceptualizations have been investigated in several studies. A study by Thommen et al. (1988) on how therapists regulate their behavior and by Schmitt et al. (2003) on the effects of Plan Analysis-based interaction training with doctors have already been mentioned. Grawe et al. (1990) found that in a comparison of client-centered therapists and broad-spectrum behavior therapists using traditional functional behavior analysis versus Plan Analysis, on average all forms of therapy produced good results. The latter therapists, however, had better achievements related to individually important patient goals, and they had, above all, a strikingly better therapeutic relationship, along with lower dropout rates. Our fear that patients could feel that their therapists think more about them than they say, that they speak in a too complicated way, or that they pay too little attention to patient feelings turned out not to be justified. Overall, Plan Analysis-based therapies are somewhat better in important outcome measures and, above all, are superior in a broad spectrum of process measures. An aspect of high importance is that therapists were, just as their patients, much more satisfied with what they did. Another surprising result was not the fact but the degree to which the therapeutic procedure in Plan Analysis-based therapies was richer in terms of the types of techniques used: The use of Plan Analysis seems to lead to significantly more ideas how to proceed than traditional behavioral analyses.

NOTE

1. A text, which is more explicit in this respect, can be requested from the author.

REFERENCES

Argyle, M. (1969). *Social interaction*. London: Methuen.

Averill, J. R. (1980). A constructivist view of emotion. In R. Plutchik & H. Kellerman (Eds.), *Emotion: Theory, research, and experience* (Vol. 1, pp. 305–339). New York: Academic Press.

Beck, A. T., Rush, J. A., Shaw, B. F., & Emery, G. (1979). *Cognitive therapy of depression*. New York: Guilford Press.

Berger, T. (2005). *Die Dynamik psychischer Störungen: Strukturen und Prozesse aus der Perspektive neuronaler Netzwerkansätze*. Dissertation. Retrieved December 20, 2005, from http://www.freidok.uni-freiburg.de/volltexte/1968/.

Beutler, L., & Clarkin, J. (1990). *Systematic treatment selection*. New York: Brunner/ Mazel.

Beutler, L., & Harwood, M. (2000). *Prescriptive psychotherapy: A practical guide to systematic treatment selection*. New York: Oxford University Press.

Beutler, L. E., Malik, M., Alimohamed, S., Harwood, T. M., Talebi, H., Noble, S., et al. (2003). Therapist variables. In M. J. Lambert (Hrsg.), *Bergin & Garfield's Handbook of psychotherapy and behavior change* (5th ed., pp. 227–306). New York: Wiley.

Carver, C. S., & Scheier, M. F. (2002). Control processes and self-organization as complementary principles underlying behavior. *Personality and Social Psychology Review, 6,* 304–315.

Caspar, F. (1984). *Analyse interaktioneller Pläne*. Unpublished dissertation, Universität Bern.

Caspar, F. (1987). Anxiety: A complex problem calling for flexible therapy planning. In J. P. Dauwalder, M. Perrez, & V. Hobi (Eds.), *Controversial issues in behavior modification* (pp. 139–147). Amsterdam: Swets & Zeitlinger.

Caspar, F. (1988, June). *The dangers of standardizing the elements of dynamic formulations*. Paper presented at the annual meeting of the Society for Psychotherapy Research, Santa Fe, NM.

Caspar, F. (1995). *Plan analysis: Towards optimizing psychotherapy*. Seattle, WA: Hogrefe.

Caspar, F. (1998). A connectionist view of psychotherapy. In D. J. Stein & J. Ludik (Eds.), *Neural networks and psychopathology* (pp. 88–131). Cambridge, UK: Cambridge University Press.

Caspar, F. (2000). Therapeutisches Handeln als individueller Konstruktionsprozess. In J. Margraf (Hrsg.), *Lehrbuch der Verhaltenstherapie*, Bd.1 (2. Auflage) (S. 155–166). Göttingen: Hogrefe.

Caspar, F. (2003). Psychotherapy research and neurobiology: Challenge, chance, or enrichment? (SPR presidential address Santa Barbara). *Psychotherapy Research, 13,* 1–23.

Caspar, F., & Berger, T. (2006). Struktur und Dynamik psychischer Störungen: Was tragen neuere Modelle zu einem Verständnis bei? In H. Lang & H. Faller (Hrsg.), *Struktur—Persönlichkeit, Persönlichkeitsstörung*. Würzburg: Königshausen & Neumann.

Caspar, F., & Grawe, K. (1981). Widerstand in der Verhaltenstherapie. In H. Petzold (Ed.), *Der Widerstand: Ein strittiges Konzept in der Psychotherapie* (pp. 349–384). Paderborn: Junfermann.

Caspar, F., Grossmann, C., Unmüssig, C., & Schramm, E. (2005). Complementary therapeutic relationship: Therapist behavior, interpersonal patterns, and therapeutic effects. *Psychotherapy Research, 15,* 91–102.

Caspar, F., Koch, K., & Schneider, F. (2004). Psychotherapie und ihre neurobiologischen Voraussetzungen. In W. Senf & M. Broda (Hrsg.), *Praxis der Psychotherapie* (pp. 34–53). Stuttgart: Thieme.

Caspar, F., Rothenfluh, T., & Segal, Z. V. (1992). The appeal of connectionism for clinical psychology. *Clinical Psychology Review, 12,* 719–762.

Castonguay, L. G., & Beutler, L. E. (2005). (Eds). *Principles of therapeutic change that work*. New York: Oxford University Press.

Damasio, A. (1995). *Descartes' error: emotion, reason and the human brain*. London: Picador.

Gasiet, S. (1981). *Menschliche Bedürfnisse. Eine theoretische Synthese*. Frankfurt/ Main: Campus.

Grawe, K. (1980). Die diagnostisch-therapeutische Funktion der Gruppeninteraktion in verhaltenstherapeutischen Gruppen. In K. Grawe (Ed.), *Verhaltenstherapie in Gruppen* (pp. 88–223). München: Urban & Schwarzenberg.

Grawe, K. (1986). *Schema-Theorie und interaktionelle Psychotherapie* (Report 1–86). Psychologisches Institut, Universität Bern.

Grawe, K. (2004). *Psychological therapy*. Seattle & Toronto: Hogrefe.

Grawe, K., Caspar, F., & Ambühl, H. R. (1990). Differentielle Psychotherapieforschung: Vier Therapieformen im Vergleich: Die Berner Therapievergleichsstudie. *Zeitschrift für Klinische Psychologie, 19*, 294–376.

Grawe, K., Donati, R., & Bernauer, F. (1994). *Psychotherapie im wandel von der Konfession zur Profession*. Göttingen: Hogrefe.

Greenberg, L., & Safran, J. (1987). *Emotion in psychotherapy, affect, cognition, and the process of change*. New York: Guilford Press.

Grosse Holtforth, M., & Grawe, K. (2003). Der Inkongruenzfragebogen (INK)—Ein Messinstrument zur Analyse motivationaler Inkongruenz [The Incongruence Questionnaire (INC)—An assessment tool for the analysis of motivational incongruence]. *Zeitschrift für Klinische Psychologie und Psychotherapie, 32*(4), 315–323.

Halcour, D. (1997). *Die Guru Untersuchung* (Unveröffentlichter Arbeitsbericht aus dem DFG-Projekt Kulturvergleichende Untersuchung der Denk- und Handlungsstile beim Problemlösen). Bamberg.

Horowitz, L. M., Wilson, K. R., Turan, B., Zolotsev, P., Constantino, M. J., & Henderson, L. (2006). How interpersonal motives clarify the meaning of interpersonal behavior: A revised circumplex model. *Personality and Social Psychology Review, 10*, 67–86

Horowitz, M. J. (1979). *States of mind: Analysis of change in psychotherapy*. New York: Plenum Press.

Klemenz, B. (1999). *Plananalytisch orientierte Kinderdiagnostik*. Göttingen: Vandenhoeck & Ruprecht.

Klerman G. L., Weissman M., Rounsaville B. J., & Chevron, E. S. (1984). *Interpersonal psychotherapy of depression*. New York: Basic Books.

Lazarus, R. S. (1966). *Psychological stress and the coping process*. New York: McGraw Hill.

Lazarus, R. S., Kanner, A., & Folkman, S. (1972). Emotions: A cognitive–phenomenological analysis. In R. Plutchik & H. Kellermann (Eds.), *Theories of emotion* (pp. 189–217). New York: Academic Press.

Lewinsohn, P. H. (1974). A behavioral approach to depression. In R. J. Friedman & M. M. Katz (Eds.), *The psychology of depression: Contemporary theory and research* (pp. 157–185). Washington, DC: Winston Wiley.

Mandler, G. (1975). *Mind and emotion*. New York: Wiley.

Meichenbaum, D. (1974). *Cognitive behavior modification*. Morristown, NJ: General Learning Press.

Miller, G. A., Galanter, E., & Pribram, K. H. (1960). *Plans and the structure of behavior*. New York: Holt.

Ortony, A., Clore, G. L., & Foss, M. A. (1987). The referential structure of the affective lexicon. *Cognitive Science, 11*, 341–364.

Persons, J. B. (1989). *Cognitive therapy in practice. A case formulation approach.* New York: Norton.

Piaget, J. (1977). *The development of thought: Equilibration of cognitive structures.* New York: Viking Press.

Prigogine, I. (1976). Order through fluctuation: Self-organization and social system. In E. Jantsch & C. H. Waddington (Eds.), *Evolution and consciousness* (pp. 93–133). Reading, MA: Addison-Wesley.

Scherer, K. R. (2001). Appraisal considered as a process of multi-level sequential checking. In K. R. Scherer, A. Schorr, & T. Johnstone (Eds.). *Appraisal processes in emotion: Theory, methods, research* (pp. 92–120). New York & Oxford: Oxford University Press.

Schmitt, G. M., Kammerer, E., & Holtmann, M. (2003). Förderung interaktioneller Kompetenzen von Medizinstudierenden. *Psychotherapie, Psychosomatik, Medizinische Psychologie, 53*, 390–398.

Schonauer, F. (1992). Gestern traf ich Huckleberry Finn. In Herrmann-Josef-Haus Urft (Ed.), *Leben formt Leben* (pp. 157–188). Kall-Urft: Hermann-Josef-Haus.

Schütz, A. (1992). *Selbstdarstellung von Politikern. Analyse von Wahlkampfauftritten* [Self-presentation of politicians. An analysis of election campaigns]. Weinheim: Deutscher Studienverlag.

Seligman, M. E. P. (1975). *Learned helplessness.* San Francisco: Freeman.

Thommen, B., Ammann, R., & Cranach, M. (1988). *Handlungsorganisation durch soziale Repräsentationen.* Bern: Hans Huber.

Weiss, J., & Sampson, H. (1986). *The psychoanalytic process.* New York: Guilford Press.

Willi, J. (1982). *Couples in collusion.* New York: Jason Aronson.

Young, J. E. (1994). *Cognitive therapy for personality disorders: A schema-focused approach.* Sarasota, FL: Professional Resource Exchange.

Zajonc, R. B. (1980). Feeling and thinking: Preferences need no inferences. *American Psychologist, 35*, 151–175.

Chapter 10

Cognitive-Behavioral
Case Formulation

JACQUELINE B. PERSONS
MICHAEL A. TOMPKINS

This chapter describes the historical background and conceptual underpinnings of cognitive-behavioral (CB) case formulation, discusses the role of cultural factors, offers an opinion about when a case formulation is helpful (always), spells out the steps involved in developing a CB case formulation, presents a case example, discusses training issues, and briefly summarizes research.

HISTORICAL BACKGROUND OF THE APPROACH

The model of CB case formulation presented here has multiple historical origins. The most important is probably functional analysis (Haynes & O'Brien, 2000; Nezu, Nezu, Friedman, & Haynes, 1997), which itself has origins in operant conditioning theory and the tradition in psychology of the study of the single organism (Morgan & Morgan, 2001). We also rely heavily on the evidence-based formulations for particular disorders and symptoms that have been developed over the last 50 years by CB theorists. We also rely on the theories that underpin those disorder formulations, especially Beck's cognitive theory, learning theories (e.g., theories of associative learning, operant conditioning, and modeling), and theories of emotion (Lang, 1979). We also borrow from methods for formulating the case developed by other CB therapists (Beck, 1995; Koerner, Chapter 11, this volume), and from clinical writings about the case formulation by other CB therapists (Freeman, 1992; Padesky, 1996; Tarrier & Calam, 2002).

In this chapter we make several substantial changes to our earlier presentations (Persons, 1989; Persons & Davidson, 2001; Persons, Tompkins, & Davidson, 2000), including those in the previous edition of this volume (Persons & Tompkins, 1997). We present the formulation as one element of a hypothesis-testing approach to clinical work; we rely more on diagnosis, we allow for formulations based on conditioning and emotion theories (in our previous work, formulations were always based on Beck's cognitive theory), we simplify the format of the formulation, and we describe a worksheet that aids in the process of developing a case formulation. We discuss all these changes in detail below.

CONCEPTUAL FRAMEWORK

Case Formulation as One Element of a Hypothesis-Testing Approach to Clinical Work

CB case formulation is an element of an empirical hypothesis-testing approach to clinical work that has three key elements, *assessment, formulation,* and *intervention.* Information obtained during *assessment* is used to develop a *formulation,* which is a hypothesis about the causes of the patient's disorders and problems, and which is used as the basis for *intervention.* As the treatment proceeds, the therapist doubles back repeatedly to the *assessment* phase, collecting data to monitor the process and progress of the therapy and using those data to revise the formulation and intervention as needed. This chapter focuses primarily on the *formulation* piece of that model.

Qualities of a Good CB Case Formulation

A good CB formulation has several qualities. It has good *treatment utility,* that is, it contributes to the effectiveness of treatment (Hayes, Nelson, & Jarrett, 1987). It is *parsimonious;* that is, it offers the minimum detail necessary to accomplish the task of guiding effective treatment, and it is *evidence-based.* We elaborate a bit here on what we mean by an evidence-based case formulation.[1]

An *evidence-based CB case formulation* is one that is supported by evidence. Of course, all clinicians strive to develop case formulations that are supported by evidence. What distinguishes CB case formulations is the types of evidence that CB therapists value and use. CB therapists place a high value on evidence from controlled studies and on the use of objective measures to collect systematic data about the case at hand.

The CB therapist relies on several types of controlled studies in the process of case formulation, including studies of basic mechanisms under-pinning symptoms or disorders (e.g., the finding by Kring and colleagues, reviewed in Kring & Werner, 2004), that the diminished expression of emo-tion seen in individuals with schizophrenia is not accompanied by a dimin-ished experience of emotion), epidemiological findings (e.g., that bipolar disorder and substance abuse are frequently comorbid), and randomized controlled trials (e.g., the finding that panic control treatment [PCT] pro-vides effective treatment for panic disorder [Barlow, Craske, Cerny, & Klosko, 1989], a finding that provides some support for the formulation that underpins PCT, namely, that panic symptoms result from catastrophic misinterpretations of benign somatic sensations).

The CB therapist also relies on data from the case at hand, as do all cli-nicians. However, CB therapists probably rely more than other therapists on diagnosis and objective data in the process of developing and testing formulation hypotheses. For example, at our center, we frequently use self-report measures of symptoms of anxiety, depression, and obsessive–compulsive disorder to track progress in patients we treat for those prob-lems. Our waiting room holds files of measures (we use the Beck Depression Inventory [Beck, Rush, Shaw, & Emery, 1979], the Burns Anxiety Inven-tory [Burns, 1998], and the Yale–Brown Obsessive–Compulsive Scale [Goodman et al., 1989]); we ask our patients to come 5 minutes early for their therapy session, complete whichever measure or measures are being used to monitor progress, and present it to the therapist at the beginning of the session.

The Nomothetic/Idiographic Distinction

The term "nomothetic" is derived from the Greek word *nomos*, which means *law* and refers to general laws of behavior. A *nomothetic* theory, for example, describes general laws of functioning that apply to all individuals or groups of individuals (e.g., the principles of operant conditioning, or the proposal that panic disorder symptoms result from catastrophic misinter-pretations of benign somatic sensations). The word "idiographic" is de-rived from the Greek word *idios*, which means *one's own, and private,* and refers to theories that are *applicable to a particular specific case* (Cone, 1986). The method of case formulation described here emphasizes the use of evidence-based *nomothetic* formulations as the foundation for the devel-opment of *idiographic* formulations.

Levels of Formulation

Formulation occurs at several levels: the level of *symptom, disorder* or *problem,* and *case.* For example, the *symptom* of auditory hallucinations has been conceptualized by CB therapists as thoughts that are attributed by the individual to an external source (Kingdon & Turkington, 2005). A *disorder* or *problem* usually consists of a set of *symptoms* or problem behaviors. For example, *major depressive disorder* has been conceptualized as made up of automatic thoughts, negative emotions, and problem behaviors that result from the activation of negative schemas by stressful life events (Beck et al., 1979). The *problem* of treatment noncompliance experienced by John, the patient described in our case example, was conceptualized as consisting of unassertiveness and other avoidance behaviors, negative cognitions (e.g., "what's the point"), and negative emotions (e.g., dysphoria) arising from John's schemas of himself as inadequate, of others as critical, and of the future as hopeless. The formulation at the level of the *case* is a hypothesis about the causes of all of the patient's *symptoms, disorders*, and *problems*, and how they are related. We use the term "problem" in two ways: to refer to difficulties that are not symptoms or disorders (e.g., treatment noncompliance), and in a generic way that includes all *symptoms, disorders*, and *problems*. This chapter focuses primarily on formulation at the level of the *case*.

Components of the CB Case Formulation

The CB case formulation is a hypothesis that ties together, in a brief narrative or diagram, the *mechanisms* that cause and maintain all of the patient's *problems,* the *origins* of the mechanisms, and the *precipitants* that are currently activating the *mechanisms* to cause the *problems*. The formulation also describes the relationships among the *problems*. We provide a case example and then we discuss each component (problems, mechanisms, origins, precipitants) in detail.

Example: Formulation of the Case of John

John is a 37-year-old, single, second-generation Japanese American male who lives alone and is self-employed as a web designer. John, who has hepatitis C, was referred by his nephrologist for treatment of depression and poor medical adherence. His chief complaint to the therapist was: "My doctor says I'm not getting better and it's time for some new ideas."

John's therapist developed the following formulation of his case. The *origins, mechanisms*, and *precipitants* are identified in brackets [e.g., *origins*], and the problems are *italicized*.

Caused by [*origins*] a likely biological vulnerability to anxiety (as evidenced by his mother's apparent social anxiety) and by rearing in a household in which (due to his mother's shyness and her difficulty adjusting to the American culture) there were few visitors and thus few models of easy social interaction, and in which his father was largely absent but when present often brutally critical and attacking, John developed [*mechanisms*] schemas of others as critical and rejecting, of himself as weak, weird, and helpless, and of the future as hopeless. These schemas, activated by [*precipitants*] his worsening *medical problems* and increasing pressure from his physician to comply with treatment recommendations, have exacerbated John's *social anxiety* and passive, unassertive, and avoidant behaviors. John's *medical problems* also trigger [*precipitants*] his schemas by causing physical symptoms (sweating, trembling, fatigue, and dizziness) that he fears others will notice and then think him as weird or weak. In addition, John's *social anxiety* and *unassertiveness* worsen his *noncompliance*, because the symptoms block him from following some of his physician's recommendations (e.g., to attend a self-help group for hepatitis C) and even from participating fully in treatment-planning discussions with his physician. The *noncompliance*, of course, aggravates his *medical condition* and the symptoms he worries that others will notice. John's views of himself as weak and of the future as hopeless, together with all his other problems, cause *depression* and *suicidal thoughts and urges*. John copes with distress through avoidance (which leads to *social isolation* that generates evidence to support his belief that others are rejecting and he is weird), and *alcohol abuse* (which exacerbates his *liver disease, depression, and social isolation*).

Problems. We use the term "problems" to refer to overt or manifest symptoms, disorders, or difficulties the patient is having in any of the following domains: psychological/psychiatric symptoms; interpersonal, occupational, school, medical, financial, housing, legal, and leisure problems; and problems with mental health or medical treatment (Linehan, 1993; Nezu & Nezu, 1993; Turkat & Maisto, 1985). A comprehensive case formulation accounts for all of the patient's problems in all these domains; the notion is that in order to understand the case fully, the therapist must know what *all* the problems are and how they are related. The fact that the formulation includes all of the patient's problems does not mean that they will all be treated in therapy. For example, the patient illustrated here has hepatitis C, and even CB therapy does not provide effective treatment for hepatitis C! However, a comprehensive conceptualization of John's case requires attending to his medical illness.

Mechanisms. The heart of the formulation is a description of mechanisms or processes (e.g., in this case, schemas) that are causing and maintaining the patient's problems. The CB case formulation emphasizes psychological mechanisms but can also include biological and somatic mechanisms.

Origins of the Mechanisms. Here the formulation describes the distal causal factors that cause the mechanisms (in contrast to mechanisms, which can be seen as proximal or immediate causal factors of the problems). For example, if Beck's theory is used, as in the case of John, the "origins" part of the formulation describes how John learned the schemas that cause his problems. The origins section of the formulation can also identify the causes of biological mechanisms, as in the case of John, where likely genetic causes of biological mechanisms driving John's mood and anxiety disorders are identified. Cultural factors (e.g., in John's case, rearing by Japanese American parents) are also often relevant here as well as family factors, social factors (e.g., the fact that John's parents rarely entertained guests), and aspects of the physical environment, such as the fact that John's family lived in a neighborhood in which there were few other Japanese Americans.

Precipitants of the Current Problems. Most nomothetic CB formulations are diathesis–stress hypotheses, proposing that symptoms and problems result from the activation of psychological and/or biological vulnerabilities by one or more diatheses or stressors that can be internal, external, biological, psychological, or some combination of these. Sometimes the precipitants are events that cause the initial onset of a disorder or symptom (e.g., a promotion might trigger an episode of bipolar disorder) and sometimes, as in the case of John, precipitants are events that trigger an exacerbation of longstanding problems.

Tying It All Together. One purpose of a formulation is to tie together the elements of a case (origins, mechanisms, precipitants, problems) into a coherent narrative so they can be understood as a whole rather than as a list of disparate unrelated facts. The case formulation is presented in a paragraph, as in the example above, or in a diagram with arrows (for examples, see O'Brien & Haynes, 1995; Persons & Davidson, 2001).

INCLUSION/EXCLUSION CRITERIA AND MULTICULTURAL CONSIDERATIONS

Inclusion/Exclusion Criteria

CB therapy is always guided by a formulation. For example, Barlow's PCT is based on a nomothetic formulation of panic disorder as arising from catastrophic misinterpretations of benign somatic sensations (Barlow & Craske, 2001). The clinician working with a particular client individualizes this nomothetic formulation of panic by asking the client to describe the particular anxious cognitions he has, the particular bodily sensations he fears, and the particular situations he avoids. The clinician might individualize the nomothetic formulation on the fly, and for a simple case this is often sufficient.

However, we find that a complete, written individualized formulation is helpful in the treatment of clients who have multiple problems or disorders or who do not make good progress in treatment. Therapists, particularly inexperienced ones, often feel overwhelmed by complex, multiple-problem clients. The therapist wonders which problem to tackle first, how to track progress in the therapy, and how to intervene appropriately. The CB case formulation method is particularly helpful when working with these clients because of the method's emphasis on a comprehensive Problem List. The simple process of making a Problem List for a client who has many problems can be helpful to both therapist and client. In addition, the formulation provides a framework for understanding how problems are related and how they are related to the underlying hypothesized psychological mechanisms, allowing the therapist to intervene in multiple problem domains (e.g., financial, interpersonal, and personal safety) and still see the therapy as having a central theme.

Multicultural Considerations

CB therapy has long asserted the important role of context, including sociocultural context, in psychological development (Hayes & Toarmino, 1995). Sociocultural factors are the standards against which people judge their behavior as normal and expectable or pathological. For example, *taijin kyofusho* is a common form of social phobia in Japan characterized by anxiety about public self-presentation and performance and in particular by the more culture-specific concern that one's inappropriate social behavior, such as staring, will make others uncomfortable. The sociocultural expectation that it is inappropriate to make others uncomfortable reflects the importance given in Japan to harmonious interaction. As a result, symptoms of *taijin kyofusho* can be less indicative of psychopathology in Japan than they would be in other cultures. This example illustrates the way an understanding of cultural factors can affect the therapist's view of the seriousness or nature of the patient's problems and even the diagnosis. Cultural factors can also play a role in the origins of schemas or other hypothesized mechanisms, as in the example of John. Thus, to develop a comprehensive formulation of the case of a client who has been raised in another culture or by parents or caretakers who have come from another culture, clinicians would do well to consult with the client or with others knowledgeable about the culture.

In general, it is essential that CB therapists gather information regarding a client's sociocultural variables (degree of assimilation or acculturation, religious beliefs, racial identity, socioeconomic status, traditional sources of social support—e.g., the nuclear or extended family—and sociocultural values—Multicultural historical experience of client's cultural group in the United States) when developing a case formulation. John's case challenges us to consider the familial, social, and cultural factors that might influence or reinforce the problems he has with assertiveness and social anxiety. Although John was born in the United States, his parents emigrated from Japan. His therapist might wonder whether his parents expected John to adhere to Japan's cultural norms about assertiveness or those of the United States, which demand a willingness to make others uncomfortable in the service of expressing a personal wish or desire. The therapist knows that John's mother tended to spend most of her time at home and had few friends or outside interests. Is this evidence that John's mother had social phobia herself, or was it simply her difficulty acculturating? Similarly, to what degree, if any, is John's unassertiveness with his physician (or even his therapist) a reflection of the value the Japanese culture places on respecting and complying with those in authority, rather than a feature of his social anxiety? The therapist knows that John's father was critical of him. To what degree does this familial factor influence John's social anxiety and unassertiveness relative to the possible cultural factors? The answers to any of these questions not only might influence what John views as a problem, and thereby John's willingness to work with the therapist collaboratively, but also can influence therapist's views about the hypothesized psychological mechanisms that underpin John's problems.

The therapist discussed all these issues with John, taking care to be aware of cultural factors that might influence the discussion—for example, taking care not to assume that John and the therapist necessarily had the same definition of or view of the value of assertiveness. John indicated that he did not see the cultural factors as exerting as large an influence on his anxiety and difficulty with assertiveness as the familial factors (a critical and rejecting father, the absence of adequate modeling of assertive behavior, and limited exposure to social situations as a child because of his mother's social isolation), and this view is reflected in the formulation of his case.

STEPS IN CASE FORMULATION

To develop a case formulation, we suggest that the clinician carry out these steps in order: (1) obtain a comprehensive Problem List; (2) assign a five-axis DSM diagnosis; (3) select an "anchoring diagnosis"; (4) select a nomothetic formulation of the anchoring diagnosis to use as a template for the hypothesized psychological mechanisms part of the formulation; (5) individualize the template so that the formulation accounts for the details of the case at hand and for all of the problems on the Problem List and their relationships; (6) propose hypotheses about the origins of the psychological mechanisms; and (7) describe precipitants of the current episode of illness or symptom exacerbation. These steps yield the information needed to write a formulation of the case (see example of John). As he carries out these steps, the therapist may want to set up a worksheet and write down each step in turn. We strive to carry out all these steps and write a formulation after three to four sessions.

We describe here each step of the process of obtaining a case formulation. Of course, the order described here is an idealized one; in fact, lots of things happen in tandem or in a different order. For example, in the process of developing a Problem List (step 1), the therapist will be thinking about and collecting information about how the problems are related to one another and what mechanisms might be causing or maintaining them (steps 4 and 5).

1. Obtain a Comprehensive Problem List

A comprehensive Problem List describes all the problems the patient is having in all of these domains: psychological/psychiatric symptoms; interpersonal, occupational, school, medical, financial, housing, legal, and leisure problems; and problems with mental health or medical treatment. Although comprehensiveness is important, it is also important to keep the Problem List to a manageable length so the therapist can keep a grasp of it. If the list is longer than 10 items, it is a good idea to group some of the problems together in order to shorten the list to 5–8 items. It is useful to state the problems in a simple format, using a word or two to name the problem, followed by a description of the problem. It is useful when possible to describe the cognitive, behavioral, and emotion elements of problems (e.g., John's unassertiveness problem with his physician involves typical behaviors of listening to his doctor make treatment recommendations he doesn't understand but not speaking up to ask questions about them due to his following thoughts: "If I speak up my doctor will get mad and think I'm a wimp").

The main strategy most therapists use to collect a comprehensive problem list is the clinical interview. It is useful to start the interview by asking the patient to describe the problems he or she is concerned about. After this has been done, the therapist can ask for a status report on each domain that has not yet been touched on (Persons et al., 2000).

The tension the therapist always confronts is the pressure to move quickly to address the patient's current concerns while obtaining the information needed to understand how the current concerns are part of a larger context. Paper-and-pencil assessment tools are helpful in resolving this tension. We ask our patients to complete and bring to their initial interview several self-report scales, including the SCL-90-R (Derogatis, 2000), the Beck Depression Inventory (BDI; Beck et al., 1979), the Burns Anxiety Inventory (BAI; Burns & Eidelson, 1998), a modification of the CAGE for assessing substance use (Mayfield, McLeod, & Hall, 1974), and responses to questions about trauma, abuse, legal problems, and history of mental health treatment. We have also developed a brief paper-and-pencil assessment of daily functioning and satisfaction in multiple life domains (Davidson, Persons, & Valus, 2005), which is available on our website at www.sfbacct.com).

Careful observation can alert the therapist to problems that patients may not acknowledge or verbalize, such as lateness, a disheveled appearance, and, of particular importance because they are often a key reason patients seek treatment, interpersonal skills deficits such as poor eye contact. These behaviors and phenomena yield valuable information about problems and even suggest hypotheses about underlying mechanisms.

Information about past mental health problems and treatment is particularly important because it provides important information about such things as the tendency to discontinue treatment prematurely. Treatment history can also yield important diagnostic ideas that at least other therapists had (e.g., a history of treatment with lithium suggests the possibility that the patient may have bipolar disorder).

When the therapist observes problems of which the patient is unaware or which the patient does not accept (e.g., a diagnosis of bipolar disorder), the therapist might or might not wish to immediately insist that the patient endorse these as problems. To decide whether and when to do this, the nascent case formulation can be helpful. For example, patients who believe "If I have problems, I am worthless" may not be receptive to placing a new item on the Problem List until they feel more trusting of the therapist. A mutually agreed on Problem List is ideal but not always possible.

2. Assign a Five-Axis DSM Diagnosis

The role of diagnosis in CB therapy is a complex issue (Follette, 1996). We encourage the clinician to rely on diagnosis because it provides a link to evidence-based nomothetic formulations, the literature on empirically supported treatments (ESTs), and the experimental psychopathology literature. The clinician does not usually do a research-quality diagnostic assessment but might use parts of formal diagnostic interview tools in certain clinical situations (e.g., when screening for bipolar disorder); for a review of current options and their clinical utility, see Antony and Barlow (2002).

The Problem List overlaps considerably with the information provided by Axes I–IV of the DSM. The Problem List might even include one or more of the patient's Axis I disorders listed as the disorder itself (e.g., major depressive disorder or obsessive–compulsive disorder). Or, the Problem List might slice up the pie a bit differently; for example, if there are several anxiety disorders, the clinician might group them all together as one problem of anxiety. Or, if the patient has social phobia on Axis I, avoidant personality disorder on Axis II, and is socially isolated on Axis IV, all these might be grouped together as aspects of one problem on the Problem List, perhaps named social anxiety and isolation. The general rule guiding the selection and formatting of problems on the Problem List is clinical utility. Using this rule, the clinician might choose to include an important problem on the Problem List more than once; for example, John's therapist listed suicidal thoughts and urges as a problem in its own right in addition to including it as a symptom of the problem of depressive symptoms.

Again guided by the notion of clinical utility, the therapist's task is not to simply place on the Problem List all of the patient's DSM disorders (this strategy would make the Problem List unnecessary). Instead, the Problem List is a place to begin to describe problems in a way that helps the therapist develop a CB conceptualization of the case. Often this means a focus on symptoms and a description of the behavioral, cognitive, emotional, and somatic aspects of problems. Thus, for example, instead of simply placing social phobia on the Problem List, John's therapist listed some of the key behavioral, cognitive, emotional, and somatic aspects of John's social anxiety. In this way, the description of the social anxiety and isolation problem sketches out a problem or disorder-level formulation that will guide treatment of that problem and even begins to describe how the social anxiety problem is related to John's medical noncompliance problem.

It is not usually helpful to list Axis II disorders per se on the Problem List, because there are few empirically supported formulations and treatments for personality disorders and because the overlap of symptoms and problems of Axis I and Axis II disorders is so extensive. Instead, listing some of the significant symptoms and problem behaviors of a patient's Axis II disorder or disorders facilitates conceptualization and treatment from a CB vantage point.

3. Select an "Anchoring" Diagnosis

Here the clinician selects a primary or anchoring diagnosis that will be used to guide selection of a nomothetic template for the idiographic case formulation. Using the parsimony principle, a useful approach to selecting an anchoring diagnosis is to choose the diagnosis that accounts for the largest number of problems on the Problem List—that is, the diagnosis that interferes most with the patient's functioning. Practically, one implication of this rule is that if a patient has bipolar disorder, schizophrenia, or borderline personality disorder (disorders that can account for many presenting problems) the clinician may want to select this diagnosis as the anchoring diagnosis.

Sometimes it is useful to choose an anchoring diagnosis based on the current treatment goals. So, for example, if the patient has bipolar disorder under good control and wants to treat her panic symptoms, the panic disorder diagnosis might serve as the anchoring diagnosis. Even so, the clinician will want to keep the bipolar disorder in mind as treatment proceeds. Becker (2002) provides a fascinating description of her method for integrating conceptualizations and interventions from several disorders and ESTs in the treatment of a single complex case. The decision about selection of an anchoring diagnosis is a clinical and pragmatic one guided by principles of parsimony and clinical utility rather than one based on any science, as little research about this type of clinical decision making is available.

4. Select a Nomothetic Formulation of the Anchoring Diagnosis

If an evidence-based nomothetic formulation of the anchoring diagnosis is available, select one to serve as a template for the idiographic case formulation. For example, in the case presented here, the nomothetic formulations of social anxiety disorder developed by Clark and Wells (1995) and Rapee and Heimberg (1997) served as a template for the formulation of John's case. Sometimes more than one nomothetic formulation template is available (e.g., multiple evidence-based ESTs—and formulations—are available for major depressive disorder). In this situation, the therapist may want to select the one with which he or she is most familiar, the one that will be most acceptable to the patient, or the one that seems to best fit the case (Haynes, Kaholokula, & Nelson, 1999).

When no evidence-based nomothetic formulation is available, the therapist can adapt a template that has been proposed for another disorder or symptom to the case at hand, as illustrated by Opdyke and Rothbaum (1998), who used the empirically supported formulations and interventions for one impulse-control disorder (trichotillomania) as the template for a formulation and intervention plan for other impulse-control disorders for which no empirically-supported protocol is available (e.g., kleptomania and pyromania). Another option for the therapist when there is no nomothetic template to work from (e.g., none has been developed or is not easily available, and, say, the patient has psychogenic vomiting) is to develop a formulation using mainstream empirically supported theories of psychopathology, especially those that underpin many of the currently available ESTs. These general theories include Beck's cognitive theory, theories of associative and operant conditioning, and theories of emotion and emotion regulation, such as Lang's (1979) bioinformational theory and Gross's (1998) theory of emotion regulation. An elegant example is the use of operant conditioning theory as a foundation for the formulation and treatment of a child with migraine headache (O'Brien & Haynes, 1995).

5. Individualize the Template

To individualize the nomothetic formulation, the therapist must collect the details of the cognitive, behavioral, emotional, and somatic aspects of the patient's problems, as well as details about how the problems are related. Of course, not all problems result from the hypothesized psychological mechanisms that are the heart of the formulation. Some problems result entirely or in part from biological, environmental, or other nonpsychological factors, as in the case of medical problems, financial problems resulting from an employer's bankruptcy, or bipolar disorder or anxiety that has a likely biological or genetic basis (in a case in which many family members also have these problems). Also, some fears are rational!

Some problems are the consequence of other problems. For example, as a consequence of using alcohol to escape his depressed mood, John now has an alcohol problem and his liver function is worse. Often causal arrows go in more than one direction: Depression leads to alcohol use, which in turn likely exacerbates John's depression.

6. Propose Hypotheses about the Origins of the Mechanisms

Here the therapist asks and collects information to generate hypotheses about how the patient developed the schemas, how the patient learned the dysfunctional behaviors or failed to learn the functional ones, how the patient developed an emotion or emotion regulation deficit, and how the patient acquired a biological or genetic vulnerability. To do this, the clinician will collect a family history of psychiatric disorder, as well as a family and social history that identifies key events and factors in the patient's upbringing and development.

7. Describe Precipitants of the Current Episode of Illness or Symptom Exacerbation

To obtain information about precipitants and activating situations, the therapist can ask the patient and/or someone who is close to the patient to describe the sequence of events leading up to the presenting problems. As the individual does this, the therapist will be thinking about the proposed mechanism hypotheses, in an effort to tie together or link in some logical way the precipitants and the mechanisms. A. T. Beck (1983) discusses this issue very elegantly, proposing that interpersonal loss and rejection would be expected to precipitate depression in patients who have schemas relating to dependency, whereas failure would be expected to precipitate depression in patients who hold schemas relating to failure and loss of autonomy.

After walking through these seven steps, the therapist will have the information needed to write a formulation of the case.

APPLICATION TO PSYCHOTHERAPY TECHNIQUE

The case formulation guides the therapist's decision making throughout the treatment. Because as part of formulating the case the therapist collects a comprehensive Problem List, the formulation helps the therapist adapt the nomothetic evidence-based CB formulations and therapies, which usually target a single disorder, to the multiple-problem patient (most patients!). The formulation also guides intervention in the therapy session. Descriptions of John's problems using a CB format that entailed describing problems in terms of their primary emotions, cognitions, and behaviors showed that John's behavioral avoidance and passivity were aspects of most of the problems on his Problem List, including the problems of noncompliance with his medical care, social isolation and unassertiveness, depression, and alcohol abuse. The formulation thus cued John's therapist to target John's passivity and avoidance early and often.

To use the model to guide clinical decision making in the therapy session, the therapist develops a formulation of a particular instance of a problem behavior or symptom that guides intervention to address that behavior or symptom. This formulation, which might be called a situation-level formulation, is based on detailed assessment of the situation itself, but also on the symptom, disorder, problem, and/or case-level formulations developed earlier. Thus, when the therapist learned that John discontinued his antidepressant medications without discussing the matter with anyone (including the therapist), the therapist's initial hypothesis about this behavior flowed out of the case-level formulation that had already been developed, which offered the therapist the initial hypotheses that John's behavior resulted from his schema about the future as hopeless (and thus treatment as ineffectual), or from his schemas that he is a wimp if he needs medications, or that others (which may include the therapist) will attack and criticize him if he cannot recover without medications or is unhappy about side effects.

The case formulation can even help the therapist identify distortions in the self-report progress data. Self-report data such as the Beck Depression Inventory (BDI), which John's therapist collected weekly to monitor John's progress, are so transparent that they are easily manipulated. Based on the formulation's proposal that John fears being criticized and rejected by others when they are not pleased, John's therapist was aware that John might tend to underreport symptoms on the BDI in order to please the therapist and therefore evaluated his weekly BDI scores as possibly biased downward and collected additional data to assess the validity of the BDI data and to monitor John's progress in therapy.

A CB case formulation is especially helpful when the therapy is not going well. For example, John's therapy progressed in fits and starts. He failed to follow through with homework assignments, frequently canceled appointments at the last minute, was unable to suggest a single suitable treatment goal, and, in general, was not meaningfully engaged in the therapy. Upon reviewing the formulation, the therapist hypothesized that John's schema about himself ("I'm a wimp") and others ("Others are critical and rejecting") might be contributing to the therapeutic impasse. The therapist introduced to John the suggestion that perhaps he was unable to commit to a course in therapy because he feared the therapist would put him down and view John as weak and a wimp if he admitted he had some problems with which he wanted help. John acceded that this might be true. To address this issue, the therapist suggested that they examine the advantages and disadvantages of assuming the therapist would act in this way. A session spent on this exercise opened the door to some cognitive restructuring exercises focused on this problematic belief and to a plan that periodically John would "test" the therapist by stating, for example, that he was having trouble understanding the therapist (when in fact he understood him quite well) to see whether the therapist would become frustrated and impatient with John. Prescribing this behavior was particularly helpful in that John tended to test the therapist and others anyway. Using these strategies, John gradually became more engaged in the therapy and made good progress.

The CB therapist always includes the patient in the process of developing the formulation and using it to guide intervention, relying on what Padesky (1996) calls shoulder-to-shoulder case conceptualization. There is some evidence that a shared formulation contributes to therapeutic success (see the research review below). We recommend presenting the formulation and intervention plan in pieces, seeking the patient's input at each step rather than laying out the complete formulation in one fell swoop, which can be overwhelming and alienating.

CASE EXAMPLE

Here we present the information John's therapist obtained as he carried out the "Steps in Case Formulation" described previously.

1. Obtain a Comprehensive Problem List

Suicidal Thoughts and Urges

John reports suicidal thoughts (e.g., "What's the point, there's nothing that can be done for me," "I just want this whole thing to be over," "If this is life, show me the exit.") that are typically triggered by setbacks in his medical condition. The frequency and intensity of his suicidal thoughts and urges have increased over the last 6 months as his medical condition has deteriorated. A couple of times each month, John checks the Hemlock Society webpage but denies that he has decided on a plan or has means to act on his urges.

Hepatitis C

In 1990 John was injured in an automobile accident and received a blood transfusion which infected him with the hepatitis C virus. Although John is receiving interferon therapy, it does not appear that he is benefiting. His liver is moderately cirrhotic, and many days he feels quite ill. John's condition is life-threatening, and if it worsens, a liver transplant may be needed. John experiences several uncomfortable symptoms associated with his hepatitis C and interferon therapy, including flushing, dizziness, fatigue, and tremors.

Poor Medical Adherence

John has an extensive history of poor collaboration with his medical team. His nephrologist has suggested that John consider alternative therapies for his hepatitis C, some of which are experimental, but John will not discuss these alternatives with his physician, worrying that if he asks questions about them "the doc will think I'm a whiner and give up on me." In addition, John refuses to follow treatment recommendations if they involve meeting others, such as attending a hepatitis C support group, because "only losers go to those support groups" and because he experiences significant anxiety in social situations. John also refuses antidepressant medication because he believes that "it won't work" and the decision to use medications "just proves I'm a total loser." John seldom asks his physicians questions about their recommendations or directly refuses to accept the recommendations; instead, he simply fails to follow them.

Depressive Symptoms

John reports sadness, feelings of worthlessness and hopelessness, anhedonia, difficulty doing anything, fatigue, and disruptions in sleep and appetite, scoring 32 (severe depression) on the BDI (Beck, Ward, Mendelsohn, Mock, & Erbaugh, 1961). John has few contacts with others, mostly sitting at home surfing the Internet or participating in chat rooms. He does not engage in pleasurable activities because he predicts, "It won't be fun anyway," and because he is often fatigued due to his medical condition.

Social Anxiety and Social Isolation

John reports that social situations make him extremely anxious. He has never dated and has only one or two childhood friends whom he seldom sees. Because of his social anxiety, he is unwilling to join a hepatitis C support group, meet regularly with his physician and work closely with his physician, to address his medical situation or consider other medical interventions that would involve interactions with others. On several occasions, John has run out of medication but would not call his physician for a refill or even call in a refill to the pharmacy because he was too anxious to make the call. His Social Phobia Scale (Heimberg, Mueller, Holt, Hope, & Liebowitz, 1992) score = 47, and he rates as extremely true, "I fear I may blush when I am with others," "I worry about shaking or trembling when I'm watched by other people," or "I get panicky that others might see me faint, or be sick or ill." John believes that he is a "geek" and that he is a poor conversationalist, although his social skills as assessed informally in the therapist's office appear to be within normal limits. He thinks of others are far more socially skilled than he is and that they are "just waiting to call me on my stuff." Compounding John's social anxiety, he experiences a variety of physical symptoms (sweating, dizziness, flushing) secondary to the hepatitis C and interferon therapy which activate his social worries.

Unassertive Behavior

John is not assertive in his personal and professional relationships. For example, he takes on web design projects that he knows he will not be able to complete rather than negotiate an appropriate timeline with the employer. As a result, he frequently fails to complete projects on time, resulting in difficulty securing and keeping web design jobs. He is not receiving optimal care for his medical condition because he is unable to ask for changes in his treatment or to advocate for alternative treatments that he has researched. His unassertive behavior is driven by thoughts such as "they'll think I'm a whiner," or "they'll just get upset with me and it will be even worse then."

Alcohol Abuse

John drinks four to five glasses of wine each day, usually in the evenings. John denies a family history of substance abuse, blackouts, driving under the influence, or financial or legal problems as a result of his alcohol use. However, he continues to drink in spite of the fact that the physician has repeatedly pointed out that drinking is jeopardizing his liver function given his chronic illness (hepatitis C). John reports that he continues to drink because he has nothing else to do and "I'm doomed anyway, what's the point of stopping." John refuses to consider treatment for his substance abuse because it would involve anxiety-provoking social contacts; he labels people who attend Alcoholics Anonymous (AA) meetings as "a bunch of whiny losers."

2. Assign a Five-Axis DSM Diagnosis

John's DSM diagnosis is as follows:

- Axis I   Social anxiety disorder, generalized type
           Major depressive disorder, recurrent, severe
           Dysthymic disorder, early onset
           Alcohol abuse

- Axis II   Avoidant personality disorder
- Axis III Hepatitis C
- Axis IV   Inadequate social support, financial difficulties
- Axis V   45

3. Select an "Anchoring" Diagnosis

John's anchoring diagnosis is social anxiety disorder.

4. Select a Nomothetic Formulation of the Anchoring Diagnosis

The nomothetic formulation of social anxiety disorder (Clark & Wells, 1995) (Rapee & Heimberg, 1997) assumes that social anxiety results from the interplay of an individual's biological and psychological vulnerabilities with social, cultural, familial, and biological stressors. Social anxiety disorder is characterized by avoidance of social situations due to excessive and exaggerated fear of negative evaluation by others accompanied by strong physiological arousal and distress. At times, the socially anxious individual fears that his or her physical symptoms of anxiety are the focus of scrutiny, and he or she uses safety behaviors (e.g., wearing turtleneck sweaters to hide flushing) to cope. These safety behaviors and avoidance of social situations prevent the individual from obtaining evidence that would disconfirm his cognitive misappraisals.

Other relevant nomothetic formulations: None.

5. Individualize the Template

To carry out this step, the therapist spelled out details of the key biological/somatic, behavioral, and cognitive factors of John's problems.

Biological/Somatic Factors

The physical symptoms that John experiences when he's anxious and which trigger anxiety/activate his schemas include flushing, dizziness, fatigue, and tremors. Fatigue is a piece of both his anxiety and depression. These symptoms are also associated with his hepatitis C and interferon therapy.

Behavioral Factors

The key behavioral aspects of John's difficulties are avoidance behaviors, including failure to assert himself with friends, customers/clients of his web business, and physicians. He does not initiate social contacts despite loneliness; he has never dated although he would like a relationship. He avoids going to parties or speaking on the telephone. He avoids signing his name or writing in public for fear that others will notice his hand tremble.

Safety behaviors (behaviors John exhibits in order to prevent negative evaluation by others) include wearing dark shirts so that if he sweats, it is less noticeable, and holding something in his hands when he is speaking to people so that if his hand trembles, it is less noticeable.

Cognitive Factors

The cognitive aspects of John's problems are the following:

- Schema: "I'm a loser, whiner, geek, wimp, helpless."
- "Others are critical and rejecting."
- "World is bleak."
- "Future is uncontrollable and hopeless."
- Conditional assumptions: "If I ask for what I want, people will put me down."
- Typical automatic thoughts: Depression and suicidal urges are caused by thoughts such as "What's the point, there's nothing that can be done for me," "I just want this whole thing to be over," "If this is life, show me the exit." Unassertive behavior is driven by thoughts such as, "They'll think I'm a whiner," or "They'll just get upset with me and it will be even worse then," and "Other people are more socially skilled than I am and are just waiting to call me on my stuff."

6. Propose Hypotheses about the Origins of the Mechanisms

To develop hypotheses about the origins of the mechanisms, John's therapist obtained a detailed family and cultural history that emphasizes events that are likely related to the proposed mechanisms.

John is an only child, born to Japanese parents who immigrated to this country just before his birth. His father came to the United States to attend graduate school and is currently employed as an aerospace engineer and appears to have easily acculturated. John's mother, on the other hand, has not learned English, largely because she was too shy to seek help or take English-as-a-second language classes; she is largely homebound and accepts few visitors. John reports that he was a very shy child. He did not speak to anyone but his parents and a few close friends until he was 6 years old and spent much time alone playing or reading in his room. His father was seldom around, as he worked many hours and traveled extensively for his job. John remembers his father as highly critical of John, often demeaning him in an effort to motivate John to work harder at school or to go out and socialize ("If you're smart show me, otherwise shut up."). When John cried, his father would call him a "wimp" or a "whiner." John's mother was largely unable to protect him because she was very shy, depressed, and dependent on her husband. John's parents divorced when he was 10 years old and John lived with his mother. His father showed little interest in spending time with John, so John spent most of his time, when not in school, home with his mother. Because John's mother was shy and depressed, few people came into their home, and she was unable to arrange play dates or other social activities for John.

7. Describe Precipitants of the Current Episode of Illness or Symptom Exacerbation

Although John's social anxiety appears to be chronic, his current depressive episode appears to be precipitated by his deteriorating medical condition and his view that nothing can be done to help him, as well as his continued social isolation.

John's therapist used all this information to develop the formulation of John's case provided on p. 7 above.

TRAINING

Although constructing a case formulation is quite difficult, little is known about how to train clinicians to do this. Therefore, we offer observations based on our own training experiences. We find that trainees come to us for answers to two types of questions about their cases. The first type of question is a "how-to" or technique question, such as "How do I complete a Thought Record?" or "How do I design a behavioral experiment with this client?" The second type of question is a "What do I do if . . . ?" or formulation question, such as "What do I do if the client repeatedly fails to complete his therapy homework?" or "What do I do if the client refuses to set an agenda for the session?" We believe it is essential that we, as teachers, keep the distinction between these two types of questions clearly in mind, and that we teach our trainees to distinguish these two questions. Trainees who understand the distinction will ask clearer questions and thereby increase the likelihood that they will get the help they need. But even more important, trainees who are taught to distinguish between technique and formulation questions will understand the essential role of formulation in CB therapy. Too often, trainees view CB therapy as a string of techniques or strategies that the therapist throws at clients until one of them sticks. Instead, CB therapy is a way of thinking in which the therapist uses CB formulations to understand his client and as a guide to selecting interventions and trouble-shooting when obstacles arise. One of our primary training goals is to get this idea across to trainees.

We have found that training in CB case formulation happens best in a small group where therapists can work together to formulate their own and each others' cases. We have found that certain typical difficulties arise and that trainees can help one another overcome them.

Trainees often have difficulty making a Problem List, which makes it a good place to begin any discussion of a new case or review of an ongoing case. The most common problems include difficulty obtaining an exhaustive list, especially the tendency to omit medical or "nonpsychological" problems (e.g., financial or legal problems). We encourage trainees to search for problems systematically by considering the domains listed on p. x. Trainees sometimes describe problems in jargon (e.g., "codependency") or in vague terms (e.g., poor self-esteem or communication problems). The best remedy for both these difficulties is to emphasize the importance of describing the mood, cognitive, and behavioral aspects of problems. Sometimes the trainee does not seem to fully understand all the ramifications of a particular problem for the client. To flesh this out, it is useful to ask the trainee to think about why the client's problem (e.g., depressed mood) is a problem for her. In response, the therapist may learn that the client is no longer seeing his friends, is about to lose his job because of absenteeism, and has increased his alcohol intake. Surprisingly, sometimes trainees can sit with a client who has obvious problems of self-care and not think to ask about exercise, sleep, diet, or grooming. Yet another problem that trainees encounter when developing a Problem List is the failure to identify problems (e.g., self-harm behaviors or substance abuse) that the client does not wish to discuss or does not perceive as a problem.

Sometimes trainees do not recognize problems that belong on the Problem List because the client appears to have solved it. In this case, it can be helpful for the trainee to learn that some solutions are in fact problems, as in the case of the client who "solves" his problems by avoiding. For example, a trainee presented a short list of problems for a client who had been troubled by a series of panic attacks beginning 15 years earlier. The client identified no other problems. However, when the trainee was asked, "What problems do you know of that the client has already solved himself?" the Problem List expanded to include a number of long-standing avoidant "solutions" that had resulted in the loss of the client's job and the dissolution of his marriage.

We encourage trainees to generate formulation hypotheses early. This recommendation is supported by evidence collected by Elstein, Shulman, and Sprafka (1978), who, in studies of medical problem solving by physicians, found that "competent physicians begin generating hypotheses in the earliest moments of their encounter with clients" (p. ix). Trainees are often reluctant to offer hypotheses unless they are confident that they are correct. As a result, they offer too few hypotheses or delay offering hypotheses for too long. We suggest that trainees generate formulation hypotheses as early as the first telephone call from a prospective client or on first meeting him in the waiting room. How might you explain that the client took 2 weeks to return your call about setting up a consultation appointment? Why might the client be standing outside the waiting room with the waiting room door open when you go out to meet him?

In addition, trainees (and experienced therapists!) do not consider enough alternatives and can become overattached to their formulation hypotheses and have difficulty dispensing with a hypothesis that is not useful. To expand the number of alternatives considered in the formulation generation process, we recommend that each case formulation begin with a period of brainstorming in which the therapist offers as many ideas as possible, refraining from judging or editing any hypothesis offered by the group, no matter how silly it may appear. When several hypotheses are generated, the editing process can begin. Even then, it is helpful to keep several hypotheses on the table for a particular case and generate interventions based on each hypothesis. In this way, trainees are reminded that the goal is not to find the "correct" formulation but to become skilled at generating hypotheses and using them to formulate intervention strategies. To address the problem of overattachment to failing hypotheses, we encourage trainees to periodically review treatment progress with the client and to report on this to the supervisor or consultant.

Writing a complete and comprehensive case formulation for every client may not be practical for busy clinicians. However, the process of developing a written formulation is an excellent training exercise. As trainees learn to develop formulations, they may find it helpful to write down the information required for each of the items found in the section "Steps in Case Formulation Construction." The importance of this skill for trainees is highlighted by the fact that most trainees treat complex and often treatment-refractory clients.

RESEARCH SUPPORT FOR THE APPROACH

A handful of studies has examined interrater reliability of CB case formulation, with adequate but not outstanding results (Kuyken, Fothergill, Musa, & Chadwick, 2005; Persons & Bertagnolli, 1999; Persons, Mooney, & Padesky, 1995). As we indicated in our discussion of the qualities of a good CB formulation, we view treatment utility as more important than interrater reliability (in fact, different therapists might have different formulations, but those formulations might still be useful in guiding effective treatment). For that reason, we focus this brief review primarily on the treatment utility of the case formulation, that is, the degree to which the formulation contributes to a good treatment outcome (Hayes et al., 1987). Two uncontrolled trials of the method described here have shown that treatment of depressed (Persons, Bostrom, & Bertagnolli, 1999) and depressed anxious patients (Persons, Roberts, Zalecki, & Brechwald, 2005) guided by a CB case formulation and weekly progress monitoring have outcomes similar to outcomes of patients treated in manualized standardized treatments in the randomized controlled trials. Going beyond the specific format described here, several types of research designs provide relevant evidence, and we offer some highlights of those here.

A handful of randomized trials comparing outcomes of standardized CB therapy versus CB therapy guided by a case formulation shows that formulation-driven treatment is no different from or sometimes a bit better than standardized treatment on outcome of acute treatment and maintenance of gains (Jacobson et al., 1989; Schneider & Byrne, 1987; Schulte, Kunzel, Pepping, & Schulte-Bahewnverg, 1992). No studies show that formulation-driven treatment obtains worse outcomes than standardized treatment. Although the Schulte et al. (1992) finding is frequently reported as showing that patients who received individualized treatment had worse outcomes, we read it as failing to show a difference between individualized and standardized treatment. Schulte et al. (1992) randomly assigned 120 phobics to standardized exposure treatment, individualized treatment, or yoked control treatment. Although a multiple analysis of variance (MANOVA) showed that the three treatment conditions differed significantly at the $p < .05$ level for three of nine outcome measures at posttreatment, these results faded over time (appearing on only two measures at 6-month follow-up, and on none at 2-year follow-up), and no statistical tests examining pairwise comparisons of the three treatment groups, in order to identify which treatment was best and which worst, were presented.

Future studies of the treatment utility of the formulation might examine outcome variables in addition to acute and long-term outcome; we would predict that the use of an individualized case formulation ought to have effects on treatment compliance, the quality of the therapeutic relationship, dropout, and relapse. Two studies of the effects of shared formulation on compliance and dropout, however, have mixed results. Foulks, Persons, and Merkel (1986) showed that patients who viewed the causes of their illness in medical model terms (e.g., neurotransmitter derangement) were less likely to drop out prematurely and noncollaboratively (e.g., without telling the therapist of his or her intentions) than patients who endorsed non-medical model causes (e.g., the evil eye) of their psychiatric illness. Addis and Jacobson (2000), however, failed to find the predicted relationship between the patient's acceptance of the treatment rationale and homework compliance.

Addis and Jacobson (2000) and Fennell and Teasdale (1987) showed that the patient's acceptance of the treatment rationale predicts the outcome of treatment. These findings indicate that the patient's perception that the nomothetic formulation underpinning the treatment is applicable to his situation contributes to good treatment outcome. This patient–therapist agreement on the formulation is widely viewed as an aspect of the therapeutic alliance (Tracey & Kokotovic, 1989), which has of course repeatedly been shown to predict treatment outcome.

Another relevant literature is the literature on treatment matching, which investigates whether matching treatment to client characteristics leads to better outcomes. This is a large literature with a large number of negative findings (see Dance & Neufeld, 1988). Several (see Addis & Jacobson, 1996) have suggested that reasons for negative findings may include low power and the failure to examine theoretically derived predictions, and this observation is consistent with the observation (Addis & Jacobson, 1996) that prospective studies that test theoretically derived predictions have produced some more positive findings, such as the demonstrations that high-externalizing and low-resistance clients improved more in group CB therapy than did low-externalizing and high-resistance clients (Beutler, Machado, Engle, & Mohr, 1991) and the findings (see reviews by Nelson-Gray, 2003, and Haynes, Leisen, & Blaine, 1997, that functional analysis has good treatment utility in the treatment of severe behavior problems, including self-injurious behavior.

The studies reviewed here converge to provide some support for the assertion that reliance on a CB case formulation can contribute to treatment outcome. However, relatively few studies have been done to examine this question directly. For that reason, it is probably fair to say that the strongest empirical support for the treatment utility of a CB case formulation currently comes from the method's reliance on evidence-based nomothetic formulations as templates for the idiographic formulation and from the idiographic data that the therapist collects in order to test the clinical utility of the formulation.

NOTE

1. We thank the listserve of the Society for a Science of Clinical Psychology, especially Jonathan Abramowitz, John Hunsley, Howard Garb, and Drew Westen, for a helpful discussion of this topic

REFERENCES

Addis, M. E., & Jacobson, N. S. (1996). Reasons for depression and the process and outcome of cognitive-behavioral psychotherapies. *Journal of Consulting and Clinical Psychology, 64,* 1417–1424.

Addis, M. E., & Jacobson, N. S. (2000). A closer look at the treatment rationale and homework compliance in cognitive-behavioral therapy for depression. *Cognitive Therapy and Research, 24,* 313–326.

Antony, M. M., & Barlow, D. H. (Eds.). (2002). *Handbook of assessment and treatment planning for psychological disorders.* New York: Guilford Press.

Barlow, D. H., & Craske, M. G. (2001). *Panic disorder and agoraphobia.* New York: Guilford Press.

Barlow, D. H., Craske, M. G., Cerny, J. A., & Klosko, J. S. (1989). Behavioral treatment of panic disorder. *Behavior Therapy, 20,* 261–282.

Beck, A. T. (1983). Cognitive theory of depression: New perspectives. In P. J. Clayton & J. E. Barrett (Eds.), *Treatment of depression: Old controversies and new approaches* (pp. 265–288). New York: Raven Press.

Beck, A. T., Rush, J. A., Shaw, B. F., & Emery, G. (1979). *Cognitive therapy for depression.* New York: Guilford Press.

Beck, A. T., Ward, C. H., Mendelsohn, M., Mock, J., & Erbaugh, J. (1961). An inventory for measuring depression. *Archives of General Psychiatry, 4,* 561–571.

Beck, J. S. (1995). *Cognitive therapy: Basics and beyond.* New York: Guilford Press.

Becker, C. B. (2002). Integrated behavioral treatment of comorbid OCD, PTSD, and borderline personality disorder: A case report. *Cognitive and Behavioral Practice, 9,* 100–110.

Beutler, L. E., Machado, P. P., Engle, D., & Mohr, D. (1991). Predictors of differential response to cognitive, experiential, and self-directed psychotherapeutic procedures. *Journal of Consulting and Clinical Psychology, 59,* 333–340.

Burns, D. D. (1998). *Therapist toolkit.* Unpublished manuscript, Los Altos, CA.

Burns, D. D., & Eidelson, R. (1998). Why are measures of depression and anxiety correlated?—I. A test of tripartite theory. *Journal of Consulting and Clinical Psychology, 60,* 441–449.

Clark, D. M., & Wells, A. (1995). A cognitive model of social phobia. In R. G. Heimberg, M. R. Liebowitz, D. A. Hope, & F. R. Schneier (Eds.), *Social phobia: Diagnosis, assessment, and treatment* (pp. 69–93). New York: Guilford Press.

Cone, J. D. (1986). Idiographic, nomothetic, and related perspectives in behavioral assessment. In R. O. Nelson & S. C. Hayes (Eds.), *Conceptual foundations of behavioral assessment* (pp. 111–128). New York: Guilford Press.

Dance, K. A., & Neufeld, W. J. (1988). Aptitude-treatment interaction research in the clinical setting: A review of attempts to dispel the "patient uniformity" myth. *Psychological Bulletin, 104,* 192–213.

Davidson, J., Persons, J. B., & Valus, K. L. (2005). *Functioning and Satisfaction Inventory (FSI).* Available www.sfbacct.com

Derogatis, L. R. (2000). *SCL-90-R.* Washington, DC: American Psychological Association.

Elstein, A. S., Shulman, L. S., & Sprafka, S. A. (1978). *Medical problem solving: An analysis of clinical reasoning.* Cambridge, MA: Harvard University Press.

Fennell, M. J. V., & Teasdale, J. D. (1987). Cognitive therapy for depression: Individual differences and the process of change. *Cognitive Therapy and Research, 11,* 253–271.

Follette, W. C. (1996). Introduction to the special section on the development of theoretically coherent alternatives to the DSM system. *Journal of Consulting and Clinical Psychology, 64,* 1117–1119.

Foulks, E. F., Persons, J. B., & Merkel, R. L. (1986). The effect of illness beliefs on compliance in psychotherapy. *American Journal of Psychiatry, 143,* 340–344.

Freeman, A. (1992). Developing treatment conceptualizations in cognitive therapy. In

A. Freeman & F. Dattilio (Eds.), *Casebook of cognitive-behavior therapy* (pp. 13–23). New York: Plenum Press.

Goodman, W. K., Price, L. H., Rasmussen, S. A., Mazure, C., Fleischman, R. L., Hill, C. L., et al. (1989). The Yale–Brown Obsessive Compulsive Scale I: Development, use, and reliability. *Archives of General Psychiatry, 46*, 1006–1011.

Gross, J. J. (1998). The emerging field of emotion regulation: An integrative review. *Review of General Psychology, 2*, 271–299.

Hayes, S., & Toarmino, D. (1995). If behavioral principles are generally applicable, why is it necessary to understand cultural diversity? *The Behavior Therapist, 18*, 21–23.

Hayes, S. C., Nelson, R. O., & Jarrett, R. B. (1987). The treatment utility of assessment: A functional approach to evaluating assessment quality. *American Psychologist, 42*, 963–974.

Haynes, S. N., Kaholokula, J. K., & Nelson, K. (1999). The idiographic application of nomothetic, empirically based treatments. *Clinical Psychology: Science and Practice, 6*, 456–461.

Haynes, S. N., Leisen, M. B., & Blaine, D. D. (1997). Design of individualized behavioral treatment programs using functional analytic clinical case models. *Psychological Assessment, 9*, 334–348.

Haynes, S. N., & O'Brien, W. H. (2000). *Principles and practice of behavioral assessment.* New York: Kluwer Academic/Plenum Press.

Heimberg, R. G., Mueller, G. P., Holt, C. S., Hope, D. A., & Liebowitz, M. R. (1992). Assessment of anxiety in social interactions and being observed by others: The Social Interaction Anxiety Scale and the Social Phobia Scale. *Behavior Therapy, 23*, 53–73.

Jacobson, N. S., Schmaling, K. B., Holtzworth-Munroe, A., Katt, J. L., Wood, L. F., & Follette, V. M. (1989). Research-structured vs. clinically flexible versions of social learning-based marital therapy. *Behaviour Research and Therapy, 27*, 173–180.

Kingdon, D., & Turkington, D. (2005). *Cognitive therapy of schizophrenia.* New York: Guilford Press.

Kring, A. M., & Werner, K. H. (2004). Emotion regulation and psychopathology. In P. Philippot & R. S. Feldman (Eds.), *The regulation of emotion* (pp. 359–385). Mahwah, NJ: Erlbaum.

Kuyken, W., Fothergill, C. D., Musa, M., & Chadwick, P. (2005). The reliability and quality of cognitive case formulation. *Behaviour Research and Therapy, 43*, 1187–1201.

Lang, P. J. (1979). A bio-informational theory of emotional imagery. *Psychophysiology, 16*, 495–512.

Linehan, M. M. (1993). *Cognitive-behavioral treatment of borderline personality disorder.* New York: Guilford Press.

Mayfield, D., McLeod, G., & Hall, P. (1974). The CAGE questionnaire: Validation of a new alcoholism screening instrument. *American Journal of Psychiatry, 131*, 1121–1123.

Morgan, D. L., & Morgan, R. K. (2001). Single-participant research design: Bringing science to managed care. *American Psychologist, 56*, 119–127.

Nelson-Gray, R. O. (2003). Treatment utility of psychological assessment. *Psychological Assessment, 15*, 521–531.

Nezu, A. M., Nezu, C. M., Friedman, S. H., & Haynes, S. N. (1997). Case formulation in behavior therapy: Problem-solving and functional analytic strategies. In T. D. Eells (Ed.), *Handbook of psychotherapy case formulation* (pp. 368–401). New York: Guilford Press.

O'Brien, W. H., & Haynes, S. N. (1995). A functional analytic approach to the conceptualization, assessment, and treatment of a child with frequent migraine headaches. *Journal of Clinical Psychology, 1*, 65–80.

Opdyke, D., & Rothbaum, B. O. (1998). Cognitive-behavioral treatment of impulse control disorders. In V. E. Caballo (Ed.), *International handbook of cognitive and behavioural treatments for psychological disorders* (pp. 417–439). Oxford, UK: Pergamon/Elsevier Science.

Padesky, C. A. (1996). *Collaborative case conceptualization: A client session* [Videotape]. Oakland, CA: New Harbinger Press.

Persons, J. B. (1989). *Cognitive therapy in practice: A case formulation approach.* New York: Norton.

Persons, J. B., & Bertagnolli, A. (1999). Inter-rater reliability of cognitive-behavioral case formulation of depression: A replication. *Cognitive Therapy and Research, 23*, 271–284.

Persons, J. B., Bostrom, A., & Bertagnolli, A. (1999). Results of randomized controlled trials of cognitive therapy for depression generalize to private practice. *Cognitive Therapy and Research, 23*, 535–548.

Persons, J. B., & Davidson, J. (2001). Cognitive-behavioral case formulation. In K. Dobson (Ed.), *Handbook of cognitive-behavioral therapies* (pp. 86–110). New York: Guilford Press.

Persons, J. B., Mooney, K. A., & Padesky, C. A. (1995). Inter-rater reliability of cognitive-behavioral case formulation. *Cognitive Therapy and Research, 19*, 21–34.

Persons, J. B., Roberts, N. A., Zalecki, C. A., & Brechwald, W. A. G. (2005). *Naturalistic outcome of case formulation-driven cognitive-behavior therapy for anxious depressed outpatients.* Unpublished manuscript.

Persons, J. B., & Tompkins, M. A. (1997). Cognitive-behavioral case formulation. In T. D. Eells (Ed.), *Handbook of psychotherapy case formulation* (pp. 314–339). New York: Guilford Press.

Persons, J. B., Tompkins, M. A., & Davidson, J. (2000). *Cognitive-behavior therapy for depression: Individualized case formulation and treatment planning* [Videotape]. Washington, DC: American Psychological Association.

Rapee, R. M., & Heimberg, R. G. (1997). A cognitive-behavioral model of anxiety in social phobia. *Behaviour Research and Therapy, 35*, 741–756.

Schneider, B. H., & Byrne, B. M. (1987). Individualizing social skills training for behavior-disordered children. *Journal of Consulting and Clinical Psychology, 55*, 444–445.

Schulte, D., Kunzel, R., Pepping, G., & Schulte-Bahrenberg, T. (1992). Tailor-made versus standardized therapy of phobic patients. *Advances in Behaviour Research and Therapy, 14*, 67–92.

Tarrier, N., & Calam, R. (2002). New developments in cognitive-behavioural case formulation. Epidemiological, systemic and social context: An integrative approach. *Behavioural and Cognitive Psychotherapy, 30*, 311–328.

Tracey, T. J., & Kokotovic, A. M. (1989). Factor structure of the working alliance inventory. *Psychological Assessment, 1*(3), 207–210.

Chapter 11

Case Formulation in Dialectical Behavior Therapy for Borderline Personality Disorder

KELLY KOERNER

Dialectical behavior therapy (DBT; Linehan, 1993a, 1993b) is a cognitive-behavioral treatment originally developed as an outpatient treatment for clients diagnosed with borderline personality disorder (BPD) and subsequently adapted for other populations and treatment settings (see research section for more detail). Case formulation is essential to efficient, effective DBT. Skillful DBT intervention is guided by a stage theory of treatment, biosocial theory of the etiology and maintenance of BPD, behavioral principles, and ideas about common patterns that interfere with treatment. This chapter introduces the concepts and method of case formulation in DBT.

HISTORICAL BACKGROUND OF THE APPROACH

Marsha Linehan and her colleagues at the University of Washington developed DBT as a treatment for women with a history of parasuicide who met criteria for BPD. (Parasuicide is any intentional self-injurious behavior including but not limited to suicide attempts.) By watching videotapes of Linehan's therapy sessions, she and her research team identified aspects of her style and her modifications of cognitive-behavioral techniques that seemed effective. The treatment was then standardized in treatment manuals (Linehan, 1993a, 1993b).

DBT is a comprehensive treatment that integrates cognitive-behavioral interventions with mindfulness (cf. Baer's [2003] review of this literature) and shares elements in common with psychodynamic, client-centered, Gestalt, paradoxical, and strategic approaches (cf. Heard & Linehan, 1994). Dialectical philosophy influences every aspect of DBT from the rapid juxtaposition of change and acceptance techniques to the therapist's use of both irreverent and warmly responsive communication styles. Nevertheless, its guiding principle is simple. DBT is based on the theory that most "borderline" behavior regulates dysregulated emotions or is a consequence of failed emotion regulation. This emotion dysregulation both interferes with problem solving and creates problems in its own right. Maladaptive behaviors, including extreme behaviors such as parasuicide, function to solve problems. In particular, amelioration of unendurable emotional pain is always suspected as a consequence that reinforces dysfunctional behavior. Although such extreme responses are understandable given the chronic chaos and suffering experienced by many individuals with BPD, the consistent refrain in DBT is that a better solution can be found. The best alternative to suicide is to build a life that is worth living. DBT decreases maladaptive problem solving while working to enhance the capabilities and motivation needed to improve the client's quality of life.

Comprehensive treatment (1) enhances capabilities, (2) improves motivation to change, (3) ensures that new capabilities generalize to the natural environment, (4) enhances therapist capabilities and motivation to treat clients effectively, and (5) structures the environment in the ways essential to support client and therapist capabilities (Linehan, 1996). For example, clients enhance capabilities by learning skills to regulate emotions, to tolerate emotional distress when change is slow or unlikely to be more effective in interpersonal conflicts, and to control attention in order to skillfully participate in the moment. They may also enhance capabilities through pharmacotherapy. The client and therapist collaborate in individual therapy to motivate change by identifying patterns associated with problematic behavior and by addressing inhibitions, cognition, and reinforcement contingencies that interfere with solving problems in a more effective manner. To generalize new behaviors across situations in daily life, the individual therapist uses phone consultation and *in vivo* therapy (i.e., therapy outside the office). A weekly consultation meeting provides therapists with technical help and emotional support to remain able and motivated to treat clients effectively. Structuring the environment for both clients and therapists is done as needed by the clinic director, and for the client through case management, family therapy, or milieu therapy. In adapting DBT, the particular distribution of functions to modes of service delivery depends on the resources of a given setting—what is essential is that each function be in place. Typically, one primary therapist ensures that a given client has each function by providing it or acting as a service broker. Often the individual therapy has primary responsibility for crisis management and treatment planning. Case formulation influences each of these functions but is particularly relevant for the primary therapist conducting individual psychotherapy.

CONCEPTUAL FRAMEWORK

Theory-driven case formulation is the cornerstone of DBT. For some clients, the sheer number of serious (at times life-threatening) problems that therapy must address makes it difficult for therapists to establish and maintain a treatment focus. For example, it is difficult to decide what to treat first when the client has numerous problems (panics, is depressed, drinks too much, returns repeatedly to an abusive relationship, becomes mute during treatment interactions, and is chronically suicidal). Following the concern most pressing to the client can result in a different crisis management focus each week. Therapy can feel like a car veering out of control, barely averting disaster, with a sense of forward motion but not meaningful progress. With clients who have multiple serious problems, crisis management and stopgap reduction of acute problems can dominate the therapy to the extent that efficient, effective treatment becomes unlikely.

Treatment decisions are further complicated because clients with chronic parasuicidal behavior and extreme emotional sensitivity often act in ways that distress their therapists. For example, despite experience or training, it can be a struggle to manage one's emotional reactions when a client is recurrently suicidal and both rejects help that is offered and demands help that one cannot give. Even when the therapist is on the right track, progress can be slow and sporadic. All these factors can induce the therapist to make errors, including premature changes to the treatment plan. In DBT, a partial solution to this problem is to use a theory-driven case formulation to guide treatment decisions.

At an introductory level, five sets of theoretical concepts are important in DBT case formulation: (1) stage theory of treatment; (2) biosocial theory of the etiology and maintenance of BPD; (3) learning principles and ideas from behavior therapy regarding processes of change; (4) common behavioral patterns of BPD, and dilemmas created by the dialectical nature of these patterns, which interfere with efforts to change; and (5) dialectical orientation to change. These five sets of concepts can be considered the "lenses" through which any problematic behavior will be viewed. Just as one might inspect the same object through reading glasses, infrared goggles, a jeweler's eyeglass, a high-power microscope, and an orbiting satellite, these five conceptual lenses make apparent different facets of problematic behavior. The DBT therapist looks for opportunity to foster change with each lens. Theory-driven case formulation resolves confusing variability into specific hypotheses that guide assessment and intervention.

Stages of Treatment: Behavior to Target in DBT

The first conceptual lens is stages of treatment. This is the commonsense notion that the current extent of disordered behavior determines what treatment tasks are relevant and feasible. DBT's stage model of treatment (Linehan, 1993a, 1996) prioritizes the problems that must be addressed at a particular point in therapy according to the threat they pose to a reasonable quality of life. The relevance of problem behaviors is determined both by the severity and complexity of the client's disordered behavior at the moment as well as the progress of therapy. The first stage of treatment with all DBT clients is pretreatment, followed by one to four subsequent stages. The number of subsequent stages depends on the extent of behavioral disorder when the client begins treatment.

In the pretreatment stage, the primary behaviors to target are therapist and client agreement as to treatment goals and mutual commitment to treatment. Before beginning formal treatment, DBT requires that all parties agree on the essential goals and the basic format of the treatment being offered and make a verbal commitment to them. Because DBT requires voluntary rather than coerced consent, both the client and the therapist must have the choice of committing to DBT over some other non-DBT option. So, for example, in a forensic unit or when a client is legally mandated to treatment, he or she is not considered to have entered DBT until a considered verbal commitment is obtained. In pretreatment, once the therapist commits to the client, the priority is to obtain engagement in therapy.

• Stage 1 of therapy targets behaviors needed to achieve reasonable life expectancy, control of action, and sufficient connection to treatment and behavioral capabilities to achieve these ends. Treatment time is distributed to give priority to targets in the following order of importance: (1) suicidal/homicidal or other imminently life-threatening behavior; (2) therapy-interfering behavior of the therapist or client; (3) behavior that severely compromises the client's quality of life; and (4) deficits in behavioral capabilities needed to make life changes.

• Stage 2 targets posttraumatic stress responses and traumatizing emotional experiences. Its goal is to get the client out of unremitting emotional desperation.

• Stage 3 synthesizes what has been learned, increases self-respect and an abiding sense of connection, and works toward resolving problems in living.

• Stage 4 (Linehan, 1996) focuses on the sense of incompleteness that many individuals experience, even after problems in living are essentially resolved. The task is to give up "ego" and participate fully in the moment with goal of becoming free of the need for reality to be different than it is at the moment.

Although the stages of therapy are presented linearly, progress is often not linear and the stages overlap. It is not uncommon to hit a snag in stage 1 that requires a momentary return to pretreatment tasks. Indeed, with some clients this occurs repeatedly throughout therapy. The transition from stage 1 to stage 2 is usually fraught with difficulty, and it is not unusual to move back and forth between the two stages for quite some time. Stage 3 not only overlaps with stage 2 but is, at times, a review of the same issues from a different vantage point. Stage 4 is often a lifelong endeavor that requires acknowledgment and acceptance rather than completion. At termination or before significant breaks from treatment, especially if ill prepared, the client may revert briefly to stage 1 behaviors. The infrequency of stage 1 behaviors as well as the speed of reregulation (rather that the presence of any one instance of behavior) defines the differences between stages.

Across each stage of therapy, case formulation is organized by the extent of disordered behavior that determines the relevance and feasibility of treatment tasks. Although the principles of case formulation are consistent throughout all stages of DBT, the focus on case formulation does vary with the stage of therapy. The remainder of this chapter is about case formulation for stage 1 of DBT.

Biosocial Theory: The Central Role of Emotion Dysregulation

The second perspective guiding DBT case formulation is a biosocial theory of the etiology and maintenance of BPD. Linehan theorizes that the transaction of a biological vulnerability to emotion dysregulation with an invalidating environment, over time, creates and maintains borderline behavioral patterns. On the biological side, individuals with BPD are thought to be predisposed to have (1) high sensitivity to emotional stimuli (i.e., immediate reactions and allow threshold for onset of emotional reaction); (2) high reactivity (i.e., intense experience and expression of emotion and cognitive dysregulation that goes along with high arousal); and (3) a slow return to baseline arousal (i.e., long-lasting reactions that contribute to high sensitivity to the next emotional stimulus). Expanding Gottman and Katz's (1989) definition, emotion regulation requires the ability to (1) decrease (or increase) physiological arousal associated with emotion, (2) reorient attention, (3) inhibit mood-dependent action, (4) experience emotions without escalating or blunting, and (5) organize behavior in the service of external, nonmood-dependent goals. Emerging research suggests that those with borderline personality do experience more frequent, more intense, and longer-lasting aversive states (Stiglmayr et al., 2005) and that biological vulnerability may contribute to difficulties regulating emotion (e.g., Juengling et al., 2003; Ebner-Priemer et al., 2005).

Transaction with a particular social environment, termed "the invalidating environment," can create or exacerbate this biological vulnerability. In an optimally validating environment, a person is treated in a manner that strengthens those responses that are well grounded or justifiably in terms of the empirical facts, correct inference, or accepted authority, and those that are effective for reaching the individual's ultimate goals. The optimal environment treats the individual as relevant and meaningful, validates the individual's valid responses, and invalidates the invalid.

The invalidating environment, however, fails to confirm, corroborate, or verify the individual's experience and fails to teach the individual what responses are or are not likely to be effective for reaching the individual's goals. Invalidating environments communicate that the individual's characteristic responses to events (particularly emotional responses) are incorrect, inaccurate, inappropriate, pathological, or not to be taken seriously. By oversimplifying the ease of solving problems, the environment fails to teach the individual to tolerate distress or form realistic goals and expectations. By punishing communication of negative experiences and only responding to negative emotional displays when they are escalated, the environment teaches the individual to oscillate between emotional inhibition and extreme emotional communication.

Eventually, individuals learn to invalidate their own experiences and search the immediate social environment for cues about how to feel and think. The primary consequence of the invalidating environment is to punish (or fail to adequately strengthen) self-generated behavior. Self-generated behaviors are an individual's unique, uncensored responses that are not primarily under the control of immediate aversive social consequences or immediate external or arbitrary reinforcement. That is, self-generated behavior is "intrinsically motivated" or "free operant."

It could be argued that childhood sexual abuse is the prototypical invalidating environment related to BPD, given the correlation observed among BPD, suicidal behavior, and reports of childhood sexual abuse (Wagner & Linehan, 1997). However, because not all individuals who meet BPD criteria report histories of sexual abuse, nor do all victims of childhood sexual abuse develop BPD, it remains unclear as to how to best account for individual differences in etiology. Linehan's theory argues that it is the invalidating aspect of childhood sexual abuse that is most crucial to development of BPD (Wagner & Linehan, 1997). Interesting findings suggest that negative affect intensity/reactivity is a stronger predictor of BPD symptoms than childhood sexual abuse and that higher thought suppression may mediate the relationship between BPD symptoms and childhood sexual abuse (Rosenthal, Cheavens, Lejuez, & Lynch, 2005).

The transactional nature of this model implies that individuals may reach BPD patterns of behavior via very different routes: Despite only moderate vulnerability to emotion dysregulation, a sufficiently invalidating environment may produce BPD patterns. Similarly, even a "normal" level of invalidation may be sufficient to create BPD patterns for those who are highly vulnerable to emotion dysregulation. The transactional result is a disruption of the organizing and communicative functions of emotion.

The stage of treatment and the biosocial theory suggest general hypotheses (i.e., they determine "what" is to be assessed as one formulates a DBT case). In particular, the running hypothesis for any targeted problematic behavior is that it is a consequence of emotion dysregulation, an attempt to modulate emotion, or both. Behavioral principles translate these general ideas into specific hypotheses about a given individual.

Theory of Change: Learning Principles and Behavior Therapy

The third perspective used in DBT case formulation is a behavioral theory of change. In general, persistent disordered behavior is viewed as a result of deficits in capabilities as well as problems of motivation. Principles of learning and ideas from behavior therapy specify methods to analyze behavior and influence behavior change. To understand a specific problematic behavior, DBT case formulation relies on functional analysis or behavioral chain analysis. This is where the "rubber meets the road," where general hypotheses regarding problematic behavior guide the analysis of specific antecedents and consequences that maintain (motivate) current problematic behavior. Each individual is likely to have a unique pattern of variables controlling problematic behavior, and these variables may differ from one set of circumstances to another.

Careful analysis of antecedents and consequences is particularly important due to the central role of emotion dysregulation in BPD. The hallmark of emotion dysregulation is instability. Therefore, capabilities disrupted by emotion dysregulation (e.g., an abiding sense of self, resolution of interpersonal conflict, and goal-oriented action) are also likely to be unstable across settings and over time. When therapists mistakenly assume that behaviors covary, they may expect consistency beyond what the client produces. Similarly, by assuming that an observed dyssynchrony is trait like, the therapist may treat the client as overly fragile. It is useful to distinguish between capabilities in a particular context (whether a person can do something under the best possible circumstances), performance difficulty in specific contexts (ease with which a person can perform a certain response), and traits (typical or average behavior across diverse contexts) (see Paulhus & Martin, 1987, for a similar distinction). Keeping these distinctions in mind helps the therapist assess whether the client lacks an ability or has the ability but is inhibited from skilled responding.

A behavioral chain analysis is an in-depth analysis of events and situational factors before and after a particular instance (or set of instances) of the targeted behavior. The goal is to provide an accurate and reasonably complete account of behavioral and environmental events associated with the problem behavior. Close attention is paid to reciprocal interactions between environmental events and the client's emotional, cognitive, and overt responses.

A chain analysis begins with a clear definition of the problem behavior. Next, the therapist and client identify both general vulnerability factors (those factors that are the context in which precipitating events have more influence, e.g., physical illness, sleep deprivation, or other conditions that influence emotional reactivity) and specific precipitating events that began the chain of events that led to the problem behavior. Therapist and client then identify each link between the precipitating event and the problematic behavior to yield a detailed account of each thought, feeling, and action that moved the client from point A to point B. Finally, therapist and client identify the immediate and delayed reactions of the client and others that followed the problem behavior. This detailed assessment allows the therapist to identify each juncture where an alternative client response might have produced positive change and averted conditions that lead to problem behavior. When dysfunctional links occur (behaviors that interfere with achieving the client's long-term goals), the therapist assesses what alternative behavior would have been more adaptive and skillful and why that more skillful alternative did not happen.

The absence of skilled performance is due to one of the following four factors, linked to behavior therapy change procedures:

First, the client may not have the necessary skills in his or her repertoire; that is, the client has a capability deficit. DBT views specific skills deficits as particularly relevant to BPD, and therefore the therapist assesses whether clients can (1) regulate emotions; (2) tolerate distress; (3) respond skillfully to interpersonal conflict; (4) observe, describe, and participate without judging, with awareness, and focusing on effectiveness; and (5) manage his or her own behavior with strategies other than self-punishment. When clients lack these skills, skills training is appropriate.

However, if assessment revealed that the client does at times behave more effectively in similar situations, then the therapist assesses which of the three other factors interfered with more skillful behavior. The second possible reason for the lack of skilled performance is that circumstances reinforce dysfunctional behavior or fail to reinforce more functional behavior. Problem behavior may lead to positive or preferred outcomes, or create the opportunity for other preferred behaviors or emotional states. Effective behaviors may be followed by neutral or punishing outcomes, or rewarding outcomes may be delayed. If problematic contingencies are identified, contingency management interventions are appropriate.

The third possibility is that conditioned emotional responses block more skillful responding. Effective behaviors may be inhibited or disorganized by unwarranted fears, shame, guilt, or intense or out-of-control emotions. The person may be "emotion-phobic." She or he may have patterns of avoidance or escape behaviors. If this is the case, some version of exposure-based treatment is indicated.

The fourth possibility is that effective behaviors are inhibited by faulty beliefs and assumptions. Faulty beliefs and assumptions may reliably precede ineffective behaviors. The person may be unaware of the contingencies or rules operating in the environment or in therapy. If problems are identified here, cognitive modification strategies are appropriate.

BPD Behavioral Patterns and Dialectical Dilemmas

Change in primary targets (decreases in behaviors that threaten life, therapy, and quality of life, and increases in behavioral skills) is the main focus of stage 1 DBT. To successfully treat primary targets, however, other (secondary) behaviors or behavioral patterns may also need to be targeted. From clinical observation of the problems that prevent (and wreak havoc on) treatment and clinical progress, Linehan (1993a) distilled patterns organized into dialectical poles. Each pattern describes an aspect of the transaction between the experience of emotion dysregulation and a history of social consequences incurred as a consequence of emotion dysregulation. As the word "dialectical" implies, BPD individuals frequently jump from a behavioral pattern that underregulates to another that overregulates emotion, the discomfort of each extreme triggering oscillation between response patterns. These patterns perpetuate themselves and create new problems. These secondary targets are often common across behavioral chains and common across stages of treatment.

This fourth perspective orients the therapist to behavioral patterns that may destroy treatment if not directly treated. Each pattern highlights the dilemmas faced by both the client and the therapist whenever therapeutic change is initiated. DBT's aim is to help the client arrive at a synthesis or more effective balance of opposing behavioral tendencies.

Emotion Vulnerability and Self-Invalidation

Emotion vulnerability refers to the intense suffering that accompanies the experience of emotion dysregulation. By analogy, individuals with BPD can be considered the emotional equivalent of burn victims where the slightest movement causes automatic extreme pain. Because the individual cannot control the onset and offset of internal or external events that influence emotional responses, the experience itself is a nightmare of intense emotional pain and the struggle to reregulate. This unpredictability foils personal and interpersonal expectations because the person can often meet expectations in one emotional state but not another, leading to frequent frustration and disillusionment in both the client and others. Even dysregulation of positive emotions creates pain. For example, a client reported, "I got so happy and excited when I went home for the holidays, I couldn't stand it. I laughed too loud, talked too much, everything I did was too big for them!" These individuals despair that vulnerability to uncontrollable emotion will ever lessen and suicide may seem the only way to prevent further suffering. Suicide can also be a final communication to an unsympathetic public. Emotional vulnerability is an important link to parasuicide and therefore becomes a target in itself

The suffering associated with inability to regulate emotion creates numerous obstacles in therapy. Nearly any therapeutic movement evokes some emotional pain, much as debriding does in the treatment of serious burns. Sensitivity to criticism makes it painful to receive needed feedback; in-session dysregulation (dissociation, panic, intense anger) interrupts therapeutic tasks; generalization and follow-through on in-session changes and plans go awry. Therapy itself may be traumatic. An understanding of emotion vulnerability means the therapist must understand and reckon with the intense pain involved in living without "emotional skin." The DBT therapist is empathic, coaches and soothes, and, most important, treats the emotion dysregulation in session. For example, in response to intense emotional reactions during therapeutic tasks (e.g., talking about an event from the week), the therapist validates the uncontrollable, helpless experience of emotional arousal and teaches the individual to modulate emotion in session.

Self-invalidation occurs when the client responds to his or her own behavior (or the absence of needed self-generated behavior such as emotion control) as invalid, taking on the characteristics of the invalidating environment. Self-invalidation takes at least two forms. On the one hand, clients may judge themselves harshly for their vulnerability ("I should not be this way"), act in self-punitive ways, and feel self-hatred. The experience is of oneself as the agent of one's own demise. In this case parasuicide may function as punishment for transgression. On the other hand, clients may deny and ignore their vulnerability ("I am *not* this way") and hold unrealistically high or perfectionistic expectations. In doing so, the client minimizes the difficulty of solving life problems. By ignoring or blocking emotional experience, the person not only loses information needed to solve problems but disrupts the organizing and communicative functions of emotion. Self-invalidation is often a crucial link in the behavioral chain to parasuicide. Increasing self-validation and decreasing self-invalidation become essential secondary targets. The explicit focus on the necessity of appropriate self validation is a hallmark of DBT.

The intense discomfort of either extreme results in an oscillation between experiencing vulnerability and invalidation of that experience. The dilemma for June, a client, becomes who should be blamed for this predicament. She is either able to control behavior (as others believe she can) but won't, and therefore is "manipulative," or she is as unable to control emotions as she experiences herself to be, which means she will always be this way and dooms her to a never-ending nightmare of dyscontrol. June can try to fulfill expectations that are out of line with her capabilities and fail, feel ashamed, and decide she deserves to be punished or to be dead. Or, she can see her vulnerability and adjust her standards. But if others do not also change their expectations of her, she can become angry that no one offers needed help and become convinced that suicidal behavior is the only means to communicate that she cannot do what is expected.

The dilemma in therapy is that focusing on accepting vulnerability and limitations may lead June to despair that she will always have the problems she has; focusing on change, however, may lead her to panic because she knows there is no way to consistently meet expectations. Further, if she changes her problematic behavior, she may feel ashamed that she could have done what was expected all along but did not because she was "lazy" or "manipulative." To negotiate this dilemma, the DBT therapist flexibly combines, moment to moment, the use of supportive acceptance and confrontive change strategies. The therapist communicates, in word and deed, that June is doing her best yet must do better.

Active-Passivity and Apparent Competence

The second set of opposing behavioral tendencies is active-passivity and apparent competence. Active-passivity is the tendency to respond to problems passively and to regulate oneself, if one tries at all, by regulating the relevant aspects of the environment. Regulating oneself by regulating the environment is not a problem per se—the problem is that the individual with BPD is not skillful enough at regulating his or her environment.

For example, Paula, a client, returns from a psychiatric hospitalization and her roommate asks her to move out. Instead of searching for a new place to live, Paula spends the day in bed and is silent during therapy despite all efforts by the therapist to encourage active problem solving. Paula experiences herself as, and actually is, unable to do what is necessary without more help. If she had just been discharged with a broken leg, help might be forthcoming. However, without observable deficits, she may get feedback that it is socially unacceptable to need "too much" help or reassurance or to be "too" dependent. Thus, she either avoids getting the necessary help or attempts to get it in a way that is experienced as demanding by others. That is, regulation of her environment to solve her problem is deficient or unskillful and ineffective. As the situation worsens, the therapist becomes frustrated that Paula creates a crisis that could easily be solved if she would cope actively (get the newspaper, find another place). Her experience, however, is that the situation is hopeless no matter what she does. This style of problem solving—acting extremely inadequate and passive in the face of insufficient help and at times magnifying problems if they are not taken seriously—is often overlearned from repeated failure despite one's best efforts in an environment in which difficulties are minimized. Remaining passive in a manner that activates others confirms that, in fact, the problems could not have been solved without help, that in effect things are as bad as claimed. While regulating in this way can be effective, overreliance on this behavioral pattern often means problems are not solved and life gets worse. This pattern can contribute to parasuicide in many ways, including increasing life stress as problems go unsolved, alienating helpers, and making suicide one of the few means of communicating that more help is needed.

Therapeutic changes stay under the control of the therapy relationship rather than adequately generalizing to the client's natural environment unless this pattern is addressed directly. Consequently, in DBT it is as important to teach the client to solve problems as it is to get the problems solved. As one DBT therapist said to a client with active-passivity, "I can see you are working hard in therapy, but you're not working smart. You've got to be learning to create your own therapy, not just following orders." The secondary targets here are to decrease active-passivity behaviors and increase active problem solving, especially skills to more effectively manage oneself and one's environment.

Apparent competence is the sum total of behavioral responses that influence observers to overestimate and overgeneralize response capabilities. Apparent competence takes one of two forms. First, observers are likely to overgeneralize when verbal and nonverbal expressions of emotion are incongruous. Often clients verbalize extreme negative emotions but convey little, if any, distress nonverbally. Observers are likely in these instances to believe nonverbal over verbal expression when, in fact, it is the verbal channel that is the more accurate expression. Second, observers overgeneralize when they ignore the critical context needed for skilled behavior. For example, in the context of either a positive mood or positive relationship, many behaviors are more easily performed. To the extent that Paula is a relational person and has little control of her emotional state (to be expected when the core problem is emotion dysregulation), then she has little control over her behavioral capabilities. Variable and conditional competence across settings and over time may be due to behavioral capabilities that are overly mood or context dependent.

Nevertheless, the absence of expected competence is interpreted as manipulation and decreases others' willingness to help. The further implication here is that others have difficulty knowing when the person needs help, thereby creating the invalidating environment. Here the goal is to increase accurate expression of emotion and competencies and to decrease behavior that is overly dependent on mood and context.

The dilemma in therapy is that active-passivity and apparent competence make it difficult for the therapist to determine the level of help that should be offered given what Paula can do for herself. At times and for a variety of reasons, she may need more help than those in her environment are willing or able to provide. Apparent competence leads others (including the therapist) to expect more than can be delivered. The appearance of competence also desensitizes the therapist and others to low level communication of distress. "Doing for" the client when the client is passive but does have the capability to help herself reinforces the problematic learned helplessness and blocks her from learning active problem solving. But abandoning Paula to her own means without sufficient help prevents appropriate skill training, increases panic, and increases the probability of further dysfunctional behavior. The DBT therapist negotiates this dilemma by responding to low-level communication of distress with active help and coaching of more effective behavior while insisting that the client actively solve her own problems.

Unrelenting Crisis and Inhibited Grieving

Unrelenting crisis refers to a self-perpetuating behavioral pattern in which the person with BPD both creates and is controlled by incessant aversive events. Emotional vulnerability and impulsivity combine to make an initial precipitant quickly snowball into worse problems, as when a person impulsively acts to decrease distress and inadvertently increases problems. For example, yelling in anger at a case worker and impulsively ending an interview needed to complete a housing application can result in being unable to reschedule with another worker before being evicted and homeless. Incomprehensible overreactions make more sense when viewed against a backdrop of repeated experiences of helplessness. The inability to recover fully from any one crisis before the next one hits leads to a "weakening of spirit" (Berent, 1981) associated with parasuicide and other emergency behaviors. This crisis-of-the-week pattern interferes with follow-through on any behavioral treatment plan and has led DBT to separate crisis management (psychotherapy) from skills training (psychoeducation). The secondary targets are to decrease crisis-generating behavior and to increase realistic decision making and good judgment.

Inhibited grieving is an involuntary, automatic avoidance response of painful emotional experiences, an inhibition of the natural unfolding of emotional responding. The individual does not fully experience, integrate, or resolve reactions to painful events but, instead, inadvertently increases sensitization to emotion cues and reactions by avoidance and escape. Borderline individuals are constantly exposed to the experience of loss, start the mourning process, automatically inhibit the process by avoiding or distracting from relevant cues, reenter the process, and so on. The grief inhibited may be associated with childhood trauma or revictimization as an adult, or it may be evoked by the many losses that are the current consequence of maladaptive coping. Inhibited grieving is the primary target of stage 2 of DBT, but it is targeted in stage 1 when it is linked to the primary targets. The goal is to decrease inhibited grieving and increase emotional experiencing.

The dilemma in therapy is that unrelenting crisis and inhibited grieving interfere with crucial therapy tasks. Systematic behavioral interventions, particularly exposure-based therapy dealing with trauma, are not feasible when these patterns are prevalent. It is difficult to engage in "uncovering" work and, simultaneously, to inhibit grief reactions and to avoid exposure to cues that evoke memory of past loss and trauma, particularly when one is in perpetual crisis. Avoidance and escape from painful feelings with maladaptive behaviors that generate a crisis inadvertently increases exposure to crisis-induced losses, which in turn increases avoidance of cues through further maladaptive behavior, and so on. In part, this pattern differentiates a stage 1 client from one in stage 2. The DBT therapist expects oscillating expressions of extreme distress and complete inhibition of affect and teaches the client skills needed to tolerate emotional experience without engaging in behavior that worsens the situation while decreasing the behaviors that lead to further loss of relationships and other things she or he values.

Dialectics of Change: Philosophical Guiding Principles

Dialectics has been referred to as the logic of process and as a coherent system of exploring and understanding the world (Basseches, 1984; Kamenstein, 1987; Levins & Lewontin, 1985; Riegel, 1975; Wells, 1972). Within DBT (cf. Linehan & Schmidt, 1995), dialectics provides an overriding context for case conceptualization. In contrast to the four lenses reviewed so far, dialectics shifts attention from the client alone to the context within which the client interacts. The "case" that is formulated, from a dialectical perspective, is not the individual per se but rather the relationships among the client, the client's community, the therapist, and the therapist's community. Factors impinging upon the therapist become as important as those impinging upon the client.

As a world view, there are several essential tenets of dialectics. First, it is assumed that a "whole" is a relation of heterogeneous "parts" in polarity ("thesis" and "antithesis") out of whose "synthesis" evolves a new set of "parts" and, thereby, a new "whole." The parts, which hold no intrinsic or previous significance in and of themselves, are important only in relation to one another and in relation to the whole that they define. Considering phenomena to be heterogeneously composed has important implications for case formulation. The fact that parts are not merely diverse but also are in contradiction or opposition to one another focuses the observer not on a taxonomic identification of the parts but rather on the relationship or interaction of the parts as they move toward resolution.

A second tenet of dialectics states that parts acquire properties only as components of a particular whole. The same part may have different qualities when viewed as an aspect of different wholes. Parts of different wholes will embody different contradictions and dialectical syntheses. The importance of this point for case conceptualization is that no clinical phenomenon can be understood in isolation from the context in which it occurs. Because the system itself is dynamic, the ever-changing relationship between clinical phenomena and their contexts must also be a focus of assessment, conceptualization, and change.

A third tenet is that parts and wholes are interrelations, not a mere collision of objects with fixed properties and immutable boundaries. As such, the parts cannot participate in creating the whole without simultaneously being affected themselves by the whole. An important implication of this view is that it is impossible for clients not to alter the therapy system within which they interact (and which would not exist without them), even as they are simultaneously affected by the system. Attention to the "parts" other than the client, therefore, is as important as attention to the client.

Fourth, as already mentioned, dialectics recognizes change to be an aspect of all systems, and to be present at all levels of a system. Stability is the rare occurrence, not the idealized goal. Dialectics is neither the careful balance of opposing forces nor the melding of two open currents but, instead, is the complex interplay of opposing forces. Equilibrium among forces, when found, is discovered at a higher level of observation, namely, by looking at the overall process of affirming, negating, and forming a new, more inclusive synthesis (Basseches, 1984, pp. 57–59).

Examination of the root metaphors of dialectics (dialectical materialism vs. dialectical idealism) suggests how dialectics relates to DBT case conceptualization. In dialectical materialism, the "energy" or force that ultimately drives the creation and synthesis of opposites is the efforts of humans to compel change in their world. In contrast, in dialectical idealism this process is energized by the universal truth (i.e., the universe itself drives the process). DBT case formulation moves back and forth between the two views, employing human activity as the motivator in some instances (e.g., pointing out the contradiction between the ideals created and upheld in a culture and actual body types of individuals) and larger, natural contradictions in others (e.g., the interplay of chance and skill in the outcome of human interventions). While the philosophy of dialectical materialism relevant to DBT (corresponding to behavioral theory as a foundation of DBT) views humans as imposing an order on an uncaring world, dialectical idealism (corresponding to the roots of DBT in Zen psychology) believes that we can recognize and experience a unity and pattern inherent in the organization of the universe. Dialectical materialism focuses the therapy and the therapist on the application of change procedures, and the case formulation identifies both what needs to change as well as what procedures would be most effective. Dialectical idealism focuses the therapy and the therapist on radical acceptance of the whole—beginning, middle, and end.

To summarize the conceptual framework of DBT case formulation, the stage of treatment influences what problem behaviors are targeted in therapy as well as the goals one is working toward. The biosocial theory frames the key hypothesis about what variables are central to development and maintenance of the problem behaviors. Learning principles suggest both methods of behavioral analyses and change. BPD behavioral patterns and dialectical dilemmas suggest secondary behavioral patterns functionally linked to both problem behavior per se and to difficulties changing these patterns. The dialectic between change and acceptance, between dialectical materialism and dialectical idealism, is the central dialectic of DBT and informs case conceptualization at every level of treatment.

INCLUSION/EXCLUSION CRITERIA
AND MULTICULTURAL CONSIDERATIONS

DBT therapists attempt to recognize the ways in which race and ethnicity combine with other aspects of identity (gender, socioeconomic status, sexual orientation, etc.) as controlling variables of the client's behavior. At the same time, DBT practitioners start with the assumption that therapists are fallible and that uneven knowledge, biases, prejudice, and cognitive errors may interfere with accurate assessment and intervention, particularly with complicated cases in which emotions run high. Consequently, many aspects of DBT are explicitly structured to assist the therapist in overcoming biases in perception and interpretation that interfere with therapy. For example, one crucial role of the DBT consultation team is to ensure that multiple perspectives help balance and correct the therapist's phenomenological empathy. Similarly, the explicit stance taken when conducting a chain analysis is to avoid preconceptions and stay close to the idiographic controlling variables. While the steps of case formulation described here are not altered by cultural or ethnic factors, the content of the formulation itself is.

In terms of inclusion and exclusion criteria, the majority of research using this approach has been conducted with individuals who meet criteria for BPD. Yet as the research base for DBT has expanded to patient populations other than BPD, it looks as though DBT may be effective more broadly for individuals with multiple serious, chronic problems whose difficulties stem in large part from emotion dysregulation (Linehan, 2000).

STEPS IN CASE FORMULATION CONSTRUCTION

There are three steps to formulating a DBT case: (1) gathering information about treatment targets, (2) organizing information into a useful format, and (3) revising the formulation as needed.

Step I: Gather Information about Treatment Targets

Problem Definition and History

This is the essential task of DBT case formulation: In the initial sessions one must assess the range of client problems to determine the appropriate stage of treatment. A client is in stage 1 if he or she is at least minimally committed to treatment and has life-threatening and/or parasuicidal behavior, behavior that interferes with therapy, and/or behaviors that severely compromise the client's quality of life. When the client enters therapy at stage 1, collaboratively identify and obtain a history of these primary target areas.

The first target area includes five types of behavior (in descending order of priority): suicide crisis behaviors, parasuicidal acts, suicidal ideation and communications, suicide-related expectancies and beliefs, and suicide-related affect. Either before treatment or early in treatment, the therapist should obtain a thorough parasuicide history. In the University of Washington research protocol, the Parasuicide History Interview (PHI-2; Linehan, Heard, & Wagner, 1995) is used to get this history. The PHI asks for all details regarding parasuicide for the past year, including exactly what was done, the intent of the action, and whether medical attention was required. This history is essential to assess suicide risk accurately, to begin to identify situations that evoke parasuicide and suicide ideation, and to manage suicidal crises. In particular, one must identify the conditions associated with near-lethal suicide attempts, parasuicide acts with high intent to die, and other medically serious parasuicidal behavior.

The second target area, treatment-interfering behaviors, includes behavior of either the client or the therapist that negatively affects the therapeutic relationship or compromises the effectiveness of treatment. For clients this may include missing sessions, excessive psychiatric hospitalization, inability or refusal to work in therapy, and excessive demands on the therapist. For therapists this may include forgetting appointments or being late to them, failing to return phone calls, being inattentive, arbitrarily changing policies, and feeling unmotivated or demoralized about therapy. Information about these targets should be obtained from prior treatment history and prior supervision history.

The third target area, behaviors that severely compromise the client's quality of life, includes behaviors that disrupt stability or functioning and thereby curtail treatment effects. A diagnostic evaluation may help to assess the range of problems a client experiences. Structured diagnostic interviews such as the International Personality Disorder Examination (Loranger, Janca, & Sartorius, 1997) and the Structured Clinical Interview for DSM-IV Personality Disorders (SCID-II; First, Gibbon, Spitzer, & Williams, 1997; American Psychiatric Association, 1994) are useful. Mood and anxiety disorders, substance abuse, eating disorders, and psychotic and dissociative phenomena, as well as inability to maintain stable housing and inattention to medical problems, impair the client's quality of life and may also influence parasuicidal behavior and interfere with therapy.

This history will allow an operational definition of the specific target behaviors. Frequency, duration, and past and present severity of the problem should be noted—for example, "Client cuts arms with a razor, two to three times per month, in the past requiring up to 20 stitches, but in the last year requiring no medical attention"; or "Client misses one out of every four sessions and then calls in a crisis, demanding help on the phone."

Chain Analysis

The next step is to specify the controlling variables for each targeted behavior. Returning to the metaphor of viewing behavior through the lenses of stage theory of treatment, biosocial theory, behavioral principles, behavioral patterns/dialectical dilemmas, and dialectics, it is as if the therapist were a quality-control inspector examining lengths of chain for problems with individual links. Clients monitor target behaviors using a diary card that is reviewed at the beginning of each DBT session. As the therapist reviews the card, asks about the week, and observes both him- or herself and the client in session, he or she picks up those lengths of the behavior chain that end with parasuicide, therapy-interfering behavior, or behavior interfering with the client's quality of life.

Repeated chain analyses identify the precipitants, vulnerability factors, links, and consequences associated with each primary target. Each link (in session or out) is considered in light of whether the client's response is functional or dysfunctional, that is, whether it moves the client toward or away from long-term goals. This sorting process is guided by hypotheses about controlling variables suggested by biosocial theory, behavioral principles, and the behavioral patterns/dialectical dilemmas. The biosocial theory suggests that the core problem is one of emotion dysregulation; it suggests further that the conditions that have created emotion dysregulation have led to other predictable skills deficits. Common dysfunctional links might include dysregulation of specific emotions, distress intolerance, punishment and perfectionist self-regulation strategies, nondialectical thinking, crisis-generating behaviors, active-passivity, apparent competence, self-invalidation, and inhibited grieving. The behavioral principles and ideas from behavior therapy suggest searching for controlling variables in the current environment and examining ways that skills deficits, emotional responses, cognition, and contingencies interfere with more skillful responding. For example, Don, a client, may experience immediate relief from intense anxiety when he cuts his wrists and have no other reliable means for reducing anxiety. In addition, sporadically, his estranged parents take care of him after particularly serious parasuicide incidents. It is important to note that although increased care and attention follow parasuicide, this may or may not have been an intended consequence and may or may not increase the probability of suicide or parasuicide. Particularly when assessing the contingencies maintaining parasuicide, the therapist should assess (rather than assume) the functional relationship between consequences and parasuicide.

The behavioral patterns/dialectical dilemmas also suggest problematic patterns that may occur across chains and prevent therapeutic change. Maintaining a dialectical perspective reminds one to ask, "What is being left out?," thereby expanding analyses to include the effect the client has on the therapist and the influence of the therapist's own community and context on the process of therapy. As one gains information about the chain of events that leads to problematic behaviors and difficulties with change from each of these perspectives, patterns emerge.

At times a minimal intervention may replace a weak link (e.g., suggesting a solution that the client had not considered). More frequently, a problematic link will need a fair amount of work before it is replaced by more functional behavior. Then, the assessment task becomes to determine what specific functional behavior should replace dysfunctional links and what change procedure will best replace the target behavior.

Task Analysis

Identifying replacement behaviors for each target behavior and most usual dysfunctional links requires a task analysis. This means a step-by-step behavioral sequence for the particular set of circumstances needed to bypass the dysfunctional links and get to the desired behavior. The necessity of situation specific solutions can be an incredible challenge—for example, how does one, in the midst of extreme emotional arousal, inhibit the associated action urge and do what is effective for that moment? Step by step, what is needed? There are three pools to draw ideas from. First, one should consider replacing dysfunctional links with DBT skills. Staying mindful of the balance between acceptance and change, one should consider interpersonal skills to change or leave the environment, emotion regulation (emotion observing, emotion describing, emotion experiencing, attention control, self-soothing, etc.), distress tolerance (including radical acceptance), mindfulness, self-management skills, active problem-solving behaviors, congruent emotional–expressive behaviors, self-validating behaviors (acting to increase self-respect instead of active passivity and apparent competence patterns). Second, one should look to psychological literature on treatment and normal psychology for replacement behaviors. And, finally, one should consider personal experience. In similar situations, how exactly did one solve the problem?

From the situation-specific solutions of task analysis comes an understanding of the more general obstacles that interfere with replacing dysfunctional behavior. In other words, across situations, clients experience recurring problems when trying to adopt more functional behavior. Here, again, ideas from behavior therapy suggest one of four classes of problems. The client may lack the needed skills (behavioral deficits that preclude engaging in the desired behaviors), may have emotional reactions that interfere with skillful behavior or beliefs that are incompatible with being effective, or something about the situation may derail him or her (inappropriate stimulus control that elicits interfering behaviors or inhibits goal-directed behavior).

These standard steps of behavioral assessment are used to determine controlling variables and appropriate behavioral change strategies. One further step is needed, however, with many BPD clients. The question is what interferes with a straightforward use of change strategies? Here, secondary targets should be considered, and in particular the dialectical dilemmas of emotion vulnerability/self-invalidation, apparent competence/active-passivity, and unrelenting crisis/inhibited grieving. Also, attention should be paid to the transactional relationship of the individuals with the entire system—intraorganismic, within therapy, and among the individual's therapist(s) and the environment.

Step 2: Organize Information in a Useful Manner

Within the first 2 months of treatment, one should organize information on each target area into a written format. The purpose here is to create a format that helps identify areas that need further assessment, prioritize the areas that need change, and systematically consider the appropriate avenues of intervention. The content of the formulation will represent a synthesis of the five perspectives (stage of treatment, biosocial theory, behavioral theory of change, dialectical dilemmas that interfere with change, and dialectics per se) into a single statement of the problem, its controlling variables, and the behaviors required to get from problematic behavior to preferred behavior.

The written formulation should be in a format that is useful to those who will use it. A written format is particularly important with suicidal clients. The pressures and complexity of work with chronically suicidal, multiproblem clients increase the odds that a therapist will overlook, forget, or in some way miss important connections that a written format will bring to focus. For some a narrative would be most useful, whereas for others a visual representation would be best. The essential feature is that information on each target behavior be organized to guide further assessment and to keep a clear priority of targets to be treated. See Figure 11.1 in the "Case Example" section below for an illustration of one way information can be organized.

Step 3: Revise the Formulation

DBT formulations are under constant revision as more is learned about the factors influencing problematic behavior or interfering with preferred behavior. These revisions tend to be refinements of original hypotheses, but at times significant revisions may be needed. It is difficult to decide, however, whether one is working from a mistaken formulation or whether one is in the midst of slow, sporadic progress expectable with this client population. A more fundamental reassessment of the formulation, the treatment plan, or both is warranted when there is stagnation or impasse in the therapy. In DBT the emphasis is on changing the formulation or the treatment plan based on evidence from further assessment rather than based on the therapist's emotional responses to this often difficult work. The DBT therapist's first assumption is that lack of collaboration or progress is a failure in dialectical assessment (i.e., something was missed in conceptualizing the case and the treatment). The therapist's job is to figure out a reformulation that will get the client moving toward agreed-on goals.

The therapist looks for any information about the client that might be left out, and in a matter-of-fact manner raises questions regarding the formulation with the client. The therapist reviews case notes, particularly written chain analyses, and consults with other members of the treatment team to search for relevant patterns that were not noticed.

Impasses in DBT can also be caused by failure to balance technique (e.g., by too much emphasis on change or on acceptance); the therapist uses the consultation team and supervision to decide on the best means of regaining balance (Waltz, Fruzzetti, & Linehan, 1998). Where other approaches might view lack of change as resistance or lack of motivation, DBT views patterns in light of environmental determinants. In particular, the DBT therapist considers how he or she may be contributing to therapeutic impasse. Transactions between the client and therapist must be examined as well as the larger context within which the therapist is working. The transaction between a client with BPD and a therapist can lead to therapeutic impasse or actually be iatrogenic even with therapists who are very effective with other clients. Clients with BPD frequently have interpersonal behaviors that interfere with the therapist's abilities to deliver treatment. Deficient abilities to self-regulate emotions and emotion-related actions are a common source of difficulty. This is not specific to clients with BPD. Across types of treatment, "client difficulty" rather than symptom severity may be a more important influence on therapist's ability to competently deliver therapy (e.g., O'Malley, Foley, Rounsaville, & Watkins, 1988). Hostility and help rejection can be extremely difficult for therapists to respond to, and clients with BPD have more than their fair share of difficult interpersonal behaviors. As Linehan has noted, such clients often seem to reinforce iatrogenic therapist behaviors and punish effective behaviors. In addition, quite independent of the client per se, factors unique to the particular therapist, such as therapy skills deficits, stressful work or home conditions, or difficult interactions with other therapists treating the client, may make conducting effective treatment extremely difficult. Limited skills, narrow personal limits, and conflicts with other staff members affecting the therapist–client interaction must all be assessed and their role in the treatment considered in the case conceptualization.

APPLICATION TO PSYCHOTHERAPY TECHNIQUE

The case formulation guides each intervention. Usually there is no shortage of problematic behavior among chronically suicidal borderline clients, and the struggle is to choose where to intervene and how to sustain intervention in the face of slow change and extreme distress. Choosing well in stage 1 of DBT means to "pick up the correct length of chain" that leads to primary treatment targets (parasuicide, therapy-interfering behavior, and behavior interfering with the client's quality of life) and to work on change wherever the client happens to be on that chain. In the metaphor of inspecting lengths of chain for problematic links, our quality-control inspector faces an urgent task. He or she is to inspect chain that will be used as a rescue rope—in fact, the chain is already in use! For example, when a client is at imminent risk for suicide, the links that most need inspection and correction are those associated with immediate danger. In essence the inspector goes over the edge, toolkit in hand, and fixes each link within reach during the therapy hour, preferably in a manner that teaches the client to fix links for the rest of the week between sessions. When the client is further from the edge, the therapist can "inspect and repair" those links that occur earlier in the chain. An important point in DBT is that the therapist always moves for in-session change whenever the opportunity presents itself. The following case example illustrates how DBT case formulation guides intervention.

CASE EXAMPLE

Step 1

Our composite client, Mary, is a 27-year-old white female who has a history of parasuicide including two near-lethal suicide attempts. From the

PHI-2, the therapist learned that Mary has injured herself by head banging and ingesting harmful substances since age 10. Currently she uses a razor to cut her arms and legs and overdoses using prescribed medications. Due to physical abuse and neglect she was removed from the custody of her biological parents by child protective services at age 10. Through various foster care placements, she hoped that she could return to live with her family, where she hoped to receive the care and assistance she felt she needed to get her life on track. At 16 she attempted suicide after a phone call in which her mother said that she never wanted Mary to return home and would prefer that Mary stop calling. Mary cut both wrists and only by chance was found by a friend before she died. This led to the first of many subsequent psychiatric hospitalizations.

Mary was referred to the DBT program after her second near-lethal attempt. After a 6-month period of high functioning (job, romantic relationship, successful outpatient treatment for alcohol dependence), she was laid off from work. For financial reasons she moved in with her romantic partner. Mary became depressed, failed to find work, and as her unemployment compensation dwindled, argued violently with her partner until, in a state of intense anger, she stormed out. She then had a panic attack, drove to a secluded spot, and overdosed on prescribed medications (which she always carried in her purse) with the intent to die.

Mary had past diagnoses of eating disorder (not otherwise specified), major depression with psychotic features, and alcohol dependence. When she started DBT, she met criteria for BPD and dysthymia, had panic attacks but did not meet criteria for panic disorder, and was socially avoidant but met criteria for neither avoidant personality disorder nor social phobia.

By session 3, Mary and her therapist had reached agreement that their top priorities for a year would be to stop her cutting behavior and suicide attempts (parasuicide, primary target stage 1), reduce the use of psychiatric hospitalizations (both therapy-interfering and quality-of-life-interfering behavior), and reduce the frequency of panic attacks (quality-of-life-interfering behavior and also on the chain to parasuicide), and to replace these with more skillful coping. After 4 months in the DBT program of individual therapy and group skills training, Mary and her individual therapist had identified the most typical sequence of events that led to both cutting and increased suicidal ideation. A chain analysis of suicidal crisis behavior gathered about 2 months into therapy is representative. In the late evening, Mary called her therapist (who had just arrived back from vacation that night), sobbing, "It's over," and stating she wanted to die and it was all she could do not to slash her throat. As the therapist began to assess imminent suicide risk, Mary had a call on the other line. She returned to the therapist to say it had been her partner, crying, saying she was sorry they fought. Mary said she would be able to make it through the night and agreed to a session early the next morning.

In the behavioral chain analysis during the next session, they identified the vulnerability factors (difficulties at work) and immediate precipitating event (an argument with her partner about whether Mary should or should not quit her new part-time job). At work Mary was asked to take on a project that had been clearly stated in her job description but which she had no idea how to do. Rather than ask for help or ask that the task be modified, she set unrealistic standards for her performance (self-invalidation). As the week of orientation continued, she began to fail at the task but never communicated effectively that she was having difficulty (apparent competence). She left work early Thursday with a migraine and called in sick on Friday. Over the weekend, she lay on the couch fighting a migraine, ruminating about work. During a conversation with her partner about her work problems, Mary said she was thinking about quitting and her partner said, "I hope you're not thinking I'm going to support you. I can't take you quitting anymore." Panic at the thought of being on her own to handle a problem she experienced as overwhelming and out of her control ensued but within seconds changed to fury at her partner for withdrawing help and pressuring her not to quit. As the argument and anger escalated, Mary began to have vivid images of cutting her wrists and of blood pouring out. In session she was unable to label the emotion other than to say she felt "incredibly tense, wound up," desperately wanted someone to help her, and thought, "You don't understand. I can't stand this." The argument ended with her partner's parting comment, "This is not going to work out." Mary then sat alone in their dark apartment. She began invalidating her disappointment in her partner and her legitimate work difficulties, planning to kill herself by cutting her wrists, imagined the process of dying, of being met by her nurturing grandmother who had died 2 years ago, and kept repeating to herself that she had failed again, things would never get better, and being dead would stop the pain. As this continued, the anger decreased and tearfulness, sadness, emptiness, and apathy increased. As she got out the razors, she thought of her therapist and called the answering service.

During the session, as the therapist and client reviewed the elements of the chain analysis, Mary again experienced self-invalidation and emotional vulnerability as she had the night before. This in-session occurrence provided the opportunity to directly treat two of the key links leading to increased urges to suicide. The therapist oriented Mary to the opportunity to practice skills she'd learned *now in session* to reregulate and reengage in the chain analysis and linked this in-session practice to the goal of being able to do it out of session.

Step 2

Figure 11.1 shows a more general summary of the events leading to Mary's suicide crisis behavior.

SUICIDE ATTEMPT JUST PRIOR TO ENTERING THERAPY

Vulnerability Factors	Precipitating Event(s)	Links	Problem Behavior	Consequences
Laid off—failing to find new job	Argument w/romantic partner	Intense anger, storms out	Takes OD (carried prescribed meds in purse at all times)	?? Further assessment needed
Depressed		Panic attack		
		Drives to secluded spot		

SUICIDE CRISIS 2 MONTHS INTO THERAPY

Vulnerability Factors	Precipitating Event(s)	Links	Problem Behavior	Consequences
Migraine	Discussing work problems with partner, partner says "I can't take you quitting anymore."	Intense fear—"She's not going to help"— quickly turns to fury at partner	Planning to kill self by cutting wrists, images of dying and being met by grandmother	Tearful, sad, empty, apathy, anger decreases
Deficits in assertiveness, *self-invalidation*, and apparent competence lead to work problems.		Argument escalates image of cutting her wrists and blood pouring out	Gets out razors	Calls therapist
		"She doesn't understand, I can't stand this." Partner says, "This is not going to work out" and leaves apartment Ruminating, *"I've failed again," *"Things will never get better," "Being dead will stop the pain" *Intense shame		

Initial Task Analysis

Remove means: commitment with follow through to get rid of "stash" in home and purse; throw out razors.

Treat key links: Increase distress tolerance in context of relationship conflict. Treat rumination about past failures (activity scheduling on weekends, exposure, skills training, and cognitive restructuring to modify/cope with overwhelming shame).

Reduce vulnerability factors: remedy skills deficits that contribute to problems at work (assertiveness and self-invalidation that interfere with getting sufficient help); adequate pain management for migraines.

*Occurs in session also.

FIGURE 11.1. Chain analysis and task analysis snapshot for target 1: Life-threatening behavior at 2 months.

341

First, her vulnerability to emotion dysregulation was heightened by recurrent migraines. Second, she had a variety of problems that resulted from not keeping a job. Most work problems originated from not being appropriately assertive and from an appearance of competence, both of which kept her from obtaining needed help. Third, unstructured time alone regularly resulted in ruminative thoughts about past failures and a downward mood spiral that culminated in overwhelming shame, anxiety, and limited-symptom panic attacks. Finally, when the situation was further complicated by conflict with a partner, she had panic, anger, and intense urges to cut herself and to escape. The best predictor of a chain ending with increased suicidal ideation or a suicide attempt was her interpretation of the likelihood of reconciliation with her partner versus being alone forever.

Even a brief task analysis suggests many possibilities of what could change to reduce Mary's suicide crisis behavior. Adequate pain management of migraines would lower her vulnerability to emotion dysregulation. The skills deficits that contribute to problems at work (a lack of appropriate assertiveness and apparent competence) would be remedied by skills group attendance and systematic work in individual therapy to apply these new skills to the work setting. Further, the individual therapist could watch for Mary's tendency to minimize problems and discrepancy between emotional experience and expression in-session and encourage change whenever these behaviors occurred. Another dysfunctional link to parasuicide is the pattern of rumination about past failures. The therapist could use a variety of strategies, from activity scheduling during the weekends to exposure and cognitive restructuring to modify the overwhelming shame evoked by thoughts of past failures. In addition to the emotion regulation and distress tolerance skills taught in the group sessions, the therapist also might teach basic panic management techniques. Practical measures such as removing razors and not keeping a lethal dose of any medications in her home or purse would decrease her risk of impulsive self-injury (self-management skills and contingency management). A final area for further assessment highlighted by this chain analysis is to identify exactly what it is about the loss of a love relationship that leads to suicide attempts. For example, Mary believed that if she makes someone who loved her reject her, she deserves to be dead; that if she were dead the other person would regret leaving her; that she was unwilling to exist unless she was loved intensely; and that she was incapable of making it on her own. Again, there are many potential strategies to break the link between the threat of interpersonal loss and suicidal behavior, including cognitive modification of beliefs that maintain suicide as an effective solution, strengthening distress tolerance and reality acceptance skills, strengthening the therapeutic relationship to provide another source of love and regard, increasing other sources of social support, and increasing skills (and recognition of those skills) for coping with everyday problems in living.

The written formulation helps the therapist select, from all these potential areas of change, those most likely to reduce parasuicide. Because Mary's suicide attempts had been so nearly lethal, the therapist's foremost goal was to break the link between threat of interpersonal loss and suicidal behavior. This included increasing Mary's skills at maintaining good relationships, couple work, practical agreements about not keeping lethal means available, and active use of distress tolerance skills during relationship conflicts. The other target selected as central was to stop rumination about past failures and to increase Mary's ability to self-validate and regulate shame reactions. While the therapist watched for opportunities for change in each of the areas in the task analysis, these two areas of change became the primary focus of the first stage of therapy.

Step 3

As therapy proceeded, it became clear that part of Mary's social avoidance was due to worries that if she increased her interactions with others, she would lose her temper and become physically violent. She reduced that possibility by limiting social interactions, placing few demands on the environment to avoid frustration and anger, and limiting her emotional expressiveness in general. Given her history of physical aggression toward others, these worries were realistic. Consequently, anger management techniques were added as a central intervention. The consultation team also helped the therapist see that she was responding to Mary's hostile statements and suicide threats by decreasing demands on the client, inadvertently reinforcing these behaviors and increasing their frequency over time. Analyses indicated that the therapist was experiencing a hostile work environment as well, which decreased her tolerance for client hostility and stress. The therapist was also unskilled in how to assess for and treat credible suicide threats. By problem solving with the therapist about her own work environment and its effects on the treatment, as well as by providing support, encouragement, and skills training (regarding response to suicidal behaviors), the team helped the therapist to decrease the rate of therapist reinforcement of hostile and suicidal behavior and to tolerate the resulting "behavioral burst" that occurred before the behavior decreased.

TRAINING

Training in DBT case conceptualization can be a complex task, depending on the previous training and experience of the therapist to be trained. Because DBT integrates behavior therapy with an Eastern psychological approach drawn from Zen, the therapist must think like a behaviorist and experience like a Zen student. In addition, the empirical-minded, hypotheses-generating and -verifying frame that DBT case conceptualization sits within requires a flexible mind and skill at logical and scientific testing of hypotheses. The necessity of using one's reactions to the client but not letting one's own emotional reactions control the case formulation requires therapists who are able to think clearly under stress and regulate emotions in situations in which almost anyone would have a reasonable level of emotional arousal. The emphasis in the treatment on use of basic psychological principles as well as behavior therapy procedures suggests that DBT training should begin after an individual is already reasonably well trained in behavior therapy. To date, our primary method of training research therapists has been to combine the following into an ongoing training/supervision program: an intensive formal didactic seminar (approximately 100 hours), individual case supervision (1 hour weekly), ongoing didactic training in principles of DBT case conceptualization, observing and discussing videos of expert treatment, group outlining of case conceptualization of various training cases (1 hour weekly), DBT peer team consultation (1 hour weekly), and various readings via e-mail communications and journal articles.

RESEARCH SUPPORT FOR THE APPROACH

The efficacy of DBT has now been evaluated in seven well-controlled randomized clinical trials by four independent research teams (Koons et al., 2001; Linehan, Armstrong, Suarez, Allmon, & Heard, 1991; Linehan et al., 1999; Linehan, Dimeff, et al., 2002; Turner, 2000; Verheul et al., 2003, van den Bosch, Koeter, Stijnen, Verheul, & van den Brink, 2005; Linehan, Comtois, et al., 2002). In addition it has demonstrated efficacy in randomized controlled trials for chronically depressed older adults (Lynch, Morse, Mendelson, & Robins, 2003) and eating-disordered individuals (Telch, Agras, & Linehan, 2001). DBT has been adapted for other populations and settings (cf. Dimeff & Koerner, 2000) and has been examined for a variety of clinical problems in several uncontrolled or nonrandomized trials (i.e., Bohus et al., 2000; Comtois, Elwood, Holdcraft, & Simpson, 2002; Koons, Betts, Chapman, O'Rouke, & Robins, in press; Rathus & Miller, 2002). Across studies, DBT has resulted in reductions in self-injurious behaviors, suicide attempts, suicidal ideation, hopelessness, depression, substance abuse, and bulimic behavior.

As yet, there is no research on whether the adequacy of case conceptualization actually affects treatment outcomes.

SUMMARY AND CONCLUSIONS

In this chapter we have introduced the basic concepts and method of case formulation used in DBT individual therapy for stage 1. DBT is guided by the etiological theory that "borderline" behavior is a function of emotion dysregulation. In attempts to regain emotional equilibrium, clients oscillate between extreme behavioral patterns that are self-perpetuating and present significant obstacles to change. Stage 1 of DBT seeks to decrease parasuicide and behaviors that interfere with therapy and the client's quality of life. Repeated and detailed review of particular instances of problematic behavior identifies the unique antecedents and consequences that maintain the chain of environmental and experiential events leading to the problematic behavior. Through this process, the therapist identifies skills deficits, cognition, emotional responses, and contingencies that interfere with more functional behavior. The therapist uses this information to select the appropriate change strategies (skill training, cognitive modification, exposure therapy, and contingency management). Noncollaboration and therapeutic impasse are to be expected and should occasion further review of how both parties contribute to problems in therapy. The formulation is a "work in progress," under constant revision, yet maintaining coherence with respect to targeted behaviors and the conceptual framework within which they are analyzed.

Case formulation is a crucial element of effective, efficient DBT. Despite the time it takes, case formulation should be a standard of care with multiproblem interpersonally difficult clients. Case formulation helps direct focused activity, even when the therapist is under duress, and serves as a reference point for thoughtful changes in the treatment plan.

ACKNOWLEDGMENTS

Thanks to Dr. Marsha M. Linehan for her contribution to an earlier version of this chapter and to Thomas Winter for help preparing the manuscript.

REFERENCES

American Psychiatric Association. (1994). *Diagnostic and statistical manual of mental disorders* (4th ed.) Washington, DC: Author.

Baer, R. A. (2003). Mindfulness training as a clinical intervention: A conceptual and empirical review. *Clinical Psychology: Science and Practice, 10,* 125–143.

Basseches, M. (1984). *Dialectical thinking and adult development.* Norwood, NJ: Ablex.

Berent, I. (1981). *The algebra of suicide.* New York: Human Sciences Press.

Bohus, M., Haaf, B., Stiglmayr, C., Pohl, U., Bohme, R., & Linehan, M. (2000). Evaluation of inpatient dialectical behavior therapy for borderline personality disorder—A prospective study. *Behaviour Research and Therapy, 38,* 875–887.

Comtois, K. A., Elwood, L. M., Holdcraft, L. C., & Simpson, T. L. (2002, November). *Effectiveness of dialectical behavior therapy in a community mental health cen-*

ter. Paper presented at the annual meeting of the Association for Advancement of Behavior Therapy, Reno, NV.

Ebner-Priemer, U. W., Badeck, S., Beckmann, C., Wagner, A., Feige, B., Weiss, I., et al. (2005). Affective dysregulation and dissociative experience in female patients with borderline personality disorder: a startle response study. *Journal of Psychiatric Research, 39,* 85–92.

First, M. D., Gibbon, M., Spitzer, R. L., & Williams, J. B. W. (1997). *Structured Clinical Interview for DSM-IV® Axis II Personality Disorders (SCID-II).* Washington, DC: American Psychiatric Press.

Fruzzetti, A. E., Waltz, J. A., & Linehan, M. M. (1998). Supervision in dialectical behavior therapy. In C. Watkins (Ed.), *Handbook of psychotherapy supervision.* New York: Wiley.

Gottman, J. M., & Katz, L. F. (1989). Effects of marital discord on young children's peer interaction and health. *Developmental Psychology, 25*(3), 373–381.

Heard, H. L., & Linehan, M. M. (1994). Dialectical behavior therapy: An integrative approach to the treatment of borderline personality disorder. *Journal of Psychotherapy Integration, 4,* 55–82.

Juengling, F. D., Schmahl, C., Hesslinger, B., Ebert, D., Bremner, J. D., Gostomzyk, J., et al. (2003). Positron emission tomography in female patients with borderline personality disorder. *Journal of Psychiatric Research, 37,* 109–115.

Kamenstein, D. S. (1987). Toward a dialectical metatheory for psychotherapy. *Journal of Contemporary Psychotherapy, 17,* 87–101.

Koerner, K., & Dimeff, L. A. (2000). Further data on dialectical behavior therapy. *Clinical Psychology: Science and Practice, 7,* 104–112.

Koons, C., Betts, B., Chapman, A. L., O'Rourke, B., & Robins, C. J. (in press). Dialectical behavior therapy adapted for the vocational rehabilitation of significantly disabled mentally ill adults. *Cognitive and Behavioral Practice.*

Koons, C., Robins, C. J., Tweed, J. L., Lynch, T. R., Gonzalez, A. M., Morse, J. Q., et al. (2001). Efficacy of dialectical behavior therapy in women veterans with borderline personality disorder. *Behavior Therapy, 32,* 371–390.

Levins, R., & Lewontin, R. (1985). *The dialectical biologist.* Cambridge, MA: Harvard University Press.

Linehan, M., Comtois, K., Brown, M., Reynolds, S., Welch, S., Sayrs, J., et al. (2002). *DBT versus nonbehavioral treatment by experts in the community: Clinical outcomes.* Symposium presentation for the Association for Advancement of Behavior Therapy, Reno, NV.

Linehan, M., Dimeff, L., Reynolds, S., Comtois, K., Shaw-Welch, S., Heagerty, P., et al (2002). Dialectical behavior therapy versus comprehensive validation plus 12 step for the treatment of opioid dependent women meeting criteria for borderline personality disorder. *Drug and Alcohol Dependence, 67,* 13–26.

Linehan, M., Schmidt, H., Dimeff, L., Craft, C., Kanter, J., & Comtois, K. (1999). Dialectical behavior therapy for patient with borderline personality disorder and drug-dependence. *American Journal of Addictions, 8,* 279–292.

Linehan, M. M. (1993a). *Cognitive-behavioral treatment of borderline personality disorder.* New York: Guilford Press.

Linehan, M. M. (1993b). *Skills training manual for treating borderline personality disorder.* New York: Guilford Press.

Linehan, M. M. (1996, August). *Treatment development, validation and dissemina-*

tion. Invited address at the Conference on Drug Abuse, American Psychological Association Meeting, Toronto, Ontario, Canada.

Linehan, M. M. (2000). Commentary on innovations in dialectical behavior therapy. *Cognitive and Behavioral Therapy, 7*, 478–481.

Linehan, M. M., Armstrong, H. E., Suarez, A., Allmon, D., & Heard, H. (1991). Cognitive-behavioral treatment of chronically parasuicidal borderline patients. *Archives of General Psychiatry, 48*, 1060–1064.

Linehan, M. M., Heard, H., & Wagner, A. (1995). *Parasuicide History Interview: Development, reliability and validity.* Unpublished manuscript.

Linehan, M. M., & Schmidt, H., III (1995). The dialectics of effective treatment of borderline personality disorder. In W. O. O'Donohue & L. Krasner (Eds.), *Theories in behavior therapy: Exploring behavior change* (pp. 553–584). Washington, DC: American Psychological Association.

Loranger, A., Janca, A., & Sartorius, N. (1997). *Assessment and diagnosis of personality disorders: The ICD-10 International Personality Disorders Examination (IPDE).* Cambridge, UK: Cambridge University Press.

Loranger, A. W. (1988). *Personality Disorder Examination (PDE) manual.* Yonkers, NY: DV Communications.

Lynch, T. R., Morse, J., Mendelson, T., & Robins, C. J. (2003). Dialectical behavior therapy for depressed older adults: A randomized pilot study. *American Journal of Geriatric Psychiatry, 11*, 33–45.

O'Malley, S. S., Foley, S. H., Rounsaville, B. J., & Watkins, J. T. (1988). Therapist competence and patient outcome in interpersonal psychotherapy of depression. *Journal of Consulting and Clinical Psychology, 56*, 496–501.

Paulhus, D. L., & Martin, C. L. (1987). The structure of personality capabilities. *Journal of Personality and Social Psychology, 52*, 354–365.

Rathus, J. H., & Miller, A. L. (2002). Dialectical behavior therapy adapted for suicidal adolescents. *Suicide and Life Threatening Behavior, 32*, 146–157.

Riegel, K. R. (1975). Toward a dialectical theory of development. *Human Development, 18*, 50–64.

Rosenthal, M. Z., Cheavens, J. S., Lejuez, C. W., & Lynch, T. R. (2005). Thought suppression mediates the relationship between negative affect and borderline personality disorder symptoms. *Behavioral Research and Therapy, 9*, 1173–1185.

Spitzer, R., Williams, J., Gibbon, M., & First, M. (1988). *Structured Clinical Interview for DSM-III-R: Patient version (SCID-P).* New York: Biometrics Research Department, New York State Psychiatric Institute.

Stiglmayr, C. E., Grathwol, T., Linehan, M. M., Ihorst, G., Fahrenberg, J., & Bohus, M. (2005). Aversive tension in patients with borderline personality disorder: A computer-based controlled field study. *Acta Psychiatrica Scandinavica, 111*, 372–379.

Telch, C. F., Agras, W. S., & Linehan, M. M. (2001). Dialectical behavior therapy for binge eating disorder. *Journal of Consulting and Clinical Psychology, 69*, 1061–1065.

Turner, R. (2000). Naturalistic evaluation of dialectical behavior therapy-oriented treatment for borderline personality disorder. *Cognitive and Behavioral Practice, 7*, 413–419.

van den Bosch, L. M. C., Koeter, M. W. J., Stijnen, T. C. R., & van den Brink, W.

(2005). Sustained efficacy of dialectical behavior therapy for borderline personality disorder. *Behaviour Research and Therapy, 43,* 1231–1241.

Verheul, R., van den Bosch, L. M. C., Koeter, M. W. J., de Ridder, M. A. J., Stijnen, T., & van den Brink, W. (2003). Dialectical behavior therapy for women with borderline personality disorder. *British Journal of Psychiatry, 182,* 135–140.

Wagner, A. W., & Linehan, M. M. (1997). A biosocial perspective on the relationship of childhood sexual abuse, suicidal behavior, and borderline personality disorder. In M. Zanarini (Ed.), *The role of sexual abuse in the etiology of borderline personality disorder* (pp. 203–223). Washington, DC: American Psychiatric Association.

Waltz, J., Fruzzetti, A. E., & Linehan, M. M. (1998). The role of supervision in dialectical behavior therapy. *The Clinical Supervisor, 17,* 101–113.

Wells, H. K. (1972). Alienation and dialectical logic. *Kansas Journal of Sociology, 3,* 7–32.

Chapter 12

Case Formulation for the Behavioral and Cognitive Therapies
A Problem-Solving Perspective

Arthur M. Nezu
Christine Maguth Nezu
Travis A. Cos

HISTORICAL BACKGROUND OF THE APPROACH

We begin by noting that cognitive-behavioral therapy is not a single therapeutic strategy but, rather, the umbrella term for an expanding group of
behavioral and cognitive treatment techniques and approaches that share a
common history and world view. As such, the term "cognitive-behavioral
therapy" can be misleading to those individuals who are unfamiliar with
the breadth of scope represented by scores of differing techniques. For
example, O'Donohue, Fisher, and Hayes (2003) include over 65 differing
behavioral and cognitive therapy techniques in their "encyclopedic" compendia (see also Freeman, Felgoise, Nezu, Nezu, & Reinecke, 2005). As
such, a more accurate label, as noted in our chapter title, would be *behavioral and cognitive therapies* (or cognitive and behavioral therapies).[1]
Therefore, the acronym *CBT* used throughout this chapter will refer to the
myriad such treatment strategies and not a specific singular approach. Note
that the order C-B-T, rather than B-C-T, is used for convention sake, rather
than suggesting the primacy of one type of strategy over the other.

Definition of CBT

We define CBT as a world view that emphasizes an empirical approach to clinical case formulation, intervention, and evaluation regarding human problems (Nezu, Nezu, & Lombardo, 2004). It is a conceptual framework geared to understand, based on scientific findings, both "normal" and abnormal aspects of human behavior, as well as to articulate a set of empirically based guidelines by which behavior can be changed. During its birth and adolescence, behavior therapy was defined as the application of "modern laws of learning" (e.g., Hersen, Eisler, & Miller, 1975) and was represented by clinical interventions based on operant (e.g., token economies) and classical (e.g., systematic desensitization) conditioning paradigms. It initially grew out of the philosophical framework of behaviorism, which focused exclusively on events and behaviors that were observable and objectively quantifiable. A major hallmark of this approach was its insistence on the empirical verification of its various interventions.

During the early 1970s, behavior therapy, along with psychology in general, underwent a partial paradigm shift, whereby a "cognitive revolution," in part, influenced traditional behavioral researchers and clinicians to underscore the mediational role that cognitive processes could play regarding behavior. This suggested that cognitive mechanisms of action in their own right should serve as meaningful targets for change. Such cognitive processes included self-control mechanisms, self-efficacy beliefs, social problem solving, negative self-schemas, and irrational beliefs. As such, during the past 20–30 years, the domain, concepts, and methods of this overarching approach have continued to expand greatly to incorporate myriad behavioral and cognitive therapy strategies (Nezu, Nezu, & Lombardo, 2004). More recently, behavior therapy has experienced the emergence of a "third wave" of treatment strategies, such as acceptance and commitment therapy, which are characterized "by openness to older clinical traditions, a focus on second order and contextual change, an emphasis of function over form, and the combination of flexible and effective repertoires" (Hayes, 2004, p. 639).

Our approach to CBT falls within an experimental clinical framework and incorporates a broad definition of human functioning that includes overt actions, internal cognitive phenomena, the experience of affect, underlying biological phenomena, and social interactions (e.g., marriage, family, friendships, and overlaying culture). These components range in complexity from molecular (i.e., lower-level) events (e.g., smoking a cigarette, hyperventilation, or a critical comment made during a dyadic interaction) to more molar (i.e., higher-level) pluralistic and multidimensional constructs (e.g., complex social skills or coping with acculturation stress).

CBT and Case Formulation

Historically, the preponderance of early empirical efforts extended by CBT clinicians and researchers was aimed at developing, improving, and validating assessment and treatment protocols rather than at the process of clinical judgment invoked when designing such protocols for a particular client (Haynes, 1994; Nezu & Nezu, 1989). Specifically, as noted previously, a multitude of efficacious CBT interventions have been developed for the treatment of a wide range of psychological disorders. CBT-oriented theorists have also participated greatly in the advancement of empirically based assessment protocols for such disorders. However, few scholarly attempts have addressed the *translation* of assessment data into treatment design recommendations. Unlike the omnibus treatment guidelines that are often associated with other theoretical orientations, CBT endorses the concept that treatment be applied *idiographically*, focusing on the unique characteristics of a given case across various patient and environmental variables. However, unless significant attention is paid to this decision-making process, a particular case formulation, and the treatment plan it is based on, can be erroneous (Nezu & Nezu, 1989). The need for systematic approaches to clinical decision making becomes especially important given the body of literature documenting the vulnerability that even professional decision makers have toward making ubiquitous human reasoning errors (Garb, 1998).

Although the movement toward developing empirically supported interventions for specific psychological disorders has made strides in regard to identifying efficacious clinical protocols (Chambless & Hollon, 1998), practicing clinicians would agree that it is the rare patient who represents a "textbook case," where he or she fits the exact inclusion and exclusion criteria required by the randomized controlled trial (RCT). In other words, significant variations exist regarding both patient- and environment-related factors (e.g., race, age, religion, socioeconomic status, comorbid diagnoses, and marital status) even among individuals coming to therapy for the same presenting problems. Conversely, we would argue that evidence-based interventions supported by internally valid RCTs have much to offer clinicians (Nezu & Nezu, in press). In fact, it is the accumulation of such research data that CBT is actually based on. Collectively, this duality suggests that whereas "high-quality garments do exist, one size does not fit all." As such, therapists need to creatively apply evidence-based clinical protocols in a tailored fashion.

Models of CBT Case Formulation

In recent years, to address the aforementioned concerns, four differing models of CBT-related case formulation have been developed (Nezu, Nezu,

Peacock, & Girdwood, 2004). The model by Persons (see Persons & Tompkins, Chapter 10, this volume) is more aligned with traditional Cognitive Therapy (with a capital *T*) as initially developed by Beck (e.g., Beck, Rush, Shaw, & Emery, 1979), rather than broad-based CBT, thereby placing primacy on those cognitive factors contained in such a model (e.g., cognitive distortions) when conceptualizing psychopathology and identifying key etiological variables. Linehan's approach (see Koerner, Chapter 11, this volume) was developed to address the case formulation process when conducting dialectical behavior therapy, a form of CBT originally designed for the treatment of persons with borderline personality disorder. A third approach, one developed by Haynes (e.g., Haynes & Williams, 2003), is termed "functional analytic clinical case models," which helps guide the process of matching treatment mechanisms to causal variables, in part, by quantifying the strength of the relationships between hypothesized etiological factors and psychological problems. Our model advocates the use of certain problem-solving principles as a means of fostering the process of creatively applying an evidence-based approach to case formulation.

Although these four models vary in the emphasis they place on various factors, several similarities are also evident. These include (1) emphasizing the role that a functional analysis plays in understanding human behavior, (2) espousing the belief that behavioral problems are likely to have multiple causes that can be dynamic over time, (3) acknowledging that biased clinical judgment can negatively influence treatment decisions, and (4) being amenable to a constructional approach, thereby including positive treatment goals (Nezu, Nezu, Peacock, & Girdwood, 2004). The remainder of this chapter focuses on our problem-solving model of case formulation.

CONCEPTUAL FRAMEWORK

Our model of CBT case formulation is predicated on three general principles: (1) conceptualizing human functioning and psychopathology within the framework of a functional analysis; (2) relying on the empirical literature for identifying meaningful clinical targets specific to a given psychological problem, as well as clinical interventions geared to impact meaningfully on such problems; and (3) casting the CBT clinician in the role of "problem solver."

Functional Analysis

A CBT case formulation involves conducting a *functional analysis,* which is the clinician's assessment-derived integration of the important functional relationships among variables (i.e., the effects of a given variable on others). It is a meta-judgment and a synthesis of several judgments about a client's problems and goals, their effects, related causal and mediating variables, and the functional relationships among such variables (Haynes & O'Brien, 2000).

In conceptualizing treatment goals, we advocate adopting the distinction between ultimate outcome and instrumental outcome goals initially made by Rosen and Proctor (1981). *Ultimate outcome goals* are general therapy goals that represent the reason why treatment is initially undertaken (e.g., improve a marital relationship or decrease phobic behavior) and reflect the objectives toward which treatment efforts are actually directed. These goals are differentiated from *instrumental outcome* (IO) goals (also termed "intermediate outcomes," e.g., Mash & Hunsley, 1993), which are those effects that represent the instruments by which other outcomes can be attained. IOs, depending on their functional relationships to other variables, can have an impact on ultimate outcomes (e.g., increasing one's self-esteem can reduce depression) or on other IOs within a hypothesized causal chain (e.g., improving individuals' coping ability can increase their sense of self-efficacy, which in turn may decrease depression).

Clinically, IOs reflect the therapist's hypotheses concerning those variables that are believed to be causally related to the ultimate outcomes. IOs can be viewed as *independent variables* (IVs), whereas ultimate outcomes represent *dependent variables* (DVs). IO variables can serve as *mediators*, which are those elements that account for or explain the relationship between two other variables, similar to a causal mechanism (i.e., the mechanism of action by which the IV influences the DV). They can also serve as *moderators*, or those types of factors (e.g., patient characteristics) that can influence the strength and/or direction of the relationship between two or more other variables (Haynes & O'Brien, 2000). In general, the underlying assumption of this approach is that attaining the various IOs will, either directly or indirectly, lead to achieving the ultimate outcomes. In this manner, *IO variables denote potential targets for clinical interventions.*

Making the distinction between IO and ultimate outcome goals can help guide the process of treatment planning, implementation, and evaluation (Nezu, Nezu, Friedman, & Haynes, 1997). In addition, it can help to identify when treatment is *not* working. Mash and Hunsley (1993), for example, suggest that a primary goal of assessment should be early corrective feedback, rather than a simple evaluation at an endpoint of the successful or unsuccessful achievement of a patient's ultimate goal. For example, if a problem-solving intervention is found to be ineffective in engendering actual changes in a given depressed patient's coping ability, then such information provides for immediate feedback that this particular treatment, as implemented, may not be working. Therefore, in order to reduce the likelihood of treatment failure, assessment of success in achieving IOs (e.g., improvement in problem-solving ability) should *precede* an evaluation of whether one's ultimate goals were attained (e.g., decrease in depression).

Evidence-Based Approach

A CBT orientation has traditionally aligned itself with an evidence-based approach to understanding and treating human problems. For example, a CBT conceptualization regarding the etiopathogenesis of a particular psychological disorder is based less on clinical experience and theoretical conjecture, and more on well-controlled research studies involving actual patient populations. This is not to suggest that noncontrolled research sources of information are meaningless; rather, a CBT world view extends primacy to the validity of information if derived from empirical venues.

However, the extant empirical literature regarding the etiopathogenesis of psychological disorders, as well as their treatment, is unable to currently provide idiographic prescriptions for *all* patients experiencing all types of problems. Further, differing causal hypotheses exist regarding various IO–ultimate outcome relationships for a given clinical disorder. For example, several cognitive-behavioral theories exist regarding the etiopathogenesis of major depression. These theories differ in the degree to which they emphasize potential IO variables, such as *cognitive distortions* (e.g., Beck et al., 1979), *decreased levels of positive social experiences* (e.g., Hoberman & Lewinsohn, 1985), *ineffective problem-solving ability* (e.g., Nezu, Nezu, & Perri, 1989) and *deficient social skills* (e.g., Hersen, Bellack, & Himmelhoch, 1980). Although these particular IO–ultimate outcome relationships are all supported by research, studies have demonstrated individual differences in causal factors—that is, no independent variable can account for 100% of the variance in explaining why a given individual becomes depressed.

Second, RCTs, due to the requirement that they be internally valid (e.g., inclusion criteria necessitate homogeneous patient samples), are currently characterized by substantial gaps in knowledge regarding the efficacy of a given CBT strategy across various patient characteristics. For example, even though Cognitive Therapy has been found to be an effective approach for ameliorating adult depression, few studies exist focusing on its efficacy for depression among populations differing in various patient characteristics (race, age, religious background, socioeconomic status, presence of comorbidity, etc.).

Given the foregoing limitations of the extant empirical literature, the CBT clinician needs to translate existing evidence-based nomothetic knowledge idiographically for multitudes of differing patients in a meaningful way. We argue that casting the therapist in the role of problem solver can facilitate the effectiveness of this translation, the third major precept of our model.

Therapy as Problem Solving

In viewing the clinician as problem solver, we define a "therapist's problem" as one in which he or she is presented with a set of complaints by an individual seeking help to reduce or minimize such complaints. In addition, therapists' problems can also involve helping patients attain positive goals, such as developing a new career, becoming more assertive, or obtaining a promotion. This situation is considered a problem because clients' current states represent a discrepancy from their desired state, whereby a variety of impediments (i.e., obstacles or conflicts) prevent or make it difficult for them to reach their goals without a therapist's aid. Such impediments may include characteristics of the patient (e.g., behavioral, cognitive, or affective excesses or deficits) and the environment (e.g., lack of physical or social resources).

Within this paradigm, the clinician's "solution" is represented by those treatment strategies that assist patients to achieve their goals. Identifying the most efficacious treatment plan for a given client who is experiencing a particular disorder, given his or her unique history and current life circumstances, by a certain therapist, becomes the overarching goal of therapy.

The Problem-Solving Process

Our approach to cognitive-behavioral case formulation and treatment design draws heavily from the prescriptive model of social problem solving developed by D'Zurilla, Nezu, and their colleagues (e.g., D'Zurilla & Nezu, 2006; Nezu, 2004). Adapted for the current purpose, our model of CBT case formulation focuses on two major problem-solving processes— problem orientation and rational problem solving.

Problem orientation refers to the set of orienting responses (e.g., general beliefs, assumptions, appraisals, and expectations) one engages in when attempting to understand and react to problems in general. In essence, this represents a person's *world view* regarding problems. In the present context, a *clinician's world view* involves the cohesive framework that guides attempts to understand, explain, predict, and change human behavior. A CBT world view underscores the importance of two major themes—planned critical multiplism and general systems.

Planned critical multiplism is the methodological perspective that advocates the use of "multiple operationalism" (Shadish, 1993). With regard to case formulation, this espouses the notion that a particular symptom can result from many permutations of multiple causal factors and multiple causal paths. For example, when developing a case formulation for a depressed client, the CBT therapist should engage in a search for both confirming *and* disconfirming evidence regarding the relevance to this particular person regarding a variety of empirically supported causal variables, such as cognitive distortions (e.g., overgeneralizations of negative feedback or dichotomous thinking), medical-related difficulties (e.g., hypothyroidism or iatrogenic effects from medications), poor self-control skills (e.g., difficulty establishing realistic goals or being overly self-critical), ineffective problem solving (e.g., inability to predict consequences of one's actions or diminished self-efficacy beliefs) and low rate of reinforcement (e.g., ineffective social skills to obtain positive social reinforcement, or decrease in resources to engage in pleasurable activities).

A *general systems* perspective emphasizes the notion that IO and ultimate outcome variables can relate to each other in mutually interactive ways, rather than in a simple unidirectional and linear fashion (Nezu et al., 1997). For example, various biological, psychological, and social factors can interact with each other in initiating and maintaining various nonbiologically caused distressing physical symptoms (e.g., noncardiac chest pain or fibromyalgia) in the following manner (Nezu, Nezu, & Lombardo, 2001)—early imitative learning within a family, where a parent responds to stress with undue physical symptoms, can serve as a psychological vulnerability factor that influences the manner in which a child interprets the experience of physical symptoms (i.e., gastrointestinal distress) under stressful circumstances. Such cognitive factors then can influence his or her behavior (e.g., avoiding stress, seeking out his or her parents' reassurance or focusing undue attention on the distress "caused" by the symptoms). This in turn can lead to parental reinforcement of the behavior and an exacerbation of the symptoms, which can then lead to an intensification of the child's beliefs concerning appropriate behavior under certain circumstances, and so forth.

As such, the CBT clinician should assess the manner in which such pathogenically involved variables reciprocally interact with one another in order to obtain a more complete and comprehensive picture of a patient's *unique network or set of behavioral chains*. This allows one to better identify those IO variables that play a key causal role in order to prioritize such variables as initial treatment targets. In addition, this approach enables the therapist to delineate *numerous* potential targets simultaneously (e.g., changing negative thinking, decreasing maladaptive behavior, or improving negative mood), thereby increasing the likelihood of success if a group of such variables become targets of effective interventions.

Rational problem solving entails a set of specific cognitive and behavioral operations that help to solve problems effectively. These include (1) *problem definition and formulation* (i.e., delineating the reasons why a given situation is a problem, such as the presence of obstacles, as well as specifying a set of realistic goals and objectives to help guide further problem-solving efforts); (2) *generation of alternatives* (i.e., brainstorming a large pool of possible solutions in order to increase the likelihood that the most effective ideas will be ultimately identified); (3) *decision making* (i.e., conducting a systematic cost–benefit analysis of the various alternatives by identifying and then weighing their potential positive and negative consequences if carried out, and then, based on this evaluation, developing an overall solution plan); and (4) solution evaluation (i.e., monitoring and evaluating the effectiveness of a solution plan after it is implemented in order to determine if the outcome is satisfactory). It is these specific problem-solving operations that should be applied by the CBT clinician when conducting a case formulation, as described later in the section "Steps in Case Formulation."

INCLUSION/EXCLUSION CRITERIA AND MULTICULTURAL CONSIDERATIONS

One strength of both the CBT construct system and our case formulation model is the potential widespread applicability across populations, behavior problems and disorders, assessment settings, and ages. The major constraints are imposed only by the lack of empirical data that exist for various patient-related variables. Further, because it emphasizes a scientific approach to understanding human behavior, the problem-solving model of case formulation is especially useful at such times when little is available in the literature to guide the therapist's decision making (Nezu, Nezu, & Lombardo, 2004). Therefore, we view our model to be appropriate for all types and ranges of client problems and for all types of patient populations. Last, this approach is particularly helpful with complex or complicated cases, as such cases are composed of a multitude of possible causal variables and intervention targets.

The gap in knowledge noted previously is particularly acute regarding minority populations, such as those with differing cultural backgrounds (Tanaka-Matsumi, Seiden, & Lam, 1996). In particular, the evidence-based literature is sparse with regard to information concerning empirically supported interventions for ethnic minority individuals (Hall, 2001). Thus it is important in any case formulation approach to incorporate a set of guidelines regarding the role of diversity with regard to both etiological considerations and treatment guidelines on *an individual basis for each patient*.

Our model considers multicultural diversity to be an individual difference variable that always needs to be considered when conducting a case formulation. We would argue that a similar perspective be adopted when working with gay and lesbian individuals, persons who identify strongly with a particular religious or spiritual philosophy (be it traditional or non-traditional), and individuals of extreme socioeconomic status (SES) backgrounds (either poor or wealthy). In this manner, we are better able to understand what might be considered "normal" within the parameters of a given patient's "world," as well as to identify problems that might exist simply due to differences between the person's cultural status and other groups in society, be they dominant or minority in nature. As such, the following factors should also be investigated in order to assess their etiopathogenic relevance for a given patient: (1) self-defined ethnic/racial/cultural identity; (2) self-identified cultural group; (3) immigration history; (4) acculturation status; (5) perceived minority status; (6) poverty level; (7) experience of discrimination; and (8) cultural-based values.

STEPS IN CASE FORMULATION

In general, the goals of CBT case formulation are to (1) obtain a detailed understanding of the patient's presenting problems, (2) identify those variables that are functionally related to such difficulties, and (3) delineate treatment targets, goals, and objectives. In this section, we briefly describe the steps in conducting such a formulation, which primarily entails applying specific problem-solving operations throughout the process in order to achieve such goals (for additional details regarding the conceptual underpinnings of these steps, see Nezu, Nezu, & Lombardo, 2004).

Step 1: Identify Ultimate Outcomes

In keeping with the critical multiplism approach, clinicians use a "funnel approach" to assessment (Mash & Hunsley, 1993), whereby they initially conduct a broad-bandwidth investigation across a multitude of areas and eventually narrow it down to those variables that are specifically relevant to a given client. With regard to ultimate outcomes, this entails identifying possible difficulties that a patient is experiencing across a wide range of life domains, such as interpersonal relationships (e.g., marital, family, parent–child, and friends), career, job, finances, sex, physical health, education, leisure, religion, and personal goal attainment. As accumulating evidence indicates that no problems exist in a given domain, the focus of the assessment process narrows ("going down the funnel").

Note that ultimate outcomes can be *patient*-defined (e.g., patients states, "I'm feeling really sad and I want to feel better," "I have a lot of difficulty having good relationships with the opposite sex") or the therapist's *translations* of the patient's presenting complaints. These can involve a formal diagnosis (e.g., obsessive–compulsive disorder or major depression) or a series of statements regarding specific objectives (e.g., "improve interpersonal relationships," "increase self-confidence and self-esteem" or "reduce pain"). It should be noted that as a function of changes that can occur due to treatment, ultimate outcome goals may be discarded or modified, or new ones may be added by the patient or therapist.

Step 2: Identify Potentially Relevant Instrumental Outcomes

Next, the therapist begins to identify those IO variables that are likely to be causally related to the delineated ultimate outcome goals. To increase the likelihood that clinicians are able to conduct a comprehensive review of the representative domains of potentially relevant IO variables, we recommend that they address the following broad-based dimensions: (1) *patient-related* variables (i.e., factors relating to patients themselves, including behavioral, affective, cognitive, biological, and socio/ethnic/cultural background variables); and (2) *environment-related* variables (i.e., IO factors related to one's physical or social environment). Table 12.1 contains a list of various categories and examples within these domains.

In addition, clinicians also use the generation-of-alternatives (GOA) approach in order to increase the probability that the most important and salient IO variables are ultimately identified. The GOA strategy involves a two-step process: (1) searching the evidence-based literature, and (2) applying the brainstorming method of idea production.

Initially, the therapist searches the evidence-based literature to identify those IO variables that have been found to be etiologically associated with a given ultimate outcome goal. As an example, a comprehensive search of the literature regarding common major IO goals for social anxiety might produce the following list: (1) decrease heightened physiological arousal; (2) decrease dysfunctional beliefs; (3) enhance interpersonal skills; (4) de-

TABLE 12.1. Domains and Categories of Potentially Relevant Instrumental Outcome Variables

Patient-related variables

- Behavioral factors
  - Behavioral deficits (e.g., social skills deficits, unassertiveness)
  - Behavioral excesses (e.g., compulsive behavior, aggression)
- Affective factors
  - Negative emotions (e.g., anxiety, depression, anger)
- Cognitive factors
  - Cognitive deficiencies (e.g., inability to predict consequences)
  - Cognitive distortions (e.g., misinterpretations of meaning of events)
- Biological factors
  - Biological vulnerabilities (e.g., heightened arousal to stress)
  - Medical illness (e.g., obesity)
  - Physical limitations (e.g., nonambulation)
  - Demographic characteristics (e.g., gender, age)
- Socio/ethnic/cultural factors
  - Ethnicity (e.g., self-identification with a particular subculture)
  - Sexual orientation (e.g., gay, lesbian, and bisexual)
  - Religion/spirituality (e.g., self-identification with a particular religious/spiritual faith)
  - Socioeconomic status (e.g., poor and rich)

Environment-related variables

- Physical environment (e.g., housing, crowding, and climate)
- Social environment (e.g., spouse/partner, family, friends, and coworkers)

crease general stress; (5) improve specific social skills deficits; (6) decrease focus on bodily sensations; and (7) address related comorbid disorders if present (Nezu, Nezu, & Lombardo, 2004).

The CBT clinician also identifies additional IO variables that may be relevant to a *specific* patient not found in the extant literature (e.g., if little research exists regarding cultural factors related to a given disorder) using brainstorming guidelines. Brainstorming advocates adoption of the following three general problem-solving principles: (1) *quantity is important* (i.e., the more ideas that are produced, the more likely that the potentially most effective ones are generated); (2) *defer judgment* (i.e., more high-quality alternatives can be generated if evaluation is deferred until after a comprehensive list of possible solutions has been compiled); and (3) *think of strategies and tactics* (i.e., identifying solution strategies, or general approaches, in addition to specific tactics, increases idea production).

Related to case formulation, the strategies–tactics principle refers to the notion of response classes. *Functional response classes* are those groups of behaviors that on first glance may appear very different in form but are similar in their functional relationships to the ultimate outcome (Haynes, 1996). For example, there are many ways that a person can obtain money—investing in stocks or real estate, working for a paycheck, begging, stealing, selling possessions, prostituting, or borrowing money from a bank (i.e., various tactics). These behaviors are all topographically different, yet the effects of these behaviors may be similar—all lead to obtaining money (i.e., a functional strategy).

Step 3: Conduct a Functional Analysis

Next, the clinician conducts a functional analysis, being certain to address both distal (e.g., early trauma and developmental milestones) and proximal (e.g., recent stressful events) factors within this analysis. A functional relationship refers to the covariation that exists between two or more variables. Note that this association can signify causation (i.e., A "caused" B), as well as a simple reciprocal relationship without invoking causality (i.e., A changes when B changes and vice versa). In this latter case, the covariation might describe a functional relationship whereby one variable serves as a *maintaining* factor of the second variable. For example, B may not be the original "cause" of A but serves as the reason A continues to persist (e.g., B might serve as a stimulus that triggers A, or B serves to increase the probability of A persisting because of its reinforcing properties in relation to A).

The acronym *SORC* can be a useful means to summarize various functional relationships among variables. For example, if the presenting problem (e.g., phobic behavior) is identified as the *response* to be changed (i.e., the ultimate outcome), then assessment can determine which variables function as the *antecedents* (e.g., phobic object), which serve as *consequences* (e.g., increase in anxiety and subsequent avoidance of object), and which function as organismic *mediators or moderators* of the response (e.g., presence of comorbid problems). In this framework, a variable can be identified as a *stimulus* (S; intrapersonal or environmental antecedents), *organismic variable* (O; biological, behavioral, affective, cognitive, or socio/ethnic/cultural variables), *response* (R), and *consequence* (C; intrapersonal, interpersonal, or environmental effects engendered by the response).

To illustrate this SORC chaining, consider the case of Paul, a patient who came into treatment because he has been feeling "really down during the past several months." A potential case formulation, following a comprehensive assessment approach, might be as follows: Paul experiences depressed mood (R) when he is alone (e.g., in his bedroom at night or alone and inactive in the evenings), feels tired and thinks about his past failures and recent breakup with his girlfriend, which trigger thoughts of self-blame and hopelessness (S). His depressive reaction usually involves a sad mood, increased fatigue, thoughts of loneliness, hopelessness, and despair, and slight sensations of anxiety (topography of the overall response). When Paul begins to feel depressed, it becomes difficult for him to get out of bed and attempt to counteract the depressive mood (C). Often, when friends call to cheer him up, he tends to focus on his internal state (O) and generally refuses to socialize with them. This behavior usually irritates his friends, who then cease to call him (another C), which in turn reinforces his feelings of rejection and isolation. Note that this is only one causal chain—there are likely to be multiple causal chains operating concurrently.

To illustrate how case formulation and treatment design are inextricably tied together, note that intervention strategies can be identified to address each of the variables within this causal chain. For instance, (1) the amount of time Paul spends in isolation can be decreased (focus on the stimulus); (2) Paul can be trained in self-control skills in order to redirect his attention toward positive events and skills (focus on the "organism"); (3) he can be taught relaxation skills to counteract feelings of depression when he is alone (focus on the response); (4) Paul can be taught problem-solving skills to facilitate his ability to identify alternative ways to react in response to depressive feelings, such as developing new social relationships (focus on the consequence); and (5) he can be helped to develop new pleasurable activities (focus on the stimulus).

Step 4: Select Treatment Targets

Selecting IO variables that will serve as treatment targets can be accomplished by applying certain decision-making guidelines. The goal here is to select IO variables that, when targeted, can maximize treatment success. Effective decision making is based on an evaluation of the *utility* of alternatives, which in turn is determined by both (1) the *likelihood* that an alternative will achieve a particular goal, and (2) the *value* of that alternative.

Likelihood Estimates

Estimates of likelihood involve two probability assessments: (1) that an alternative will achieve a particular goal, and (2) that the person implementing the alternative will be able to do so optimally. With regard to CBT case formulation, this translates into answering the following questions with specific relevance to the patient at hand:

- Will achieving this IO goal lead to the desired ultimate outcome either directly or by means of achieving another related IO goal?
- Based on the empirical literature, can this IO goal be achieved successfully?
- Do I as the therapist have the expertise to implement those interventions that are geared toward changing this target problem?
- Is the treatment necessary to achieve this IO goal actually available?

Value Estimates

The value of ideas is estimated by addressing the following four specific dimensions:

1. *Personal consequences* (regarding both the therapist and patient)
   - Time, effort, or resources necessary to reach the IO
   - Emotional cost or gain involved in reaching this outcome
   - Consistency of this outcome with one's ethical values
   - Physical or life-threatening effects involved in changing this target problem
   - Effects of changing this problem area on other target problems.
2. *Social consequences* (i.e., effects on others, such as a spouse/significant other, family members, larger community)
3. *Short-term effects* (e.g., immediate consequences)
4. *Long-term effects* (e.g., long-range consequences)

By using these criteria in order to evaluate the utility of a given alternative, the CBT clinician actually conducts a cost–benefit analysis for each potential target problem previously generated. In essence, IO variables associated with a high likelihood of *maximizing positive effects* and *minimiz-*

ing negative effects should be selected as initial target problems. Thus, the likelihood and value criteria are used to guide the selection of target problems and to prioritize which areas to address early in therapy.

Step 5: Develop a Clinical Pathogenesis Map

The next step in CBT case formulation involves developing a *clinical pathogenesis map*, or CPM (Nezu & Nezu, 1989; Nezu, Nezu, & Lombardo, 2004), which is a graphic depiction of those variables hypothesized to contribute to the initiation and maintenance of a given patient's difficulties, specifying the functional relationships among each other using SORC nomenclature. It can be viewed as a path analysis or causal modeling diagram idiographically developed for a particular patient (Nezu et al., 1997). In essence, the CPM offers a concrete statement of the therapist's initial causal hypotheses against which to test alternative hypotheses. As new information is obtained, and various predictions are confirmed or disconfirmed, the CPM can be altered.

A CPM incorporates the following five elements: (1) distal variables; (2) antecedent variables; (3) organismic variables; (4) response variables; and (5) consequential variables.

Distal Variables

These include those historic or developmental variables that have potential etiological value regarding the initial emergence of particular vulnerabilities or for the psychological disorders or distressing symptoms themselves. Examples include severe trauma (e.g., rape or combat), early learning experiences, lack of appropriate social models for responsible behavior, and negative life events. Identifying these distal IOs can help to predict various responses to certain stimuli (e.g., early childhood experiences of being ridiculed in public might predict anxiety responses as an adult in public settings).

Antecedent Variables

This set of elements includes the various *patient-related* (i.e., behavioral, cognitive, affective, biological, socio/ethnic/cultural) and *environment-related* (i.e., social and physical environmental) variables that can serve as proximal *triggers* or *discriminative stimuli* for other IO factors, or with regard to the distressing symptoms themselves. An example of the first type of situation involves the environmental variable of social isolation, which can trigger certain negative thoughts (e.g., "I am such a loser because I am once again home alone on a Saturday night having nothing to do!") which can then trigger feelings of sadness and hopelessness. An example of the latter situation is the social factor of "being rejected" when asking someone for a date, which may serve to trigger strong feelings of depression.

Organismic Variables

These include any of the various types of patient-related variables. Such factors can represent response *mediators,* (i.e., variables that help explain why a given response occurs in the presence of certain antecedent variables) or response *moderators* (i.e., variables that influence the strength and/or direction of the relationship between an antecedent factor and a response). Examples of mediating variables include poor social skills (behavioral variable), cognitive distortions related to mistrust of other people (cognitive variable), heightened arousal and fear (emotional variable), coronary heart disease (biological variable), and ethnic background concerning one's understanding of the meaning of a particular set of symptoms (socio/ethnic/cultural variable). An example of a organismic moderator variable is problem-solving ability, which has been found to decrease the likelihood of experiencing depression under circumstances of high stress (Nezu, 2004).

Response Variables

This category refers to either certain patient-related IO variables that are very closely associated with one of the patient's ultimate outcome goals (e.g., suicide ideation is strongly associated with suicidal behavior), or the set of distressing symptoms that constitute the ultimate outcomes themselves (e.g., depression, pain, substance abuse, or a distressed marriage).

Consequential Variables

These involve the full range of both patient-related and environment-related variables that occur in reaction to a given response variable. Depending on the nature and strength of the consequence, the response–consequence relationship can serve to either increase or decrease the probability of the response occurring in the future (via the process of positive and negative reinforcement and punishment). For example, avoidance behavior (the response) in reaction to a feared stimulus (antecedent variable) can serve to decrease a mediating organismic variable (heightened arousal to high places), thus leading to a decrease in fear and anxiety (consequence) via a negative reinforcement paradigm. Such consequential variables are often a major reason why various maladaptive behaviors continue to persist (e.g., a decrease in phobia-related anxiety that results from avoidance behavior serves to negatively reinforce such a response, thereby increasing the likelihood that such a response will persist in the future).

Step 6: Evaluate the Validity of the CPM

Having constructed a CPM, the therapist next seeks to determine its validity. This can be accomplished in two ways: social validation and hypothesis testing.

Social validation involves having the CBT clinician share the initial CPM with the patient (and significant others if they are involved). Patient feedback can be sought regarding the relevance, importance, and salience of the selected target problems and goals. Having the CPM in pictorial form makes this process much easier.

Second, *testable hypotheses* that are based on the original case formulation can also be used to verify the CPM. Specifically, the therapist can evaluate the outcome by attempting to confirm and disconfirm CPM-generated hypotheses. For example, if an initial CPM indicates that a patient's major presenting problem involves anxiety related to interpersonal difficulties and fears of social rejection, then the therapist can delineate certain predictive statements. One prediction might suggest that this patient would have high scores on a measure of social avoidance. Another hypothesis might suggest that during a structured role play involving a social situation (e.g., meeting new people), he or she would experience anxiety, display visible signs of tension, and report feeling distressed. Confirmations *and* disconfirmations of such predictions can aid the clinician to evaluate the veracity and relevance of the initial CPM.

A second set of hypotheses can occur at a later time. This involves assessing the effects of treatment strategies implemented on the basis of the CPM (see Nezu, Nezu, & Lombardo, 2004, for a detailed description of how case formulation drives treatment planning). This particular form of validation provides a powerful source of feedback about the validity of the CPM. If the hypothesized CPM is valid, modification of important causal variables identified in the model should be associated with predicted changes in the associated behavior problems and goal attainment. If successful intervention with instrumental variables is not associated with expected effects, the content validity of the CPM becomes questionable.

APPLICATION TO PSYCHOTHERAPY TECHNIQUE

Case formulation and intervention strategies in CBT are specific to each client. There is no generic form of treatment or "cookbook" to follow based on the outcome of the therapist's hypotheses. Rather, the individuality of the functional analysis leads to goals and potential routes to reach those goals that are specific to each client. That is, CBT is predicated on the idiographic application of nomothetic principles; it is not an omnibus "one size fits all" therapeutic approach. Therefore, our case formulation model is integrally attached to the treatment plan. In essence, the CPM provides the groundwork for a treatment map that can facilitate overall goal attainment.[2]

The CPM is often shared with the client in order to obtain initial feedback about its veracity. Further, it is used collaboratively by the therapist and client as a means of identifying the specific goals of therapy and the impediments to the attainment of those goals. However, not all clients will benefit from the presentation of the CPM. Therapists may choose to share their hypotheses and ideas about treatment subgoals and obstacles in a less formal manner. Each client will have different desires, expectations, and cognitive abilities that may affect decisions about how much or how little should be directly shared. On the one hand, sharing the CPM with the patient may be useful as a means of education and motivation enhancement. When this formulation is shared, the patient can become more motivated to "work hard in therapy" as he or she is able to more concretely understand the process. Alternatively, the number and severity of behavioral difficulties that have been identified as obstacles to goal attainment might be too discouraging for certain patients. In general, it is advisable to use common-sense language when presenting CPMs to patients.

CASE EXAMPLE

To illustrate the application of our model, we present the case of Sandra, a 56-year-old, white female of Italian descent and Catholic faith. Sandra was a recent widow who worked in the human resources department of a local hospital. She is a mother of three children, ranging in ages from 20 to 30 years. At the time of her initial session, one child was away at college, whereas the other two were married and living several hours away. Sandra's initial presenting complaints consisted of symptoms of depression and anxiety, chronic worries, fears of death, and medically unexplained chest pain (i.e., chest pain without known underlying cardiovascular or gastrointestinal disease). Due to these problems, she reported that she felt increasingly limited in what she could accomplish at home and at work. She came to therapy stating that she felt very distressed, although not suicidal, and confused as to what to do.

Initial Presentation

During the first session, Sandra reported several ongoing stressful events in her life that she believed to contribute to her feelings of depression and anxiety. Foremost was the recent death of her husband, John, who died of a heart attack approximately 18 months previously. Since that time, Sandra felt she was chronically depressed. She also reported feeling significant guilt for feeling this way as she believed she "must be strong" for her children and extended family, as they were also still struggling with John's untimely death. However, she further experienced a sense of "being trapped" in the role of caregiver with regard to this extended family at a time when it was she who had lost her own primary means of emotional and practical support. Moreover, the death of her husband had led to significant worries about her future.

Another major symptom complaint concerned periodic episodes of acute chest pain during the past 6 months. However, results of extensive testing for underlying cardiovascular or gastrointestinal problems were negative. As a result, Sandra stated that "doctors can't seem to find a medical explanation and more than one has suggested that it is all in my head." She reported that the chest pain has caused her to miss work, has kept her from doing activities she enjoys, and has led to a number of worries about her health.

In addition, Sandra reported that her job was extremely stressful. She indicated that she had a very demanding supervisor, who although at times was sensitive to Sandra's medical problems and concerns surrounding the death of her husband, often set unrealistic deadlines which became overbearing for Sandra. Further, there were frequent rumors of cutbacks at the hospital which exacerbated her financial concerns and worries about holding a job given the frequent absences due to chest pain and physician appointments.

A final major stressor for Sandra involved her interactions with her extended family. Her husband's nuclear family lived in an Italian American community and had close ties to their extended family in Naples, Italy. Sandra reported that they held strong religious beliefs associated with the "culture of the family" (e.g., there were two nuns and a priest in this family). During the time when her children were growing up, as well as when her husband first died, John's family provided practical support to Sandra. For example, there was always someone from the family at her house after John's death, they often provided meals, and were ever present to "lend a hand." However, Sandra reported that her extended family had always been "too involved in our relationship" and had a history of high expectations for John and Sandra to continually be at family functions (e.g., first communions, birthdays, weddings, and holidays). She often felt that sacrificing her choices in order to appease John's family was unfair. She reported that over the past year, these family members grew increasingly intrusive following John's death, often turning to her for emotional support and sympathy given that she had appeared "so strong" at the funeral. Recently, however, when her son brought home a girlfriend from college who was African American and non-Catholic, the negative reaction of her in-laws increased her resentment of their intrusion and caused her to have arguments with various family members. Sandra also reports that such family disagreements have led to her questioning her spiritual and religious beliefs, which gets entangled with her loyalty to her husband's family, her Catholic faith, her love for her son, and the desire to support his new relationship.

Historically, Sandra sought counseling for panic attacks shortly after returning home from college to care for her mother who was diagnosed with breast cancer at that time. She indicated that she interrupted her studies in order to return home, and while caring for her mother during the daytime, she took evening classes to finish her business degree. She reported that the supportive therapy she received at that time through the school's counseling center was helpful in reducing the panic attacks and helping her cope with caregiver stress.

Assessment Plan and Results

Ultimate Outcome Goals

According to our model, the major areas of assessment should first focus on identifying possible ultimate outcome goals. Sandra's initial symptom picture suggested that the more crucial treatment goals were likely to include reducing symptoms of depression, anxiety, and chest pain. One particular diagnostic issue involved determining whether the anxiety and chest pain was actually part of a panic disorder symptom cluster, especially in light of her history of panic attacks during her college years. In addition, to ensure that the therapist would not overlook anything crucial, it would be important to collect information about problems that might exist in other areas of her life. Therefore, consistent with the "funnel approach," the therapist continued to conduct a clinical interview, in addition to administering several inventories, in order to (1) obtain additional information about her medical, family, and psychosocial background (i.e., Multimodal Life History Questionnaire: Lazarus, 1980); (2) assess the intensity of her distress symptomatology (i.e., Beck Depression Inventory–II [BDI-II]: Beck, Steer, & Brown, 1996; Beck Anxiety Inventory [BAI]: Beck, Epstein, Brown, & Steer, 1988); and (3) better determine the nature and scope of her chest pain (i.e., Panic Attack Questionnaire—Revised [PAQ-R]: Cox, Norton, & Swinson, 1992; rating scale of pain intensity and frequency; test results from EKG studies, blood assays, and heart imaging results during a stress-test procedure). Last, her oldest daughter, who frequently visits Sandra, agreed to fill out collateral ratings of depression and anxiety.

On the BDI-II, Sandra obtained a score that was clinically significant (i.e., 28). Some of the major concerns that she endorsed included loss of pleasure, loss of interest in previously enjoyed activities, feelings of sadness, profound feelings of guilt, indecisiveness, concentration difficulties, and sleep problems. However, she did not endorse any items indicating that she had any suicidal thoughts or intentions. On the BAI, Sandra reported the following symptoms of anxiety at a moderate to intolerable level: heart pounding, fear of dying, abdomen discomfort, and several symptoms of heightened physiological arousal. Responses from Sandra during the clinical interviews, as well as from her daughter, essentially confirmed these results, as well as identifying decreased motivation and a recent increase in tension and irritability.

In terms of her chest pain, Sandra described it as an acute pain at the chest level. She stated that although it occurs infrequently (a couple of times a month), when it does, it is intense (i.e., ratings of "8 or 9" on a scale of 1–10 where 10 = very intense pain). Moreover, this symptom causes her to worry whether it is undiagnosed heart disease and she fears that it may, in fact, kill her, given her familial background (i.e., father's death from heart disease). The medical reports obtained from Sandra's primary care physician and cardiologist with her written consent indicated no evidence of any underlying cardiovascular disease. In fact, her results were indicative of her being in overall good physical health. Last, results from both the interviews and the PAQ-R indicated that Sandra was not currently suffering from a panic disorder. In fact, she adamantly reported that she knew the difference between both types of experiences.

The semistructured interviews and responses to the Multimodal Questionnaire yielded considerable additional information about Sandra's background and current life experiences. She describes her family of origin as particularly isolative and made worse by her mother's long-term abuse of alcohol and her father's health problems. Following her father's death from heart failure when she was 15 years old, Sandra was "forced" into the role of family caregiver and had to make considerable personal sacrifices. She stated that the caregiver role was a "double-edged sword" for her—on one hand, she received approval and affection when she was sacrificing herself to help others, but on the other hand, she perceived herself as alone and left to take on problems without support. She was able to gain some independence from this role when she went away to college, but was soon forced to return home to resume her caregiving responsibilities when her mother became seriously ill.

With regard to her husband, John, Sandra reported that she was initially attracted to him because "he was the first person in my life who seemed to really take care of me." She indicated that their marriage was very strong and relatively harmonious, where the few marital arguments were triggered by pressures associated with the demands and expectations placed on them by John's family. With his death, Sandra stated she experiences guilt, often dwelling on negative thoughts, such as "I should have been able to prevent his death, knowing the warning signs; if I only took better care of him and didn't cook all that food I know was bad for him."

Potential Instrumental Outcome Goals

Based on a review of the overall assessment results, Sandra and her therapist jointly decided to delineate three initial overall treatment goals: (1) decrease depression, (2) decrease anxiety and worries, and (3) decrease chest pain. Having identified these ultimate outcome goals, the next step in the problem-solving model of case formulation is to identify those IO variables that are functionally related to these three treatment goals.

According to our model, the search for such etiopathogenically involved variables should be conducted using the problem-solving orientation that espouses a critical multiplism world view and extends priority to evidence-based research findings. It also should be conducted using brainstorming principles in order to prevent therapist oversight. With regard to Sandra, this involved continuing to collect data via clinical interviews, as well as having her complete various self-report inventories to assess the relevance of various possible evidence-based IO dimensions.[3] Factors that may possibly be causally related to Sandra's depression would include (1) dysfunctional thinking patterns, (2) ineffective problem-solving ability, (3) poor self-control skills, (4) lowered rates of reinforcement, and (5) ineffective social or interpersonal skills (Nezu, Nezu, & Lombardo, 2004). With regard to her anxiety, such possible IO variables might include (1) dysfunctional thinking, (2) high levels of intolerance of uncertainty, (3) avoidance of anxiety-provoking situations, (4) heightened physiological reactions to stressful situations, (5) catastrophic interpretations of negative physiologic arousal, (6) heightened sensitivity to experiencing anxiety, especially negative physical symptomatology, (7) use of inappropriate "safety" behaviors (i.e., those behaviors that are thought to decrease panic or anxiety, but actually serve as an avoidance mechanism, such as being accompanied by a "safe person"), and (8) ineffective coping and problem-solving skills (Nezu, Nezu, & Lombardo, 2004). Some of these same factors might also be functionally related to her chest pain (e.g., heightened anxiety sensitivity, poor coping skills), given that there was no evidence of underlying cardiovascular disease (Nezu et al., 2001). An additional potential mechanism of action regarding the presence of the noncardiac chest pain, as well as with regard to other forms of medically unexplained physical symptoms (e.g., fibromyalgia), involves emotional and thought suppression or the tendency to strongly avoid or deny one's feelings which paradoxically leads to an increase in the intensity of such emotions (Nezu et al., 2001). As such, Sandra was also requested to complete the White Bear Suppression Test (Wegner & Zanakos, 1994), a measure of one's general tendency to suppress one's emotions.

Last, in the spirit of "brainstorming principles," based in part on the frequency with which the topic of her religious beliefs arose during the various interviews, as well as the need to consider the role of cultural factors (e.g., the differences in cultural beliefs and background between her ethnicity and that of her extended family), it was decided to further explore Sandra's religious and spirituality beliefs and activities using the Brief Multidimensional Measure of Religiousness/Spirituality (Fetzer Institute, 1999).

Selecting Initial Treatment Targets

To illustrate this decision-making process with regard to Sandra's case, take one potential treatment target previously identified during the problem definition phase—heightened sensitivity to physical anxiety symptoms. This IO variable was previously identified, via a search of the evidence-based literature, as an important possible mechanism of action for anxiety symptoms per se, as well as with regard to the noncardiac chest pain. In terms of initially assessing various likelihood estimates, the therapist's answers were "yes" to the following relevant criterion questions:

1. Will achieving this IO (i.e., reducing Sandra's sensitivity to negative physical sensations of anxiety) directly or indirectly achieve an ultimate outcome goal?
2. Is this target amenable to treatment (e.g., does the evidenced-based literature provide data to suggest that certain treatment protocols exist that are effective in reducing this heightened sensitivity)?
3. Is the therapist at hand able to treat this given target (note that this requires a self-assessment by the therapist regarding competency)?
4. Is this treatment actually available?

Note that if treatment can be successful in changing this problem, the potential impact it might have simultaneously on two ultimate outcome goals (i.e., anxiety and noncardiac chest pain) suggests that its value is especially high as an initial treatment target.

The specific criteria used to assess the value of a given alternative would be applied next in order to evaluate this choice, as well as all alternative choices (i.e., potential treatment targets). Specifically, the therapist would now assess the value of choosing heightened sensitivity to anxiety symptoms as a treatment target focusing on dimensions of personal, social, short-term, and long-term consequences or treatment effects. Based on such a cost–benefit analysis, the therapist's next task is to develop an initial CPM.

Sandra's CPM

Sandra's CPM is contained in Figure 12.1. In developing any CPM, the therapist attempts to graphically depict how various distal, antecedent, organismic, response, and consequential variables functionally interact with

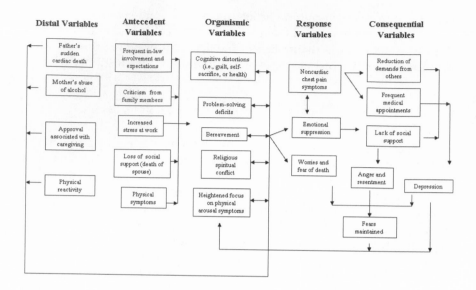

FIGURE 12.1. Sandra's hypothesized CPM.

each other in order to maintain the presence of a patient's symptoms and problems.

Based on the broad-based assessment previously described, the therapist identified several distal factors that appeared to be etiologically tied to Sandra's current worries, depressive symptoms, and medically unexplained symptoms. These include (1) her father's death resulting from a heart attack at the age of 15 years; (2) receipt of positive attention and affection primarily as a function of her caregiver duties; (3) her role as family caregiver which required her to make considerable personal sacrifices; and (4) a heightened vigilance and strong physical reactivity when her own attempts for approval were ignored or refused.

Such early learning experiences were functionally related to certain organismic variables as they were hypothesized to have created a variety of emotional vulnerabilities: (1) heightened sensitivity to extensive caregiving demands and expectations; (2) strong physical reactions to stressful events; (3) significant conflict when relationships provided love and support but placed unwanted demands on her; (4) feelings of guilt involving the possibility of "God's punishment" when she failed to provide care or support for others; and (5) a negative orientation toward problems, where she assumed responsibility for day-to-day stressors, leading to frequent avoidance and emotional suppression when overwhelmed.

In developing a CPM, it is also important to determine which situations serve as stressors that trigger an individual's vulnerabilities (i.e., antecedent variables). In other words, these would be factors that when they occur, increase the likelihood that an individual will engage in maladaptive behavior or cognitions. For Sandra, the following events and stimuli served in this capacity: (1) the loss of her husband, particularly with regard to financial and emotional support, (2) financial and work stress, including the high expectations of her supervisor; (3) demands and criticism from her husband's family; and (4) John's family's negative reaction to her son's interracial, interfaith relationship. Furthermore, Sandra often experienced a variety of physical symptoms including muscle aches, tightening of the chest, and shortness of breath, which she feared was an undiagnosed cardiac condition. These more recent stressors also served to trigger continued bereavement and religious/spiritual conflict.

The multidimensional assessment also indicated that Sandra's presentation of "being strong" and suppressing her feelings were critical components of her case formulation. Although her provision of support and care to family members had frequently led to decreases in her concerns about receiving love and acceptance, it, in fact, negatively reinforced the perceptions of others that Sandra was able to handle all these additional responsibilities and that she needed little emotional support in return. This frame usually led Sandra to worry more about her health and financial security, as well as to experience considerable feelings of anger and frustration at her extended family for their unrelenting expectations and lack of compassion toward her struggles. Such factors (i.e., response variables) were further magnified by her ineffective coping attempts of ignoring these problems, suppressing her feelings, and not seeking support from others. As such, her depressive symptoms increased and her worries and fears were maintained.

Sandra's chest pain was hypothesized to be functionally related to a number of ongoing events in her life. The chest pain symptoms frequently led Sandra to consult with various physicians and specialists to determine the medical cause for her recurring chest pain. Similar to other patients with noncardiac chest pain, she held catastrophic explanations for her chest pain and experienced a sense of frustration that no one could diagnosis or truly understand what she was going through (Nezu, Nezu, & Lombardo, 2001). However, she did often experience reduced demands from her supervisor and extended family, as well as increased social support and compassion from her friends (i.e., reinforcement). Sandra did worry though that these health concerns and frequent absences from work would eventually lead to her losing her job, which increased her fears of economic instability and exacerbated her symptoms of depression.

Sandra's spiritual beliefs, depending on the focus, were functionally related to distress symptoms such as guilt but also served to have her view others as worthy of God's love without discrimination. If the compassionate beliefs she held toward others could be directed toward herself, she might be able to reduce the pressures she placed on herself concerning her responsibility for others' happiness.

Note that the overall CPM for Sandra could change as various IOs are (or are not) achieved as a function of either treatment or inadvertent changes in her social environment (e.g., rumors of downsizing at the hospital turn out to be false).

Once a working CPM is agreed on between the therapist and client, the CBT clinician would then use this case formulation to develop an overall treatment plan. In essence, he or she would use similar problem-solving activities to first identify and then choose among groups of evidence-based cognitive and behavioral treatment strategies that would be hypothesized to optimally achieve each of the IO goals specified in the CPM (see Nezu, Nezu, & Lombardo, 2004, for a detailed explanation of this process) in order to reach each of the ultimate outcome goals. It should be noted that Sandra's CPM allowed her therapist to develop an overall effective and accepted treatment plan that ultimately led to successful achievement of the ultimate outcome goals. For example, relaxation training was able to have a significant impact on Sandra's worries, anger, and noncardiac chest pain. Cognitive restructuring strategies were applied to change her distortions regarding guilt, self-sacrifice, and unconfirmed fears of death. In addition, training Sandra in problem solving led to major changes in the manner in which she related more assertively and satisfactorily with her extended family as well as with her boss.

TRAINING

The following are crucial areas relevant to CBT case formulation:

1. *Behavioral assessment.* A fundamental knowledge of the theory and procedures of behavioral assessment is crucial to conducting a functional analysis and CBT case formulation. This involves a familiarity with the relevant literature concerning the process of understanding human behavior from a cognitive-behavioral perspective, as well as various behavioral assessment methods unique to this orientation (e.g., behavioral observation, behavioral avoidance tests, or role-play assessments).

2. *Cognitive and behavior therapy strategies.* Similarly, a familiarity with the vast literature base regarding cognitive and behavioral interventions is considered crucial to conducting a valid case formulation (see Freeman et al., 2005; Nezu, Nezu, & Lombardo, 2004; and O'Donohue et al., 2003, as examples).

3. *Psychopathology.* Fundamental knowledge of adult and child psychopathology is also considered essential. Familiarity with DSM-IV-TR (American Psychiatric Association, 2000) is also considered advisable.

4. *Psychometrics.* The concepts of reliability and validity of any assessment procedure, be it objective or projective testing, behavioral observation, or a structured interview procedure, play an essential role in the accurate formulation of any patient's specific case. As such, a basic understanding of these issues is viewed as important parts of training in case formulation (see Haynes & Heiby, 2004).

5. *Multivariate statistics.* In keeping with the planned critical multiplism tenet of our problem orientation, it is important to be able to understand various assumptions inherent in multiple causal modeling. Familiarity with path analysis or structural causal modeling is particularly useful (see also Haynes, 1992).

6. *Problem-solving principles.* A basic familiarity with the general problem-solving model (Nezu, 2004), especially as it applies to clinical decision making and judgment (Nezu & Nezu, 1989, 1993; Nezu, Nezu, & Lombardo, 2004), is particularly helpful.

7. *Clinical judgment.* Knowledge of research on the process and errors in clinical judgment is helpful. These issues are discussed in Nezu and Nezu (1989).

Having a basic knowledge in each of the aforementioned areas is a beginning point to learning this approach. However, as is the case with any skill, the key component is concerted practice. Although this approach is based heavily on the precepts of the scientific process, because of the ubiquity of human error (Nezu & Nezu, 1989), as well as the slipperiness of the "art" inherent in the *application* of anything scientific (see Nezu & Nezu, 1995), such practice is essential.

RESEARCH SUPPORT FOR THE APPROACH

The commitment to an empirical and scientific methodology is often cited as a major cornerstone of a broad-based CBT approach to assessment and clinical interventions. In fact, this argument has been often used in support of its clinical superiority over more traditional models. However, as noted earlier, this empiricism was more evident in terms of developing and evaluating CBT assessment and intervention strategies than in the process of translating these assessment data into case formulations and treatment implications. In fact, research has pointed to various discrepancies between broad-based CBT as it is practiced and the empirical rigor with which its attempted validation is espoused in the literature (Nezu & Nezu, 1993).

It was in response to this gap that our model was developed. Whereas a plethora of research exists underscoring the effectiveness of teaching individuals problem-solving principles in order to improve their overall decision making (Nezu, 2004), our problem-solving model of case formulation awaits empirical validation. However, as this approach delineates a set of processes that is parallel with a scientific reasoning model of conducting empirical research, we suggest that its conceptual foundation is strong.

NOTES

1. An example of the movement by the profession to make such clarifications is provided by the recent name change of the major North American organization representing professionals and students who espouse this orientation from the Association for Advancement of Behavior Therapy (AABT) to the Association of Behavioral and Cognitive Therapies (ABCT). In addition, the national credentialing organization that awards the diplomate (i.e., board certification) in this area of applied psychology, the American Board of Behavioral Psychology, recently changed its name to the American Board of Cognitive and Behavioral Psychology.

2. The problem-solving model of case formulation is actually half of an overall approach to CBT where the second part involves treatment design. As indicated earlier, these two activities are inextricably tied together in that one's case formulation should drive one's treatment design. Similar to developing a CPM that graphically depicts a patient's case formulation, we suggest that the therapist further constructs a goal attainment map (GAM), which would be a graphic representation of an overall treatment plan whereby specific intervention strategies are delineated to address the various IO variables (see Nezu, Nezu, & Lombardo, 2004). In essence, the GAM is a roadmap that outlines how a planned treatment protocol will help overcome a patient's obstacles to achieving his or her ultimate outcome goals.

3. Due to space limitations, we are unable to describe the various possible measures that could be applied to this endeavor. The reader is referred to Nezu, Ronan, Meadows, and McClure (2000) and Antony, Orsillo, and Roemer (2001), for compendia of depression-related and anxiety-related measures, respectively. In addition, elsewhere we have described a problem-solving approach to selecting assessment measures in clinical and research settings (Nezu & Nezu, 1989; Nezu, Nezu, & Foster, 2000).

REFERENCES

American Psychiatric Association. (2000). *Diagnostic and statistical manual of mental disorders* (4th ed., Text rev.). Washington, DC: Author.

Antony, M. M., Orsillo, S. M., & Roemer, L. (2001). *Practitioner's guide to empirically based measures of anxiety.* New York: Kluwer Academic/Plenum Press.

Beck, A. T., Epstein, N., Brown, G., & Steer, R. A. (1988). An inventory for measuring clinical anxiety: Psychometric properties. *Journal of Consulting and Clinical Psychology, 56,* 893–897.

Beck, A. T., Rush, A. J., Shaw, B. F., & Emery, G. (1979). *Cognitive therapy of depression: A treatment manual.* New York: Guilford Press.

Beck, A. T., Steer, R. A., & Brown, G. K. (1996). *Manual for the BDI-II*. San Antonio, TX: Psychological Corporation.

Chambless, D. L., & Hollon, S. D. (1998). Defining empirically supported therapies. *Journal of Consulting and Clinical Psychology, 66*, 7–18.

Cox, B. J., Norton, G. R., & Swinson, R. P. (1992). *Panic Attack Questionnaire—Revised*. Toronto, Ontario, Canada: Clarke Institute of Psychiatry.

D'Zurilla, T. J., & Nezu, A. M. (1996). *Problem-solving therapy: A positive approach to clinical intervention* (3rd ed.). New York: Springer Publishing Company.

Fetzer Institute. (1999). *A multidimensional measurement of religiousness/spirituality for use in health research: A report of the Fetzer Institute/National Institute on Aging Working Group* [Online]. Available: www.fetzer.org.

Freeman, A., Felgoise, S. H., Nezu, A. M., Nezu, C. M., & Reinecke, M. A. (Eds.). (2005). *Encyclopedia of cognitive behavior therapy*. New York: Springer.

Garb, H. N. (1998). *Studying the clinician: Judgment research and psychological assessment*. Washington, DC: American Psychological Association.

Hall, G. C. N. (2001). Psychotherapy research with ethnic minorities: Empirical, ethical, and conceptual issues. *Journal of Consulting and Clinical Psychology, 69*, 502–510.

Hayes, S. C. (2004). Acceptance and commitment therapy, relational frame theory, and the third wave of behavioral and cognitive therapies. *Behavior Therapy, 35*, 639–665.

Haynes, S. N. (1992). *Models of causality in psychopathology: Toward synthetic, dynamic and nonlinear models of causality in psychopathology*. Boston: Allyn & Bacon.

Haynes, S. N. (1994). Clinical judgment and the design of behavioral intervention programs: Estimating the magnitudes of intervention effects. *Psicologia Conductual, 2*, 165–184.

Haynes, S. N. (1996). The changing nature of behavioral assessment. In M. Hersen & A. Bellack (Eds.), *Behavioral assessment: A practical guide* (4th ed.). Boston: Allyn & Bacon.

Haynes, S. N., & Heiby, E. M. (Eds.). (2004). *Behavioral assessment*. New York: Wiley.

Haynes, S. N., & O'Brien, W. H. (2000). *Principles and practice of behavioral assessment*. New York: Kluwer Academic/Plenum Press.

Haynes, S. N., & Williams, A. E. (2003). Case formulation and design of behavioral treatment programs: Matching treatment mechanisms to causal variables for behavior problems. *European Journal of Psychological Assessment, 19*, 164–174.

Hersen, M., Bellack, A. S., & Himmelhoch, I. M. (1980). Treatment of unipolar depression with social skills training. *Behavior Modification, 4*, 547–556.

Hersen, M., Eisler, M., & Miller, P. (1975). *Progress in behavior modification*. New York: Academic Press.

Hoberman, H. M., & Lewinsohn, P. M. (1985). The behavioral treatment of depression. In E. E. Beckham & W. R. Leber (Eds.), *Handbook of depression: Treatment, assessment, and research* (pp. 39–81). Homewood, IL: Dorsey.

Lazarus, A. A. (1980). *Multimodal Life History Questionnaire*. Kingston, NJ: Multimodal Publications.

Mash, B. J., & Hunsley, J. (1993). Assessment considerations in the identification of failing psychotherapy: Bringing the negatives out of the darkroom. *Psychological Assessment, 5*, 292–301.

Nezu, A. M. (2004). Problem solving and behavior therapy revisited. *Behavior Therapy, 35,* 1–33.

Nezu, A. M., & Nezu, C. M. (Eds.). (1989). *Clinical decision making in behavior therapy: A problem-solving perspective.* Champaign, IL: Research Press.

Nezu, A. M., & Nezu, C. M. (1993). Identifying and selecting target problems for clinical interventions: A problem-solving model. *Psychological Assessment, 5,* 254–263.

Nezu, A. M., & Nezu, C. M. (Eds.). (in press). *Evidence-based outcome research: A practical guide to conducting randomized controlled trials for psychosocial interventions.* New York: Oxford University Press.

Nezu, A. M., Nezu, C. M., Friedman, S. H., & Haynes, S. N. (1997). Case formulation in behavior therapy: Problem-solving and functional analytic strategies. In T. D. Eells (Ed.), *Handbook of psychotherapy case formulation* (pp. 368–401). New York: Guilford Press.

Nezu, A. M., Nezu, C. M., & Lombardo, E. R. (2001). Cognitive-behavior therapy for medically unexplained symptoms: A critical review of the treatment literature. *Behavior Therapy, 32,* 537–583.

Nezu, A. M., Nezu, C. M., & Lombardo, E. R. (2004). *Cognitive-behavioral case formulation and treatment design: A problem-solving approach.* New York: Springer Publishing Company.

Nezu, A. M., Nezu, C. M., Peacock, M. A., & Girdwood, C. P. (2004). Case formulation in cognitive-behavior therapy. In S. N. Haynes & E. M. Heiby (Eds.), *Behavioral assessment* (pp. 402–426). New York: Wiley.

Nezu, A. M., Nezu, C. M., & Perri, M. G. (1989). *Problem-solving therapy for depression: Theory, research, and clinical guidelines.* New York: Wiley.

Nezu, A. M., Ronan, G. F., Meadows, E. A., & McClure, K. S. (Eds.). (2000). *Practitioner's guide to empirically based measures of depression.* New York: Kluwer Academic/Plenum Press.

Nezu, C. M., & Nezu, A. M. (1995). Clinical decision making in everyday practice: The science in the art. *Cognitive and Behavioral Practice, 2,* 5–25.

Nezu, C. M., Nezu, A. M., & Foster, S. L. (2000). A 10-step guide to selecting assessment measures in clinical and research settings. In A. M. Nezu, G. F. Ronan, E. A. Meadows, & K. S. McClure (Eds.), *Practitioner's guide to empirically based measures of depression* (pp. 17–24). New York: Kluwer Academic/Plenum Press.

O'Donohue, W., Fisher, J. E., & Hayes, S. C. (Eds.). (2003). *Cognitive behavior therapy: Applying empirically supported techniques in your practice.* New York: Wiley.

Rosen, A., & Proctor, E. K. (1981). Distinctions between treatment outcomes and their implications for treatment evaluations. *Journal of Consulting and Clinical Psychology, 49,* 418–425.

Shadish, W. R. (1993). Critical multiplism: A research strategy and its attendant tactics. In L. Sechrest (Ed.), *Program evaluation: A pluralistic enterprise* (pp. 13–57). San Francisco: Jossey-Bass.

Tanaka-Matsumi, J., Seiden, D., & Lam, K. (1996). The Culturally Informed Functional Assessment (CIFA) Interview: A strategy for cross-cultural behavioral practice. *Cognitive and Behavioral Practice, 3,* 215–233.

Wegner, D. M., & Zanakos, S. (1994). Chronic thought suppression. *Journal of Personality, 62,* 615–640.

Chapter 13

Case Formulation
in Emotion-Focused Therapy

LESLIE S. GREENBERG
RHONDA GOLDMAN

HISTORICAL BACKGROUND OF THE APPROACH

Emotion-focused therapy (EFT) also known as process–experiential therapy
(PE), is a neohumanistic experiential approach to therapy reformulated in
terms of modern emotion theory and affective neuroscience (Greenberg,
2002; Elliott, Watson, Goldman, & Greenberg, 2004; Greenberg & Johnson, 1988; Greenberg, Rice, & Elliott, 1993; Greenberg & Watson, 2005).
This model is informed by both humanistic–phenomenological theory
(Rogers, 1951, 1957; Perls, Hefferline, & Goodman, 1951), emotion and
cognition theory (Arnold, 1960; Fridja, 1986; Pascual-Leone, 1984, 1991;
Leventhal, 1986; Greenberg & Safran, 1987), affective neuroscience (Le
Doux, 1996; Davidson, 2002; Lane & Nadel, 2000), and dynamic and
family systems theory (Thelen & Smith, 1994). EFT focuses on moment-
by-moment awareness, regulation, expression, transformation and reflection on emotion in the practice of therapy with the goal of strengthening
the self and creating new meaning.

The EFT approach to case formulation is very much embedded within
the humanistic tradition, specifically client-centered and Gestalt therapy.
Neither of these therapy theories, however, originally developed a case formulation approach. Gestalt therapy (Perls et al., 1951) did not directly use
case formulation, but it did identify certain problem determinants such as
interruptions to contact with self and other or neurotic self-regulation. In-

terruptions such as projection, confluence, retroflection, introjection, and deflection were identified as producing current unhealthy functioning and these concepts were implicitly used to guide formulation and treatment as were concepts such as unfinished business and splits. Rogers (1951) could be seen as having one universal formulation, that of incongruence between self-concept and experiencing, although the concept of depth of experiencing can also be seen as a way of making process formulations about the client's current level of functioning. Rogers (1951) was also opposed to most forms of assessment and wrote that "psychological diagnosis as usually understood is unnecessary for psychotherapy and may actually be detrimental to the therapeutic process" (p. 220). Rogers (1951) expressed concern about the imbalance of power created when the therapist is in the position to diagnose. He was concerned about "the possibility of an unhealthy dependency developing if the therapist plays the role of expert, and the possibility that diagnosing clients places social control of the many in the hands of the few" (p. 224).

While we are largely in agreement with Rogers's concerns, that expertness creates too great a power imbalance and interferes with the formation of a genuine relationship, we do hold the view that developing a focus in therapy, which involves some type of formulation, is beneficial. We believe that differential process formulations in our therapy help guide interventions and in so doing facilitate the development of a focus for treatment that ultimately enhances the healing process. The focus that develops is tantamount to a case formulation. Our particular approach to the case formulation approach, however, stays very much within the bounds of the experiential therapy tradition from which it emerges. In EFT, formulations are *never* performed a priori (i.e. based on early assessment) as we do not attempt to establish what is dysfunctional or presume to know what will be most salient or important for the client. We believe that that which is most problematic, poignant, and meaningful emerges progressively, in the safe context of the therapeutic environment, and that the focus is co-constructed by client and therapist.

Furthermore, we, like Rogers, believe that assuming an authoritative position of deciding for ourselves on, or definitively informing clients as to, the source of their problems can be problematic. It can (1) rupture the delicate interpersonal nature of the therapeutic bond, and (2) create situations wherein clients are prevented from discovering, through attention to their own emerging experience, that which is idiosyncratically meaningful and relevant for them. Self-organization is seen as a powerful experiential learning process (i.e., key to change in this type of therapy).

Given this view, it is imperative in experiential therapy that formulations are co-constructed collaboratively by client and therapist and are reformed continuously to stay close to client's momentary experience or current states rather than being made about a person's character. Our major means of formulation involves "process diagnoses," about how people are currently experiencing their problem and impeding or interfering with their own experience. In relation to diagnoses, we believe that knowledge of certain nosological categories or syndromes can be helpful to experiential therapists but are best conceived of as descriptions of patterns of functioning rather than of types of people. Thus, for example, we prefer to think about anxious, obsessive, or borderline processes rather than people.

A fundamental tenet underlying this emotion-focused approach is that the organism possesses an innate emotion-based system that provides an adaptive tendency toward growth and mastery; a corollary of this is that clients are viewed as experts on their own experience in that they have closest access to it. In the therapeutic hour, the therapist therefore encourages the client to attend to momentary experiencing and nurtures the development of more adaptive functioning by continuously focusing clients on their felt sense and emotions. The I–thou relationship based on principles of presence, empathy, acceptance, and congruence is at the center of the approach (Buber, 1960; Rogers, 1951). This type of relationship permits a focus on adaptive needs and validates the client's growth toward adaptive flexibility. The growth tendency is seen as being embedded in the adaptive emotion system (Greenberg et al., 1993; Rogers, 1951; Perls et al., 1951). Clients are consistently encouraged to identify and symbolize internal experience and bodily felt referents in order to create new meaning. Therapy is seen as facilitating conscious choice and reasoned action based on increased access to and awareness of inner experience and feeling.

CONCEPTUAL FRAMEWORK

In this view, the self is seen as an agent, constantly in flux, manifesting itself at the contact boundary with the environment (Perls et al., 1951). The person is a dynamic system constantly creating and synthesizing a set of internal schemes evoked in reaction to the situation, thereby reforming a "self-in-the-situation." (Greenberg & van Balen, 1998; Greenberg & Watson, 2005). Overly repetitive experiences of painful emotions across situations and occasions imply lack of flexibility in the processing system and dysfunction; chronic enduring pain often represents rigid patterns of schematic activation and limited access to creatively adaptive responses to situations. Psychological health is seen as the ability to creatively adjust to situations and to be able to produce novel responses and experiences. The goal of treatment, therefore, is to overcome blocks to creative adjustment and to reinstate a "process of becoming."

As well as having biologically based inwired emotion, people are viewed as living in a constant process of making sense of their emotions. We have proposed a dialectical–constructivist view of human functioning to explain this process (Greenberg & Pascual-Leone, 1995, 2001; Greenberg et al., 1993; Pascual-Leone, 1991; Watson & Greenberg, 1996a; Greenberg & Watson, 2005). In our view the self is a multi-process, multilevel organization emerging from the dialectical interaction of many neurochemical, physiological, affective, motivational, and cognitive component elements within the self, and from interaction between self and other. In this view meaning is created by the dialectical synthesis of ongoing, moment-by-moment implicit experience influenced by biology and experience, and higher-level explicit reflexive processes influenced by culture and language that interpret, order, and explain elementary experiential processes. In addition to possessing biologically based inwired affective meaning and expressive systems, individuals thus are active agents constantly constructing meaning and creating the self they are about to become.

Affectively toned, preverbal, preconscious processing is seen as a major source of self-experience. This itself is a function of many dialectical processes at many levels that produce affective experience. Articulating, organizing, and ordering this experience into a coherent narrative, however is another major element. This too involves many dialectical processes that generate cognition. In our view two-way communication then occurs between the implicit and explicit systems. In addition, the self is construed as modular in nature with different voices in dialogue constituting a dialogical self (Hermans & Kempen, 1993; Whelton & Greenberg, 2004; Stiles, 1999). The goal of the complex self-organizing process is both affect regulation and adaptive flexibility.

Dysfunction can arise through various mechanisms: through the creation of meanings and narrative that are overly rigid or dysfunctional (meaning creation); from incoherence or incongruence between what is reflectively symbolized and the range of experienced possibilities (disclaimed or unsymbolized experience); from the maladaptive experience that is generated by the schematic syntheses formed on the basis of prior negative experience (learning); and from problematic shifts between a plurality of self organizations or lack of fit or integration between them (conflict or splits) (Greenberg & van Balen, 1998).

Emotion Schematic Processing

The emotion schematic system is seen as the central catalyst of self-organization, often at the base of dysfunction and ultimately the road to cure. For simplicity, we refer to the complex synthesis process in which a number of coactivated emotion schemes coapply to produce a unified sense of self in relation to the world as the emotion schematic process (Greenberg & Pascual-Leone, 1995; Greenberg & Watson, 2005). The experiential state of the self at any one moment will be referred to as the current self-organization. In depression, for example, the self generally is organized experientially as unlovable or worthless and helpless or incompetent because of the activation of emotion–schematic memories of crucial losses, humiliation, or failure in prior experience (Greenberg & Watson, 2005). These emotion memories are evoked in response to current losses or failures and cause the self to lose resilience and collapse into powerlessness. This state is symbolized by clients and reported as feeling hopeless or worthless or anxiously insecure.

We also refer to a level of organization of self, higher than the schematically based self-organization that generates the feeling of who one is as a narrative identity (Whelton & Greenberg, 2000, 2004; Greenberg & Angus, 2004). This identity involves the integration of accumulated experience and of various self-representations into some sort of coherent story or narrative. Identity cannot be understood outside these narratives. To assume coherence and meaning, human lives must be "emplotted" in a story. In this process, events are organized by narrative discourse such that disparate actions and experiences of a human life are formed into a coherent narrative. These stories are influenced by different cultures that have complex rules about the form meaningful narratives can take. The stories that tell us who we are emerge in a dialectical interaction between the experiencing and the explaining aspects of self-functioning.

Emotional change in EFT is seen as occurring through the processes of emotion awareness and expression, regulation of emotion, making sense of emotion by reflecting on it, and finally transformation of maladaptive emotion (Greenberg, 2002; Greenberg & Watson, 2005). Self-acceptance and the ability to integrate various disowned aspects of self as well as the need for restructuring maladaptive emotional responses are the central means of overcoming psychological dysfunction. Reowning involves overcoming the avoidance of disowned internal experience and disclaimed action tendencies and shifting from the negative evaluation of one's experience toward a more self-accepting stance. With the reowning of affect and associated action tendencies comes an increased sense of self-coherence and volition and the development of a sense that one is the agent of one's own experience. With the development of a coherent, agentic sense of self comes a greater sense of efficacy and mastery over one's psychological world.

In this approach, empathic attunement to affect and meaning is the therapist's primary medium of engagement. At all times, the therapist tries to make psychological *contact* with and convey a *genuine* understanding of the client's internal experience (Rogers, 1951, 1957). The therapist continually tracks what is important to the client throughout the session, constantly responding to what appears to be the client's central meanings. The approach involves the therapist actively entering into the client's internal frame of reference, resonating with the client's experience, and guiding the client's attentional focus to what the therapist hears as most crucial or poignant for the client at a particular moment (Rice, 1974; Vanaerschot,

1990). This helps get to the underlying determinants of, or conditions generating, the presenting problem.

Our approach to case formulation involves identifying the client's core pain and using that as a guide to the development of a focus on underlying determinants generating the presenting concerns. This is the case formulation aspect of this treatment. Clients' presenting problems, or symptomatic distress, are seen as manifestations of underlying emotional–schematic processing difficulties. These core painful experiences are articulated as concerns such as a deep fear of abandonment or a shame-based sense of unworthiness.

A defining feature of our approach is that it is process diagnostic (Greenberg et al., 1993) rather than person diagnostic. Thus it is clients' manner of processing, in-session markers of problematic emotional states, and co-evolving therapeutic themes that are attended to as ways of helping to develop a focus on underlying determinants. Although the person in treatment may have been diagnosed as depressed or as having an anxiety disorder, this in itself is not the necessary information to help form a focus. The focus depends much more on the establishment in therapy of the underlying determinants of this person's problems and the collaborative development of an understanding of the person's core pain. In our process-oriented approach to treatment, case formulation is ongoing, as sensitive to the moment and the session context as it is to an understanding of the person as a case. This is both because of the egalitarian relationship one wishes to maintain and because people are seen as active agents who constantly create meaning. People's current momentary states and accompanying narratives are more determining of who they are than any conceptualization of more enduring patterns or reified self-concepts that may be assessed early in treatment. Therefore, in a process-diagnostic approach there is a continual focus on the client's current state of mind and current cognitive/affective problem states. The therapist's main concern is one of following the client's ongoing process and identifying markers of current emotional concerns more than developing a picture of the person's enduring personality, character, or core pattern.

In formulating a focus the therapist therefore attends to a variety of different markers at different levels of client processing as they emerge. Markers are client statements or behaviors that alert therapists to various aspects of clients' functioning that might need attention as possible determinants of the presenting problem. It is these that guide intervention more than a diagnosis or an explicit case formulation. It is the client's presently felt experience that indicates what the difficulty is and whether problem determinants are currently accessible and amenable to intervention. The early establishment of a focus and the discussion of determinants or generating conditions of the depression act only as a broad framework to initially focus exploration. The focus is always subject to change and development, and process diagnosis of in-session problem states always acts as a major means of focusing each session.

INCLUSION/EXCLUSION CRITERIA
AND MULTICULTURAL CONSIDERATIONS

Given that we do not assume a generic or unitary view of "normal" human functioning and dysfunction this approach is seen as appropriate for clients from ethnically and culturally diverse backgrounds. As emphasized, this therapy adopts an empathic and egalitarian relationship and is thus sensitive to inherent power imbalances that may exist between therapists of the monoculture and their culturally different clients. Cultural empathy as well as individual empathy is needed. Therapists therefore resist applying preconceived diagnostic labels that may not reflect the cultural meaning frameworks of clients from racially and ethnically different backgrounds or may in fact pathologize culturally different value systems. When working with clients with social, economic, racial, sexual, or ethnic backgrounds different to their own, therapists are encouraged to be careful not to automatically impose assumptions that may reflect their own culture-bound value systems. Therapists educate themselves about the client's cultural background if it is unfamiliar to them, being careful to assess degree of acculturation into the mainstream culture. Potential issues of difference are directly addressed through the therapeutic relationship early in the therapy if clients express discomfort in any form or fear of potential power differentials.

We also recognize that there may be ways in which this therapy has not extended its theoretical understanding and therapeutic practice to accommodate cultural differences and we acknowledge that some underserved populations may not feel comfortable with the therapeutic format. They may prefer a less traditional setting, for example, other than the therapist's office such as the church or the school. On the other hand, EFT therapy can be adapted to clients of different cultural backgrounds with different rules and norms surrounding emotional experiencing and expression.

It is important in this approach to understand how emotion functions in other cultures. For example, some cultures are less likely to show emotions readily (Lam & Sue, 2001), and the therapist must be sensitive to this, openly discuss a rationale for emotional expression with clients, provide high degrees of safety, allow for a slower pace, and understand cultural assumption related to emotion. For example, showing disrespect for parents is taboo in many cultures that follow traditions of ancestor worship, and thus expressing anger toward a parent in an empty-chair dialogue may violate these beliefs. A strong alliance will be needed and more of a rationale provided and permission given for emotional expression before clients from these cultures will express any negative emotion toward parents. On the other hand with some African and some more expressive Latin-based cultures, emotions are often expressed more somatically. In expressive cultures further degrees of internal bodily based focusing and symbolizing may need to be attended to more than emotional expression. Formulation, however, is still the same regardless of cultural differences, but given that formulation and intervention are so intertwined it will take longer to develop a focus and more directiveness may be needed to get to a formulation with certain cultural groups.

In terms of inclusion/exclusion criteria, before therapy begins, a global assessment is conducted in which the client's appropriateness for this therapy is evaluated. If strong biological factors (i.e. a biochemical disorder) or systemic factors (that would deem the person more appropriate for marital or couple therapy) are judged as being primary problem determinants, the client is considered inappropriate for this treatment. This therapy is most suitable for dealing with moderate affective disorders or traumatic life events as well as interpersonal, identity, and existential problems. In addition, people who meet the following criteria are judged as not suitable for short-term EFT treatment (16–20 weeks): high suicidal risk; long-term alcohol or drug addiction; three or more depressive episodes; psychotic; and schizoid, schizotypal, borderline, and antisocial personality disorders. Long-term EFT treatment is not appropriate with schizoid, schizotypal, and antisocial personality disorders or with psychotics. Beyond an initial assessment that the client satisfies the inclusion/exclusion criteria, that the problems are appropriate for individual psychotherapy, and that the client desires treatment, no other formal assessment is conducted. The person's ability to form an alliance is informally assessed at the outset and in an ongoing manner throughout treatment.

STEPS IN CASE FORMULATION

A strong therapeutic relationship needs to be formed to allow the formulation process to proceed. Through the empathic process, client and therapist are continually negotiating the terms of the working relationship, clarifying what the problems are, and developing an agreement on the tasks, immediate goals, and responsibilities of treatment. In the initial stages, while the therapist may apply some of the steps of case formulation, such as an assessment of focusing capacity and manner of affective–cognitive processing, the initial phase emphasizes making contact with and responding to the client and does not involve actively collecting information or intervening.

In our view, formulations are always co-constructions that emerge from the relationship rather than being formed by the therapist. The establishment of a problem definition is tantamount to the agreement on treatment goals in the formation of the initial alliance (Bordin, 1994). This important aspect of alliance formation involves the collaborative identification of core issues and the establishment of a thematic focus. An important aspect of the initial alliance also involves the client perceiving the tasks of the treatment as relevant (Horvath & Greenberg, 1989). The initial tasks that the client needs to perceive as relevant in the treatment are those of disclosure, exploration, and deepening of experience. Once the client is engaged in these, the exploration for a focus begins.

Identifying and articulating the problematic cognitive–affective processes underlying and generating symptomatic experience is a collaborative effort between therapist and client. The establishment of agreement on the determinants of the person's problem helps alliance development in that it implicitly suggests that the goal of the treatment is to resolve this issue. Sometimes this agreement is implicit or so clear that no explicit goals are discussed. Generally, however, an explicit agreement is established that treatment goals involve addressing the underlying determinants and the connection between the determinants and the presenting problem is discussed. Sometimes for very fragile clients, however, it is the establishment of a validating relationship itself that is the goal. For some clients who are unable to focus inward and be aware of their experience, the very ability to attend to their emotions and make sense of them may become the focus of treatment. A focus and a goal for another client might be to acknowledge and stand up to his overly hostile critic who produces feelings of inadequacy. For another client with low self-esteem, the focus and goal might be to become more aware of, and more clearly able to express, her feelings and needs. For another dependent client the focus and goal might be to assertively express and resolve her resentment at feeling dominated by her husband. For an anxious client it might be to develop a means of self-soothing and self-support; for another to restructure a deep fear of abandonment and insecurity based on trauma or losses in the past.

As well as the collaborative process of establishing a focus in each session and in the treatment as a whole, the therapist also is constantly making "process diagnoses," or formulations, of what is occurring in the client at the moment, and how best to proceed with productive emotional exploration at this time. Process diagnoses involve attending to different client markers, which helps develop a formulation of the client's difficulties and focus the treatment. These markers include clients' emotional processing style, task markers, markers of clients' characteristic styles of responding and micromarkers of client process. Any formulation is held very tentatively and is constantly checked with the client for relevance and fit, with clients' moment-to-moment processing in the session remaining the ultimate guide. It is important that therapists' frame their interventions in a manner that is relevant to their clients' goals and objectives and that there is agreement about the behaviors and interactions that are contributing to the client's problems. Formulation and intervention are, in the final analysis, inseparable and they span the entire course of treatment. They also occur constantly at many levels. There is no discrete initial formulation or assessment phase. The therapist, rather, gets to know the client over time but never comes to know definitively what is occurring in the client. Formulation thus never ends.

The following steps have been identified to guide clinicians in the development of case formulations (Greenberg & Watson, 2005).

1. Identify the presenting problem.
2. Listen to and explore the client's narrative about the problem
3. Gather information about client's attachment and identity histories and current relationships and concerns
4. Observe and attend to the client's style of processing emotions.
5. Identify and respond to the painful aspects of the client's experiences.
6. Identify markers and when they arise suggest tasks appropriate to resolving problematic processes.
7. Focus on thematic intrapersonal and interpersonal processes
8. Attend to clients' moment-by-moment processing to guide interventions within tasks.

Initial Steps

The first steps in developing a case formulation involve the identification of the presenting problem, listening to the related narrative, and gathering information regarding attachment and identity histories as it pertains to current relationships. As clients report their view of their presenting problem(s), the therapist empathically reflects and explores how clients fit problems into their wider life narrative. At this point, therapists are also gathering information about relevant life circumstances in order to assess client's current levels of functioning and outside support. Throughout all of this, therapists seek to understand the core of clients' relationships and attachment and identity histories.

Attending to Moment-by-Moment Style of Processing Emotions

In parallel with the initial steps and throughout the process, therapists attend to the manner in which clients process emotions from moment to moment. This is a hallmark of this approach. Initially, this provides essential information to therapists about what to focus on. As therapy progresses, therapists continue to attend to a momentary style of processing to make process diagnoses about how best to intervene to facilitate emotional processing.

In each session, the therapist both follows and guides the client in a focused exploration of internal experience. In-session, process-diagnostic formulations are made in response to the current material presented by the client. In some sessions, this involves continued exploration of momentary cognitive–affective processing, encouraging awareness of internal experiencing, while in other sessions, a marker might emerge that will lead to a formulation that it would be most productive to introduce a specific task. There is generally no definite plan that particular contents should be focused on in future sessions. In each session, the therapist waits to see what emerges for the client. As the self is seen to be reforming freshly in each moment, it is assumed that clients reorganize themselves differently each session, having reintegrated new information that may have emerged in the previous session and throughout the week. Any formulation is held very tentatively and is constantly checked with the client for relevance and fit, with clients' moment-to-moment processing in the session remaining the ultimate guide. As all clients have a tendency, in a facilitative environment, to work toward mastery, it is assumed that by closely attending to clients' current phenomenology, their efforts at resolving their problems and their blocks or interruptions to this will emerge. The different ways in which therapists attend to emotional processing initially and throughout therapy are outlined below.

As therapists build the relationship, they begin, from the first session, to formulate the person's type of global processing style. They note whether the client is emotionally overregulated or underregulated and engaged in conceptual or experiential processing and note the depth of the client's experiencing, the client's vocal quality, and the degree of emotional arousal. The therapist assesses whether clients have the capacity to assume a self-focus and are able to turn attention inward to their experience. For this, therapists attend not only to clients' content but also to the manner and style in which they present their experiences. Attention is paid to *how* clients are presenting their experiences in addition to *what* they are saying. To aid therapists in reading such paralinguistic cues, they are trained to evaluate vocal quality (Rice & Kerr, 1986), the current depth of experiencing (Klein, Mathieu, Gendlin, & Kiesler, 1969), and the concreteness, specificity, and vividness of language use and different types of emotional processing.

Four vocal styles relevant to experiential processing have been defined: focused, emotional, limited, and external (Rice & Kerr, 1986). For example, a therapist will notice when a client's voice becomes more focused. This is an indication that the client's attentional energy is turned inward and the person is attempting to freshly symbolize experience. Alternatively, a highly external voice that has a premonitored quality involving a great deal of attentional energy being deployed outward may indicate a more rehearsed conceptual style of processing and a lack of spontaneity. While this may initially give an impression of expressiveness, the rhythmic intonation pattern conveys a "talking at" quality. It is unlikely that content being expressed in this voice is freshly experienced. A high degree of external vocal quality suggests that the person does not have a strong propensity to self-focus (Rice & Kerr, 1986). Clients who demonstrate little or no focused or emotional voice are seen as less emotionally accessible and needing further work to help them process internal experiential information. Clients with a high degree of external vocal quality need to be helped to focus inward, whereas those with a high degree of limited vocal quality, indicating a wariness, need a safe environment to develop trust in the therapist and allow them to relax.

Another indicator of current capacity for self-focus is the client's initial depth of experiencing (Klein et al., 1969). The Experiencing (EXP) scale defines clients involvement in inner referents and experience from the impersonal (level 1) and superficial (level 2) through externalized or limited references to feelings (level 3) to direct focus on inner experiencing and feelings (level 4) to questioning or propositioning the self about internal feelings and personal experiences (level 5) to experiencing an aspect of self from a new perspective (level 6), to a point where awareness of present feelings is immediately connected to internal processes and exploration is continually expanding (level 7). Momentary formulations, with clients' processing at a low level of EXP, suggest facilitating deeper experiencing, sometimes by conjecturing empathically as to what clients are presently experiencing and at other times, by guiding attention inward to focus directly on bodily felt experience.

Narrative style, whether clients are external (talking about what happened), internal (what it felt like), or reflexive (what it meant), is also attended to with the goal being to encourage a focus on internal to promote later reflection (Greenberg & Angus, 2004). Noticing the clients' expressive stance, indicating whether clients are observers of their experience, speaking about the self, or expressers, speaking from the self, and whether they are differentiating or global, descriptive, or evaluative in their processing is also important. Attention also is paid to vividness of language use, such as the poignancy and aliveness of images and feelings that are conjured up by the material. A high degree of concreteness, specificity, and vividness of language use indicates a strong self-focus and high involvement in working. The therapist also is attending to other micromarkers, such as deflections, rehearsed descriptions, rambling, silence, and many other indicators of the person's manner of processing affect. These alert therapists to clients' moment-by-moment processing to enable them to adjust their interventions in order to be maximally responsive to their clients. In summary, formulation at this general level involves evaluations of the nature of current emotional processing style and process diagnoses of how to best facilitate a focus on internal experiencing.

Degree of emotional awareness and expressiveness, whether emotion is under- or overregulated and whether the person is able to reflect on and make sense of emotion, is also assessed. To aid in formulation of momentary states, therapists also are trained to distinguish between primary, secondary, and instrumental emotional responses (Greenberg & Safran, 1987; Greenberg et al., 1993). Primary emotions are immediate direct responses to situations whereas secondary emotions are reactions to more primary emotions or thoughts. These often obscure the primary generating process. Instrumental emotions are those expressions that are used in order to achieve an aim, such as expressing sadness to elicit comfort or anger in order to intimidate (Greenberg & Safran, 1989; Greenberg & Paivio, 1997). The main goal in differentiating emotional responding is to access the primary organismic emotional response that has not been acknowledged. Then therapists along with their clients ascertain whether the primary emotion is adaptive and can be utilized to provide useful information and adaptive action tendencies or is maladaptive and cannot be followed. The goal is to identify core maladaptive emotion schemes that need to be transformed. Once identified, these maladaptive schemes guide the focus.

Identifying the Pain

To formulate successfully EFT therapists develop a pain compass, which acts as an emotional tracking device for following their clients' experience (Greenberg & Watson, 2005). The therapist focuses on the most painful aspects of the client's experience and identifies the client's chronic enduring pain. Pain or other intense affects are the cues that alert the therapist to potentially profitable areas of exploration as they focus on clients' moment-to-moment experience.

The first thing EFT therapists do to develop a pain compass is to listen for what is most poignant in clients' presentations. They also immediately begin to flag the painful life events their clients have endured. Painful events provide clues as to the source of important core maladaptive emotion schemes that clients may have formed about themselves and others, providing therapists with an understanding of clients' sources of pain and vulnerability.

Therapists also observe the types and varieties of coping strategies that clients use to cope with their pain and to modulate their painful emotions and which skills might be lacking. The presence and absence of such strategies as problem-focused coping, involving the ability to think about the problem and ways of solving it, and emotion-focused coping, involving becoming aware of feelings, able to tolerate emotions, and actively reflect on the meaning and significance of feelings, are noted.

Identify Markers and Implement Tasks

The hallmark of EFT is the attention paid to specific in-session tasks. These tasks follow from the identification of specific markers consisting of statements that clients make that indicate unresolved cognitive–affective problems. As they listen to their clients' narratives EFT therapists ask themselves what specific in-session behaviors are indicators of their client's emotional processing difficulties. The focus on specific client statements is partly influenced by therapists' understanding of the painful and difficult aspects of clients' experiences that have been inadequately processed.

A focus on underlying determinants and the accessing and working through of maladaptive schemes is aided by the facilitation of client tasks that enable clients to access, explore, and reintegrate previously disallowed or muted self-information. Particular affective problem markers and tasks may become increasingly more central as therapy progresses. Research has demonstrated that particular client in-therapy states are markers of particular types of dysfunctional processing that can be resolved in specific ways (Greenberg et al., 1993; Rice & Greenberg, 1984; Greenberg, Elliott, & Lietaer, 1994). Markers signify particular types of affective problems that are currently amenable to particular interventions. The therapist therefore notices when a marker emerges and intervenes in a specific manner to facilitate resolution of that type of processing problem. The main markers and the affective tasks that we have identified and studied are (1) problematic reactions expressed through puzzlement about emotional or behavioral responses to particular situations, which indicates a readiness to explore by systematic evocative unfolding; (2) conflict splits in which one aspect of the self is critical or coercive toward another, which indicates readiness for a two-chair dialogue; (3) self-interruptive splits in which one part of the self interrupts or constricts emotional experience and expression, which indicates readiness for a two-chair enactment; (4) an unclear felt sense in which the person is on the surface of, or feeling confused and unable to get, a clear sense of his or her experience, which indicates a readiness for focusing; (5) unfinished business involving the statement of a lingering unresolved feeling toward a significant other, which indicates an opportunity for empty-chair dialogue; and (6) vulnerability in which the person feels deeply ashamed or insecure about some aspect of his or her experience, which indicates a need for empathic affirmation. A variety of markers of other important, research-based problem states and specific intervention processes such as alliance ruptures, the creation of new meaning when a cherished belief has been disconfirmed, have been identified (Elliott, Watson, et al., 2004).

Identifying the Thematic Intrapersonal and Interpersonal Processes

While therapists do not direct content from one session to the next, they do facilitate a continuing focus on internal themes that consist of underlying painful emotional issues that appear to impede healthy functioning. A focus on the main intrapersonal or interpersonal themes that are contributing to clients' pain does emerge over time. For example, in one case the therapy might focus on feelings of insecurity and worthlessness and encourage their exploration if they seem of core importance. In another, unresolved anger may emerge as a focus. Focused empathic exploration and engagement in tasks often leads clients to important thematic material. We have found that in successful cases, core thematic issues do emerge. Themes have been observed to fall into one of four major classes of determinants. Clients are seen as suffering from (1) a general inability to symbolize internal experience, (2) problems in intrapersonal relations, (3) problems in interpersonal relations, or (4) existential concerns, or from some combination of these four (Greenberg & Paivio, 1997). Intrapsychic issues generally relate to self-definition and self-esteem, such as being overly self-critical or perfectionistic, whereas interpersonal issues generally entail attachment and interdependence-related issues such as feeling too dependent or vulnerable to rejection. Existential issues relate to limit situations involving loss, choice, freedom, and death.

Attending to Moment-by-Moment Processing to Guide Interventions within Tasks

In the tasks and throughout therapists attend to and respond to clients' moment-by-moment processing to guide their interventions. The therapist attends to micromarkers such as poignancy, vividness of language, interruptions, deflections, and many other indicators of the person's manner of processing affect while the tasks are being done. Thus once tasks are engaged in therapists come full circle to attending to moment-by-moment process as the main guide to formulation and intervention. In addition, the models of the resolution process for each task described in the research section also guide differential moment-by-moment intervention during tasks.

Thus, EFT therapists pull together information from multiple levels in working with their clients. The different levels of processing to which therapists listen together constitute a sequence of comprehension. Right from the start therapists attend carefully to clients' moment-by-moment process in the session and to how clients are engaging in the work of processing their emotional experiencing. They also listen to clients' life histories to identify their characteristic ways of being with themselves and others. Therapists listen as well for markers of specific cognitive–affective tasks or problem states and for the client's main underlying problems to emerge. Once a focus has been established and the client and therapist are engaged in working on core themes the focus is on moment-by-moment experience.

While sensitized by theories of determinants of problems or disorders (e.g., for depression self-esteem vulnerability via self-criticism and dependence, loss, unresolved anger, powerlessness, shame or guilt), these theories are seen only as useful tools that provide perspective not as definitive determinants. Thus clients are understood in their own terms and each understanding of the client is held tentatively and is open to reformulation and change as more exploration takes place. Treatment is not driven by a theory of the causes of, say, depression or anxiety but, rather, by listening, empathy, following the client's process, and marker identification; a sense of the determinants are built from the ground up using the client as a constant touchstone for what is true. Treatments therefore are custom-made for each person.

APPLICATION TO PSYCHOTHERAPY TECHNIQUE

Initially and throughout therapy sessions, the therapist is empathically attuned to the client's frame of reference, listening moment by moment for that which is currently most meaningful and poignant. It is through this co-constructive meaning-making expedition that therapist's become apprised of how clients schematically organize their emotional world and eventually come to make process formulations. That is, through this continuing focus on the creation of meaning, markers that signal different types of affective–cognitive schematic processing problems arise. These markers inform the therapist on how to intervene differentially at different times. Introducing therapeutic tasks that facilitate the working through of blocks to healthy meaning construction and affect regulation does this.

Once in a mode of facilitating a particular task, the therapist is guided, both explicitly and tacitly, by a preexisting map of how such tasks tend to unfold. These maps are formulations of optimal problem-solving processes. Rather than being instructional or thinking about the steps, the therapist attends, as fully as possible, to the client's momentary experience and, in response, makes miniformulations of how to facilitate experiential exploration through to resolutions of processing difficulties. Therefore, we enter the client's meaning framework and intervene at markers of dysfunctional schematic processing that interfere with adaptive responding. Over the course of therapy, continual work on these interferences forms a coherent thematic focus

A key aspect of formulation involves helping determine whether a core experience once reached is *primary adaptive emotion* or a *maladaptive emotional experience* generated by a core dysfunctional emotion scheme (Greenberg, 2002). Clients and therapists need to decide whether a primary emotion once arrived at is a healthy experience that can be used as a guide. If it seems as if the core emotion will enhance their well-being, they can stay with this experience and be guided by the information it provides. If, however, they decide that being in this place will not enhance them or their intimate bonds, it is not a place to stay or to be guided by. When people in dialogue with their therapists decide that they cannot trust the feelings at which they have arrived as a source of good information, then the feelings need to be transformed. Now a means to leave the place they have arrived at must be found.

It is through the shift into primary emotion and its use as a resource that change occurs. Thus in some cases change occurs simply because the client accesses adaptive underlying anger and reorganizes to assert boundaries, or accesses adaptive sadness, grieves a loss and organizes to withdraw and to recover, or reaches out for comfort and support. In these situations, contacting the need and action tendency embedded in the emotion provides the motivation and direction for change and provides an alternative way of responding. Action replaces resignation and motivated desire replaces hopelessness.

In many instances, however, once a core primary emotion is arrived at it is understood to be a complex *maladaptive emotion schematic experience* rather than simply unexpressed primary *adaptive* emotions such as sadness or anger. Core schemes that are maladaptive result in feelings such as a core sense of powerlessness, or feeling invisible, or a deep sense of woundedness, of shame, of insecurity, of worthlessness, or of feeling unloved or unlovable. It is these that often are accessed as being at the core of the secondary bad feelings such as despair, panic, hopelessness, or global distress. We have found that core experiences often relate either to worthlessness or to anxious dependence (Greenberg & Paivio, 1997; Greenberg, 2002). At the core of the self-critical process is a feeling of worthlessness, of failure and of being bad, or at the core of dependence is a feeling of fragile insecurity, being unable to hold together without support. These are generated by the core emotion-based bad/weak self-schemes. In these instances the primary maladaptive feelings of worthlessness, weakness, or insecurity have to be accessed in order to allow for change. It is only through experience of emotion that emotional distress can be cured. One cannot leave these feelings of worthless or insecurity until one has arrived at them. What is curative is first the ability to symbolize these feelings of worthlessness or weakness and then to access alternate adaptive emotion-based self-schemes. The generation of alternate schemes is based on accessing adaptive feelings and needs that get activated in response to the currently experienced emotional distress. It is the person's response to their own symbolized distress that is adaptive and must be accessed and used as a life-giving resource.

The core of EFT practice thus lies in accessing primary adaptive emotions. The goal is to acknowledge and experience previously avoided or nonsymbolized primary adaptive emotion and needs. It is not only the experience of primary emotion per se but the accessing of the needs/goals/concerns and the action tendencies. Once a core primary emotion is aroused, if it is tolerated, it follows its own course, involving a natural rising and a falling off of intensity. Decrease in intensity allows for reflection.

Arousal also leads to associations and results in the activation of many new schemes, especially when attention is explicitly focused on the task of making sense of the aroused emotions. Thus it is the combination of arousing, regulating, symbolizing, and reflecting that carries forward the process of change

CASE EXAMPLE

The client begins therapy explaining her presenting problem:

> "I've been feeling quite depressed, I think, most of my life, but this has been a particularly bad year and I lost a few people who were close to me and helped me in my personal life, and I just felt that even though I had crisis in the past with depression, I've always seemed to be able to bounce back, you know, and I'm having a hard time this year and . . . "

She says that her husband also suffers from depression and was hospitalized against his will following police involvement earlier in the year. At that time her sister called the police because his behavior was unpredictable and he appeared violent. As a result of the police intervention her husband was hospitalized and prohibited from living in the home for a number of months:

> "Yes, it was very upsetting because he became violent—not so much toward me, but he would break things and smash things and his personality changed completely, because he's not that type of a person—very gentle, kind person—so that happened and I found my family very nonsupportive, and I guess that's—and because they're not like that, so basically their attitude was well get a divorce, get rid of him."

She, however, had decided to stand by her husband and support him through his difficult time, and thereby became alienated from her family. She reports her current relationship with her husband to be draining at times but solid nonetheless:

C: I'm fine with him. I find it draining because I'm not feeling good, but I go out of my way to try to—when he's having a bad day—to make him feel better and I find that he just doesn't have what it takes at this point to give it back.

T: To give it back, so sometimes you sort of maybe feel there's nothing left.

C: Right, but I'm not angry at him about that. I think I'm more angry at my family.

Historically, her family situation was so difficult that all four of the sisters left the family in their midteens. She considers her sisters the most important part of her family and has often viewed them in more of a parental role, getting much of the affection and support from them instead of her parents. In her current view of her depression, she feels most betrayed by her sisters:

C: Most of my depression I think centers around my family dynamics. I don't feel close to my family even like with my sisters. They all got married very young, they all had children, their children have children. I'm sort of like the nomad in the family, I didn't get married until I was 36. I moved around a lot and went back, took all kinds of different— you know it's just not the same—a different type of life than what they had.

T: But you felt outside.

C: Yes, they ostracized me.

T: So it's not only feeling ostracized but also criticized by them.

C: Yes, yes, my older sister didn't do it, but I felt my next older sister did it. My other sister and I used to be very close and then we're not close anymore and I don't understand that. I don't know, maybe she's tired of being around a depressed person. You know?

T: And you're saying it was hard for you that they were sort of disapproving. They were saying, yes, you should be married, you should be¾

C: Settled down.

T: And you felt kind of dumped on. And that would lead you to feeling very bad—

C: Depressed. Sometimes I feel depressed, I don't know why.

From the exploration of the first session, the therapist has a sense that throughout her childhood and into her adult life she has often experienced herself as alone and unsupported. She has internalized the critical voice of her parents and often judges herself to be a failure. Within the context of a physically and emotionally abusive past she often felt emotionally unsafe and abandoned.

In terms of her emotional processing style, the therapist observes that the client is able to focus on internal experience, particularly in response to the therapist's empathic responses that focus her internally. As she reports, however, she tends to avoid (as many people do) painful and difficult emotions. In fact, there appears to be an identifiable emotional pattern wherein she moves into states of helpless and hopeless when she starts to feel primary emotions of sadness or anger and in response to her experience of needs for closeness and acceptance. This can be seen as a form of maladaptive emotional processing.

Throughout the first session a pattern is presented where the client expresses many emotion episodes of pain, anger, or shame. During each episode her emotional arousal is fairly full, disrupting her normal speech patterns. Immediately following such intense expressions of emotion the client describes emotions of helplessness or hopelessness. In fact, hopelessness is the most predominant emotion in the first session, constituting almost 50% of all her emotion episodes. There are different points at which she demonstrates this pattern. In the first example from early in the first session, she is describing how she just cannot cope with her family anymore:

C: My sister called me and said and left a message saying, "I'd like to take you out for your birthday." And for some reason it really upset me all day yesterday and I was out in the coachhouse and I cried, I was very emotional and I thought I won't go to lunch with you because I might say something and you'll criticize me. She's very critical. She has, I guess, an ideal life and she looks at my life and she's the one who called me and told me to get a lawyer, and then I never heard from her for months when [husband] came out of the hospital. And she wonders why I don't come around. How do you think we feel? They told me to go, to leave him. Because he's mentally ill. So you're supposed to go over there and feel like everything's OK?

T: So actually it sounds you're feeling quite resentful toward them.

C: I am.

T: It's hard to sort of put on a funny face and go for a birthday lunch or whatever. It's a pretend. But it also ends up somehow in you crying and—

C: It makes me depressed. Yes.

T: Because in a way it's like you're mad at her for how's she's treated you.

C: Yes, I am.

T: And also it gets into a kind of vulnerability to, that she's going to criticize you or something—

C: I feel that I'm too sensitive. I mean sometimes when I have got angry in the past I just told her to—but I'm at the point now where I don't want to argue. Basically I want them to leave me alone. That's how I feel. And I know that's not good. Christmas is coming and I dread it.

Her relationships with family members are difficult, and often painful. Her mother is an alcoholic with whom she and her three sisters no longer have contact. Her father is a concentration camp survivor. He has always been emotionally removed from the family and is often perceived as critical and judgmental. There is a history of physical punishment throughout her childhood, particularly from her father. Talking about her parents in the first session, she says:

> "And she [mother] does things like, in the middle of the night, call you up and call you names, and once I was married, I guess I just decided I had enough. I can't take this anymore so I just cut my ties with her. And my father is just, he's just not there. Like I've been—I haven't worked for a year, my husband's had a breakdown, even my best friend died. He's never called once to touch. Not just this year, any year. Just doesn't, he just doesn't; he's not demonstrative."

The therapist, hearing a focused voice when she talked about her father just not being there, focuses her internally by selectively reflecting on her loneliness implicit in her current state: "You're feeling so alone. There's nobody really there."

Soon after this the exploration turns toward her lonely, weak, and vulnerable feelings and she moves into hopelessness. The therapist identifies this as a potential focus of therapy, marking it for later, while suggesting a rationale for an emotion-focused therapy and an alternative approach to dealing with such emotions:

C: Oh, I think I should be doing other things rather than sitting around feeling bad for myself.

T: You're saying you hate getting weak.

C: Oh, yeah, a waste of time.

T: Somehow your emotion is an important message that you're giving yourself.

C: Well, yeah, I've been doing this all my life.

T: Yes, so its here you want to—Somehow, what is this, what do you feel as you begin to cry? Do you feel so alone? Is that what—

C: I guess that's it. I just—feel tired.

T: Tired of the struggle.

C: Yeah, I'm tired of thinking about it. You know, sometimes I'm preoccupied, just like, "Oh, God like if I could turn a switch." A lot of times I like to sleep because then I don't think.

T: Yeah, yeah, but somehow whatever's going on you do think and it does go around and around.

C: All the time.

T: It's kind of like there's always unresolved feelings and then they keep coming back. Like it's a lot of emotional baggage you're carrying. We talked about quite the painful history with your family and it's as though it keeps churning, right? I guess some of what we will do is try to work with that to maybe finish it and then pack it away.

While this pattern of moving into hopelessness is clearly evident, it is also clear that the client is capable of achieving an internal focus and this augers well for developing a focus.

As the therapist listens to the client, he begins to use his "pain compass" to hear the client's chronic enduring pain. When talking about her need to be supported and accepted by her family she expresses intense emotions, feeling immediately overwhelmed by the thought that it will never happen and that, ultimately, she does not deserve such intimacy.

> "I tell myself a story over and over again to the point I believe it. I believe that it's so and that it can't be fixed. Or I don't care. I don't want it to be fixed. . . . That I'm not loved, that I'm not as good as them you know, my life is chaotic and theirs [sisters] seems to be going, you know their life seems so much easier."

The enormity of her aloneness was girded by a feeling of hopelessness. Not only did she feel she was not loved and that there was nothing she could do about it, but she felt that it was never going to change.

As the therapist listens to the client, he is attuned to possible markers that indicate openings where tasks may be undertaken. In the very first session the therapist hears two markers. Both unfinished business, around feelings of being badly treated by her family, and also a self-critical conflict between a part of herself that wants love and acceptance and another that labels her as failure and not entitled to love. As it is early in the therapy, these are simply noted and reflected on as something to return to:

C: I don't think I'm a bad. I believe I'm a bad person but deep down inside I don't think I'm a bad person. And I don't deserve all this. I haven't raped and murdered and robbed banks; I haven't done crazy things, there's no reason for them [family] to treat me this way.

T: So, in a way, it's almost like grieving for what you never had from them because you're beginning to say: "I do deserve better, I'm not a bad person, and it's like I feel really sad about what I never got. And I deserve it more."

C: Yeah, I guess so, yeah.

T: But the sadness is about all that you never got. The anger is.

C: Oh, yeah.

T: But some of part says I deserve more and how strong is that?

C: Well, I say this but then I guess we all feel we deserve more, and I don't know—yeah, I'm grieving for what I probably didn't have and know I never will have.

T: Yeah, probably that too. Because it's how much you really can believe you are deserving even if they didn't give it to you. Then somehow it's how much can I get from other people—

C: For myself. I realize now you can't depend on other people to make you happy. Not to be happy to be happy from within yourself. That's why I guess I'm doing this therapy. I figure if I can be content with myself, then that stuff won't matter to me as much. But don't forget, if you are told off enough that you're a failure, you start to believe it.

T: Yeah, so that's really an important piece to work on. And I guess that's why this disapproval is so painful, because it activates that I am a failure and being told all along that I'm a failure, that's just like her voice is almost in your head. And then it kind of diminishes you and it's hard to stand up against it.

In session 2, a marker again arises when the client is talking about possibly returning to school. She quickly becomes hopeless in the face of the further possibility of failure in the eyes of her sisters. At this point, the therapist initiates a two-chair dialogue by putting her sisters in the other chair. Although this is a dialogue with another person rather than a part of the self it is viewed as a self-critical dialogue because her hypersensitivity to her sisters' criticisms suggests that her internalized criticisms are being projected onto or attributed to the sisters. The sisters' criticisms are so damaging because they activate the client's internal critic.

"Yeah, unsupported, I feel inferior to them, I feel that I have no self-esteem left and it's like I don't want to try anymore with them. It's like OK you win, I'm not as good as you, you win and that's it. Fine. So leave me alone."

In session 3, she recounts the history of the relationship with her father. She describes not having got approval from him. In response, the therapist initiates an empty-chair dialogue to work on the unfinished business with her father:

C: I believe I'm a bad person, but deep down inside I don't think I'm a bad person . . . yeah, I'm grieving for what I probably didn't have and know I never will have.

T: Can you imagine him over here (*pointing to chair*) and tell him how he has made you feel like a bad person?

C: You destroyed my feelings. You destroyed my life. Not you completely—but you did nothing to nurture me and help me in life. You did nothing at all. You fed me and you clothed me to a certain point. That's about it.

T: Tell him what it was like to be called a devil and go to church every . . .

C: It was horrible. He made me feel that I was always bad, I guess when I was a child. I don't believe that now, but when I was a child I felt that I was going to die and I was going to go to hell because I was a bad person.

By the end of session 3, the thematic intrapersonal and interpersonal issues have emerged clearly. They are clearly embedded in what the client reports as her most painful experience. First, the client has internalized self-criticism related to issues of failure that emerge in the context of her family relationships. This voice of failure and worthlessness is initially identified as coming from her sisters but clearly has roots in earlier relationships with her parents. This becomes more evident later in therapy. Related to her self-criticism and need for approval is a need for love. Love has been hard to come by in her life. She has learned how to interrupt or avoid acknowledging this need as it has made her feel too vulnerable and alone. She has learned how to be self-reliant, but this independence has had a price as it leaves her feeling hopeless, unsupported, and isolated. This need for love is related to her unfinished business stemming from her early relationship with her father. She harbors a great deal of resentment toward her father over his maltreatment of her as a child and she has a tendency to minimize it as "being slapped was just normal." She has internalized this as a feeling of worthlessness and as being unlovable. These underlying concerns lend themselves very clearly to the emotional processing tasks of both the two-chair for internal conflict splits and to the empty-chair for unresolved injuries with a significant other.

The thematic issues of the therapy continue to be focused on through work on the emotional processing tasks.

In a self-critical dialogue in session 4, she connects her bad feelings to the criticism she heard from her parents.

C: (*speaking as internalized critic in voice of her parent*) "Well, you're wrong, you're bad, you're—you never do anything right. Every time I ask you to do something you don't do it the way I want you to do it and your marks are never good enough, and you're never on time, and you know you just—everything you do is wrong."

T: Yeah, now can you come over to this chair [experiencing chair]. It must really hurt to hear that.

C: When I'm depressed, I believe it. I believe it wholeheartedly. That I'm bad, and I'm wrong and I'm a loser. That's the big word, "loser," that goes over and over and then I'm a big loser and why can't I just have a nice simple normal life. In many ways, this is a feeling that has followed me throughout my life.

T: Tell her [critic] how she makes you feel.

C: It makes me feel horrible, it makes me feel sad. It makes me feel unloved and not able to give love you know; it makes me feel like I wish I'd never been born.

Later in the dialogue, she says to her critic:

C: I know I am loved. I've always known that, I never believed it before. So I'm starting to believe that I am loved that it's just—instead of being angry because they don't love me, I'm just accepting that they just don't have the capacity to love. It wasn't just me, it was my younger sisters too. If any, it wasn't like they loved them and didn't love me, they didn't love any of us not the way parents are supposed to love.

In this moment the core feeling of being unlovable and the articulated belief that she was not worth loving are being challenged.

The critical voice begins to soften and both her grief over having not been loved and a sense of worth emerge in a dialogue with her critic.

"Even though Mom and Dad didn't love me or didn't show me any love, it wasn't because I was unlovable, it was just because they were incapable of those emotions. They don't know how to—they still don't know how to love."

The client does not experience the hopelessness that had been so predominant in her earlier sessions again.

Later in session 7, the client and the therapist work to identify the way in which the client interrupts and prevents the feeling of wanting to be loved and protected against the pain of having her needs not met. In session 9, speaking as her "interrupter" from the other chair, she says to herself:

"You're wasting your time feeling bad cause you want them, and they are not there. So it's best for you to shut your feelings off and not need them. That's what I do in my life. When people hurt me enough I get to that point where I actually can imagine, I literally cut them out of my life like I did with my mother."

They then go on to identify the way in which needing love makes her vulnerable to hurt and pain, and how interrupting these needs have left her vulnerable to isolation and aloneness. In sessions 7 through 9, the client continues to explore the two different sides to her experience: the critic that attempts to protect her through controlling and shutting off needs and the experiencing self that wants to be loved and accepted. She continues to define and speak from both voices and expresses a range of sadness, anger, and pain/hurt. The hopelessness that was so dominant in the early sessions now is virtually nonexistent. The voice that wants love and acceptance becomes stronger and the critic softens to express acceptance of this part of her. At the same time she is feeling much better and activation of her negative feelings decrease.

The other main theme of the therapy is her interpersonal issue with her father with whom she feels hurt, angry, worthless, and unloved. In a key dialogue in session 3 she speaks to her father:

C: It hurts me that you don't love me . . . yeah . . . I guess, you know, but . . . I'm angry at you and I needed love and you weren't there to give me any love."

She later tells the image of her father about her fear:

C: I was lonely. I didn't know my father. My father—all I knew you as, was somebody who yelled at me all the time and hit me. That's all—I don't remember you telling me you loved me or that you cared for me or that you thought that I did well in school or anything. All I know you as somebody that I feared.

T: Tell him how you were afraid of being hit.

C: Yes, and you humiliated me. I was very angry with you because you were always hitting me, you were so mean and I heard Hitler was mean, so I called you Hitler.

Later in the session, she describes how she interrupts her painful sense of feeling unloved:

C: The only way I can handle it is by making a joke of it because it helps— it helps because when I'm too serious about it, I become so depressed I can't function. So I learned to laugh about it and you know I have that sarcastic humor and sort of jaded eye I guess about things.

T: Because underneath the laugh I guess there's a lot of hurt and a lot of hate.

She continues expressing her anger in an unfinished business dialogue:

C: I hate you. I hate you, there's no doubt about that in my mind. I've hated you for years. It angers me when I see you at family functions and I don't feel good being there and you act like nothing ever happened.

Later on in the session, she expresses pain and hurt at her father's inability to make her feel loved:

"I guess I keep thinking that yeah, you will never be a parent, that you would pick up the phone and just ask me how I'm doing. It hurts me that you don't love me . . . yeah . . . I guess, you know."

She ends the session with a recognition that what she needed was acceptable. "I needed to be hugged once in a while as a child or told that I was OK. I think that's normal."

By accessing both pride and anger and grieving her loss, her core shame is undone (Greenberg, 2002). The client thereby begins to shift her belief that her father's failure was not because she was not worth loving. She says to him in the empty chair:

"I'm angry at you because you think you were a good father, you have said that you never hit us and that's the biggest lie on earth, you beat the hell out of us constantly, you never showed any love, you never showed any affection, you never ever acknowledged we were ever there except for us to clean and do things around the house."

Having processed her anger and her sadness and transformed her shame she takes a more compassionate and understanding position to her father. In an empty-chair dialogue with her father in session 10 she says:

"I understand that you've gone through a lot of pain in your life and probably because of this pain, because of the things you're seen, you've withdrawn. You're afraid to maybe give love the way it should be given and to get too close to anybody because it means you might lose them. You know and I can understand that now, whereas growing up I couldn't understand."

She is also able to continue to hold him accountable for the ways that he disappointed and hurt her while also allowing her compassion to be central in the development of a new understanding of his inner struggles.

"You know [being a concentration camp victim] had a real impact on you. Instead of being a teenager, you're a prisoner of war. It obviously had a lasting impact on you and then as life went on and, you know, your marriage, ah you know, I'm sure in the beginning it was good, you know I think at one point, mom and dad did at one point really love, um, each other, but I think with my mother's drinking, and maybe with some of the anger that you had about your life, and then you lost your child, your son, that um, your way of dealing with things was to be cold. To be unfeeling, to not be supportive, not that you didn't want to be. I don't think you know how. I can really understand or I can try to feel your pain and understand that ah, you did the best you could knowing what you knew."

In talking about the dialogue at the end of the session, the client says "I feel relief that I don't have this anger sitting on my chest anymore."

The client goes on to describe how she can now accept that her father does not have more to give. This leads to emotion episodes of pride and then joy for having overcome these feelings. Her shame-based core maladaptive belief, "I am not worth loving," has shifted to include the emotional meaning that her father experienced his own pain in his life and that this pain led him to be less available to behave in loving ways toward her or her sisters. Needing to be loved no longer triggers hopelessness, and giving voice to her strong emotions has validated that she is worth loving, and that she can manage with what her father has to offer at this point in her life. A greater ability to communicate her needs, to protect herself from feeling inadequate, and to be close to her sisters has also developed.

TRAINING

Training in case formulation is embedded within training in intervention. The perceptual skills involved in process diagnosis are seen as an inherent part of intervention (Greenberg & Goldman, 1988). Therapists are trained in moment-by-moment tracking, in marker identification, and in moving toward a focus guided by process cues as described previously. Various sources such as Greenberg and Goldman (1988) and Elliott, Watson, Goldman, and Greenberg (2004) outline the steps involved in training in experiential therapy. In addition, Greenberg et al. (1993) specify many of the techniques necessary to apply the case formulation method. In addition, trainees should learn the process measures mentioned previously in this chapter, including the Client Vocal Quality (CVQ) Scale (Rice & Kerr, 1986), and the EXP scale (Klein et al, 1969). Such training helps the therapist to better assess clients' capacity for self-focus to improve his or her capacity for empathic attunement. Finally, demonstration films of have been published and are available (Greenberg, 1989, 1994, 2005) and provide a model of attention to moment-by-moment processing and markers.

RESEARCH SUPPORT FOR THE APPENDIX

The EFT tasks have been studied extensively (Greenberg, Elliott, & Lietaer, 1994; Elliott, Greenberg, & Lietaer, 2004). Manuals that guide the identification of six particular markers and tasks have been specified and studied (Greenberg et al., 1993; Elliott et al., 2004b). Each of the problematic experiential states is identified by a marker that indicates that the client is currently emotionally involved in a particular affective problem state. The marker indicates both the presence of the state and the client's current amenability to intervention. Thus, during a particular session, an emergent marker represents an opportunity for intervention of a particular kind; an intervention that will uniquely address the processing difficulty presented by the marker.

A task appropriate to the marker is then introduced. The stages involved in the resolution of the tasks have been intensively analyzed empirically and task resolution has been shown to relate to treatment outcome (Watson & Greenberg, 1996b; Greenberg & Pedersen, 2001). The resolution models offer specific guidance to therapists on how to make appropriate momentary "process diagnoses," or assessments of current cognitive–affective states, and how to determine at what point, a particular intervention would facilitate further exploration and ultimately the resolution of the particular task (Greenberg et al., 1993).

For example, working according to the model of the process of resolution of a self-evaluative conflict split (Greenberg, 1984), when an internalized self-critic has been accessed, the therapist attempts to help the person to express some of the contempt or harshness of the critic (i.e., "You make me sick"). Once the harshness of the critic has been accessed, the therapist may then make a momentary diagnosis that it would facilitate the dialogue to encourage the expression of more specific criticisms ("You do not work hard enough. You are stupid."). This work with the critic continues until such time as the underlying maladaptive emotion scheme of failure and inadequacy is accessed in the experiencing self. At this time the therapist makes another process diagnosis that it would be helpful for the client to express the underlying feelings and therefore asks the person to express feelings to the critic from the self chair (i.e. "I feel worthless when you say that, I feel like a nothing."). The therapist will continue to make such process diagnoses throughout the dialogue, facilitating the appropriate action at the appropriate moment. After accessing primary adaptive feelings, the therapist will then facilitate an assertion of needs toward the critic. Once the needs on the one hand and the values and standards underlying the criticisms on the other have been put in dialectical opposition, the therapist will continue to work to facilitate a shift or a softening of the critic. All these steps are viewed as helping the client to integrate the conflicting aspects of self (Greenberg et al., 1993). As is evident through this example, the facilitation of affective client tasks requires therapists to make specific types of moment-by-moment formulations. Each step of this process is guided by formulations informed by the model that explicates what processing proposals to offer at what point to best facilitate the next step toward task resolution.

Various research studies lend support to aspects of the method of case formulation described earlier. For example, raters can reliably agree ($r = .81$) on the client's level of vocal quality as well as on the client's depth of experiencing ($r = .75$), supporting the notion that therapists can assess the client's capacity for self-focus. In addition, studies indicate that raters can reliably distinguish between different markers for various affective tasks within therapy sessions such as unfinished business, two-chair conflict split, and problematic reaction points (Greenberg & Rice, 1991).

While EFT case formulation does not involve a priori formulations, research has shown that in successful cases, ongoing momentary formulations throughout sessions do result in particular themes emerging by the middle of therapy (Goldman, 1995). These themes form a strong focus of treatment and have been found to relate to either intrapersonal or interpersonal issues. Research also indicates that focusing on these themes through engagement in particular affective tasks repeatedly over a number of sessions and working progressively toward resolution is predictive of success in treatment. Finally, empirical support for the efficacy of EFT which operates by the approach to case formulation articulated has been documented (Paivio & Greenberg, 1995; Greenberg & Watson, 1998; Goldman, Greenberg, & Angus, 2005; Watson et al., 2003). In addition, the in-session emotional processes attended to in case formulation have been shown to relate to outcome (Pos, Greenberg, Goldman, & Herman, 2003; Missirlian, Toukmanian, Warwar, & Greenberg, 2005).

REFERENCES

Arnold, M. B. (1960). *Emotion and personality* (Vols. 1–2). New York: Columbia University Press.

Bordin, E. (1994). Theory and research on the therapeutic working alliance: New directions. In A. O. Horvath & L. S. Greenberg (Eds.), *The working alliance: Theory, research, and practice* (pp. 13–37). New York: Wiley-Interscience.

Buber, M. (1960). *I and thou*. New York: Scribner's.

Davidson, R. (2000). Affective style, psychopathology and resilience: Brain mechanisms and plasticity. *American Psychologist, 5*(11), 1193–1196.

Elliott, R., Greenberg, L., & Lietaer, G. (2004a). Research on experiential psychotherapy. In M. Lambert (Ed.), *Bergin & Garfield's handbook of psychotherapy and behavior change* (pp. 493–539). New York: Wiley.

Elliott, R., Watson, J. C., Goldman, R. N., & Greenberg, L. S. (2004b). *Learning emotion-focused therapy*. Washington, DC: American Psychological Association.

Fridja, N. H. (1986). *The emotions*. Cambridge, UK: Cambridge University Press.

Goldman, R. N., Greenberg, L., & Pos, A. (2005). Depth of emotional experience and outcome. *Psychotherapy Research, 15*, 248–260.

Goldman, R. N., Greenberg, L. S., & Angus, L. (in press). The effects of adding specific emotion-focused interventions to the therapeutic relationship in the treatment of depression. *Psychotherapy Research*.

Goldman, R. N., Greenberg, L. S., & Pos, A. E. (2005). Depth of emotional experience and outcome. *Psychotherapy Research, 15*(3), 248–260.

Greenberg, L. (1984). Task analysis of intra personal conflict. In L. Rice & L. Greenberg (Eds.), *Patterns of change: Intensive analysis of psychotherapy* (pp. 167–211). New York: Guilford Press.

Greenberg, L. (1989). *Integrative psychotherapy* [Videotape series on interactive psychotherapy]. Corona De Mar, CA: Psychological and Educational Films.

Greenberg, L. (1994). *Process experiential therapy* [Psychotherapy videotape series]. Washington, DC: American Psychological Association Press.

Greenberg, L. (2005). *Emotion-focused therapy of depression: Leslie Greenberg*. Washington, DC: American Psychological Association Press.

Greenberg, L., & Angus, L. (2004). The contributions of emotion processes to narrative change in psychotherapy: A dialectical constructivist approach. In L. Angus & J. McLeod (Eds.), *Handbook of narrative psychotherapy* (pp. 331–350). Thousand Oaks, CA: Sage.

Greenberg, L., & Johnson, S. (1988). *Emotionally focused couples therapy*. New York: Guilford Press.

Greenberg, L., & Malcolm, W. (2002). Resolving unfinished business: Relating process to outcome. *Journal of Consulting and Clinical Psychology, 70*(2), 406–416.

Greenberg, L., & Pascual-Leone, J. (2001). A dialectical constructivist view of the creation of personal meaning. *Journal of Constructivist Psychology, 14*(3), 165–186.

Greenberg, L., & Watson, J. (2005). *Emotion-focused therapy of depression*. Washington, DC: American Psychological Association Press.

Greenberg, L. S. (2002). *Emotion-focused therapy: Coaching clients to work through their feelings*. Washington, DC: American Psychological Association.

Greenberg, L. S., Elliott, R., & Lietaer, G. (1994). *Research on humanistic and experiential psychotherapies*. In A. E. Bergin & S. L. Garfield (Eds.), *Handbook of psychotherapy and behavior change* (4th ed., pp. 509–539). New York: Wiley.

Greenberg, L. S., & Goldman, R. N. (1988). Training in experiential therapy. *Journal of Consulting and Clinical Psychology, 56*, 696–702.

Greenberg, L. S., & Paivio, S. C. (1997). *Working with emotions*. New York: Guilford Press.

Greenberg, L. S., & Pascual-Leone, J. (1995). A dialectical constructivist approach to experiential change. In R. A. Neimeyer & M. J. Mahoney (Eds.), *Constructivism in psychotherapy* (pp. 169–191). Washington, DC: American Psychological Association.

Greenberg, L. S., & Pedersen, R. (2001, November). *Relating the degree of resolution of in-session self-criticism and dependence to outcome and follow-up in the treatment of depression*. Paper presented at conference of the North American Chapter of the Society for Psychotherapy Research, Puerto Vallarta, Mexico.

Greenberg, L. S., & Rice, L. N. (1991). *Change processes in experiential psychother-apy* (NIMH Grant 1R01MH45040). Washington, DC.

Greenberg, L. S., Rice, L. N., & Elliott, R. (1993). *Facilitating emotional change: The moment-by-moment process.* New York: Guilford Press.

Greenberg, L. S., & Safran, J. D. (1987). *Emotion in psychotherapy: Affect, cognition, and the process of change.* New York: Guilford Press.

Greenberg, L. S., & Safran, J. D. (1989). Emotion in psychotherapy, *American Psychologist, 44,* 19–29.

Greenberg, L. S., & Van Balen, R. (1998). The theory of experience-centered therapies. In L. S. Greenberg, J. C. Watson, & G. Lietaer (Eds.), *Handbook of experiential psychotherapy* (pp. 28–57). New York: Guilford Press.

Greenberg, L. S., & Watson, J. (1998). Experiential therapy of depression: Differential effects of client-centered relationship conditions and process interventions. *Psychotherapy Research, 8* (2), 210–224.

Greenberg, L. S., Watson, J. C., & Lietaer, G. (Eds.). (1998). *Handbook of experiential psychotherapy.* New York: Guilford Press.

Hermans, H. J. M., & Kempen, H. J. G. (1993). *The dialogical self: Meaning as movement.* New York: Academic Press.

Horvath, A., & Greenberg, L. S. (1989). Development and validation of the working alliance inventory. *Journal of Counseling Psychology, 36*(2), 223–233.

Klein, M., Mathieu, P., Gendlin, E., & Kiesler, D. (1969). *The Experiencing Scale: A research and training manual* (Vol. 1). Madison: University of Wisconsin Extension Bureau of Audiovisual Instruction.

Lam, A., & Sue, S. (2001). Client diversity. *Psychotherapy: Theory/Research/Practice/Training, 38,* 4.

Lane, R., & Nadel, L. (2000). *Cognitive neuroscience of emotion.* New York: Oxford University Press.

Le Doux, J. (1996). *The emotional brain: The mysterious underpinnings of emotional life.* New York: Simon & Schuster.

Leventhal, H. (1986). A perceptual motor theory of emotion. In L. Berkowitz (Ed.), *Advances in experimental and social psychology* (pp. 117–182). New York: Academic Press.

Missirlian, T., Toukmanian, S., Warwar, S., & Greenberg, L. (2005). Emotional arousal, client perceptual processing, and the working alliance in Experiential Psychotherapy for Depression. *Journal of Consulting and Clinical Psychology, 73*(5), 861–871.

Pascual-Leone, J. (1984). Attentional, dialectical, and mental effort: Toward an organismic theory of life stages. In M. L. Commons, F. A. Richards, & C. Amon (Eds.), *Beyond formal operations: Late adolescent and adult cognitive development* (pp. 321–376). New York: Praeger.

Pascual-Leone, J. (1991). Emotions, development, and psychotherapy: A dialectical–constructivist perspective. In J. D. Safran & L. S. Greenberg (Eds.), *Emotion, psychotherapy and change* (pp. 302–335). New York: Guilford Press.

Paivio, S. C., & Greenberg, L. (1995). Resolving unfinished business: Experiential therapy using empty chair dialogue. *Journal of Consulting and Clinical Psychology, 3,* 419–425.

Perls, F., Hefferline, R., & Goodman, P. (1951). *Gestalt therapy.* New York: Dell.

Pos, A. E., Greenberg, L. S., Goldman, R. N., & Korman, L. M. (2003). Emotional processing during experiential treatment of depression. *Journal of Consulting and Clinical Psychology, 71,* 1007–1016.

Pos, A. E., Greenberg, L. S., Korman, L. M., & Goldman, R. N. (2003). Emotional processing during experiential treatment of depression. *Journal of Consulting and Clinical Psychology, 71*(6), 1007–1016.

Rice, L. N. (1974). The evocative function of the therapist. In L. N. Rice & D. A. Wexler (Eds.), *Innovations in client-centered therapy* (pp. 289–311). New York: Wiley.

Rice, L. N., & Greenberg, L. S. (Eds.). (1984). *Patterns of change: Intensive analysis of psychotherapy process.* New York: Guilford Press.

Rice, L. N., & Kerr, G. P. (1986). Measures of client and therapist vocal quality. In L. S. Greenberg & W. Pinsof (Eds.), *The psychotherapeutic process: A research handbook* (pp. 73–105). New York: Guilford Press.

Rogers, C. R. (1951). *Client-centered therapy.* Boston: Houghton-Mifflin.

Rogers, C. R. (1957). The necessary and sufficient conditions of therapeutic personality change. *Journal of Consulting Psychology, 21,* 95–103.

Stiles, W. B. (1999). Signs and voices in psychotherapy. *Psychotherapy Research, 9,* 1–21.

Thelen, E., & Smith, L. B. (1994). *A dynamic systems approach to the development of cognition and action.* Cambridge, MA: Massachusetts Institute of Technology Press.

Toukmanian, S. (1986). A measure of client perceptual processing. In L. S. Greenberg & W. M. Pinsof (Eds.), *The psychotherapeutic process: A research handbook* (pp. 107–130). New York: Guilford Press.

Vanaerschot, G. (1990). The process of empathy: Holding and letting go. In G. Lietaer, J. Rombauts, & R. Van Balen (Eds.), *Client-centered psychotherapy in the nineties* (pp. 269–294). Leuven, Belgium: Leuven University Press.

Watson, J., & Greenberg, L. (1996a). Emotion and cognition in experiential therapy: A dialectical–constructivist position. In H. Rosen & K. Kuelwein (Eds.), *Constructing realities: Meaning-making perspectives for psychotherapists.* San Francisco: Jossey-Bass.

Watson, J., & Greenberg, L. (1996b). Pathways to change in the psychotherapy of depression: Relating Process-to Session Change and Outcome. *Psychotherapy, 33*(2), 262–274.

Watson, J. C., Gordon, L. B., Stermac, L., Kalogerakos, F., & Steckley, P. (2003). Comparing the effectiveness of process-experiential with cognitive-behavioral psychotherapy in the treatment of depression. *Journal of Consulting and Clinical Psychology, 71,* 773–781.

Whelton, W., & Greenberg, L. (2000). The self as a singular multiplicity: A process experiential perspective. In J. Muran (Ed.), *Self-relations in the psychotherapy process* (pp. 87–106). Washington, DC: American Psychological Association Press.

Chapter 14

Comparing the Methods
Where Is the Common Ground?

TRACY D. EELLS

The purpose of this concluding chapter is to compare and contrast each of the formulation methods presented earlier and to consider the future of case formulation in psychotherapy practice and research. I organize the chapter employing the standard headings used in the chapters on case formulation methods.

HISTORICAL BACKGROUND OF THE APPROACHES

By design, the *Handbook* drew chapters from the three major traditions in psychotherapy: psychoanalysis and its theoretical successors, behavioral and cognitive therapies, and the phenomenological/humanistic school. Six models trace their origins directly to the Freudian tradition: traditional psychoanalytic, the Core Conflictual Relational Theme (CCRT), configurational analysis (CA), cyclical maladaptive pattern (CMP), plan formulation method (PFM); and interpersonal psychotherapy (IPT). Two additional chapters, those on dialectical behavior therapy (DBT) and emotion-focused therapy (EFT), also credit psychoanalysis as an influence. Each of these also draws from interpersonal theories; several identify cognitive science as a theoretical foundation and identify themselves as theoretically integrative.

Three models are rooted in the behavioral and cognitive traditions—those of Persons and Tompkins (Chapter 10); Nezu, Nezu, and Cos (Chapter 12); and Koerner (Chapter 11). Each is based on operant and classical conditioning paradigms. Historical influences of these methods include functional analysis, which has origins in operant conditioning, the study of the single organism, and an explicit empirical tradition, most recently evidenced in an acknowledgment of influence by empirically supported interventions for specific psychological disorders. DBT, as described by Koerner, reaches outside behavioral and cognitive theories to psychodynamic, client-centered, Gestalt, paradoxical, and strategic approaches as well as dialectical theory and Zen psychology.

Two other models draw from other sources. The Greenberg and Goldman (Chapter 13) model of case formulation in EFT draws from a "neohumanistic experiential" approach to therapy that is informed by humanistic–phenomenological theory, emotion and cognitive theory, affective neuroscience, and dynamic and family systems theory. In accord with its primary source in client-centered theory, this approach does not involve the development of a priori case formulations but rather emphasizes formulation of therapy processes and the authority of the client rather than the therapist. Caspar's Plan Analysis draws widely from many historical traditions, although primary credit is given to the work of Klaus Grawe's schema theory.

CONCEPTUAL FRAMEWORK

In this section authors were asked to discuss, "What is formulated and why?" They were invited to address assumptions about psychopathology and healthy psychological functioning; a causal or probabilistic model underlying the method they described; assumptions about personality structure and functioning embedded in their approach; and the components of the case formulation.

These models share several features. First, they are structured in the sense that the formulation task is broken down into separate components that are then combined or sequenced into a narrative structure or are depicted in a graphical representation. Second, the methods rely on clinical judgment rather than rating scales in reaching a formulation. Third, they emphasize making relatively low-level clinical inferences, which has led to greater interrater reliability than was the case with less structured formulation that involved deeper levels of inference (Seitz, 1966).

Each method's conceptual framework flows from its historical origins. Messer and Wolitzky identify three psychoanalytic models—drive/structural, object relations, and self psychology. The first of these is based on Freud's drive reduction model; the second emphasizes internalized mental representations of self and other and their affectively tinged interactions; and the third centers on the development and maintenance of a cohesive self. Of these three models, the remaining psychodynamically based methods appear to owe their origins primarily to the object relations school. Luborsky's

(Luborsky & Barrett, Chapter 4) CCRT is consistent with an object relations perspective, drawing from Freud's conception of a "transference template" (Freud, 1912/1958a, 1912/1958b). Horowitz's (Horowitz & Eells, Chapter 5) CA also emphasizes conceptions of self and other and their interactions, as does the CMP method, which is based on the principle that people are innately motivated to search for and maintain human relatedness. The PFM, based on Weiss's (1993; Silberschatz, 2005) control mastery theory, stands apart from the other psychodynamic methods in that the primary motive it posits is a drive to disprove a pathogenic belief, not a fundamental drive to seek interpersonal relatedness.

In contrast to the explicit emphasis given to interpersonal relationships in the primarily psychodynamically rooted methods, the cognitive-behavioral methods are based on learning principles and observation of behavior in inferring maladaptive or adaptive psychological functioning. Each takes a distinct approach. Nezu, Nezu, and Cos emphasize the role of the CBT clinician as a "problem solver." In their model, the therapist identifies a patient's unique style of orienting to problems, defines ultimate and instrumental outcomes, then applies a multistep problem-solving rational strategy that is based on empirical research and aimed at achieving the defined goals. Persons and Tompkins emphasize case formulation as part of an empirical hypothesis testing process that also includes assessment and intervention. Like Nezu, Nezu, and Cos, they adapt results from studies of basic mechanisms underlying symptoms or disorders, epidemiological findings and randomized clinical trials to the specific individual being treated. DBT adds a biosocial theory of the causes and maintenance of borderline personality disorder (BPD) as well as a dialectical orientation to change.

The conceptual framework for EFT is based on a view of the psychologically healthy self as constantly in flux, creating and recreating itself, and adapting itself to environmental demands. Maladaptively, the self experiences enduring pain, is rigid, and is unable to adapt to environmental demands. Like EFT, Plan Analysis focuses on emotion, but from an instrumental standpoint in which a hierarchically organized set of Plans depict a set of motivations and means to achieve a goal. Its teleological focus is similar to the PFM model.

Although each method adheres to a primary theoretical framework, they also share a theoretical integration trend. Although they are primarily psychodynamic methods, CA, the CMP method, and the PFM have strong cognitive components in their emphasis on schematizations of self and other, core beliefs about the self and the future, and cognitive cycles. EFT draws primarily from the humanistic–phenomenology traditions, but Greenberg and Goldman also credit cognitive and emotion theory, dynamic and family systems theory, as well as dialecticism as influences. Among the primarily behavioral/cognitive methods, the DBT method is the most explicitly integrationist in its use, as noted earlier, of concepts from psychoanalysis, Zen psychology, and dialecticism. Nezu, Nezu, and Cos's concept of critical multiplism and Caspar's Plan Analysis (Chapter 9) are also integrationist through their focus on multiple causal factors and causal paths leading to symptoms and problems.

In many models, cognitive concepts are used to characterize maladaptivity. The CMP and CA models identify maladaptive cyclical patterns, which are self-perpetuating negative or positive feedback loops that maintain interpersonal relationship problems, dysfunctional concepts of the self, symptoms, and problems. EFT conceptualizes dysfunction through a number of mechanisms, including "incoherence or in-coherence between what is reflectively symbolized and the range of experienced possibilities" (p. 382).

Finally, the conceptual approach of each model focuses on understanding and formulating interpersonal experiences and relationships. The CCRT is primarily focused on identifying maladaptive interpersonal relationship patterns as revealed in relationship narratives clients relate in therapy. Similarly, CA emphasizes "role relationship models" toward the same end, as does case formulation for IPT. Drawing from the object relations model, the CMP approach is based on the assumption that people are innately motivated to search for and maintain human relatedness. Although less salient in the cognitive-behavioral methods, understanding social learning patterns is embedded in such concepts as behavioral chains in DBT, which involve interactions with others and core beliefs about the self, future and world, which are also often interpersonal in context, as described by Persons and Tompkins (Chapter 10). Similarly, EFT emphasizes the self as agent but also the self as manifesting itself through its contact with the interpersonal environment. Many of the Plans in Plan Analysis are interpersonal in focus.

INCLUSION/EXCLUSION CRITERIA AND MULTICULTURAL CONSIDERATIONS

All authors report that their case formulation model is applicable to individuals across multiple cultural backgrounds, although with the exception of Ridley and Kelly's (Chapter 2) multicultural assessment procedure (MAP), none make specific adaptations in theoretical orientation, steps taken to construct a formulation, or psychological components that are formulated to accommodate cultural data. Authors support not doing so by noting the case-specific nature of their approach, which makes it adaptable to individuals regardless of cultural background. Markowitz and Swartz note that IPT has been applied in multiple cultures throughout the world without major adaptations. Messer and Wolitzky (Chapter 3) agree that cultural, ethnic, and religious background is important in psychodynamic case formulation, and they also emphasize that the focus of this approach is

on universal themes and issues that we must all manage. Luborsky emphasizes the use of individual rather than standard CCRT categories as a way
to include cultural information. Levenson and Strupp (Chapter 6), in describing the CMP, caution about not making inferences about transference–
countertransference reenactments when the better explanation of a phenomenon in therapy would be a culturally based one. DBT case formulation includes cultural factors as controlling variables in behavior. Nezu,
Nezu, and Cos describe ethnic considerations as an individual difference
variable in cognitive-behavioral case formulation. Greenberg and Goldman
note the need for cultural empathy as well as individual empathy. Several
authors agree that research on cultural factors in case formulation is highly
limited or unavailable. Ridley and Kelly emphasizes the often unrecognized
influence of Western values on case formulation, particularly the influence
of acculturation, racial identity, and immigration on the client, the therapist, and the setting in which they meet. They emphasize culturally based
rather than universally based psychological concepts that are formulated.
They caution about the risks of both overpathologizing and underpathologizing based on a misunderstanding of culture. Their MAP includes
important steps, such as debiasing strategies, to minimize the effects of a
therapist's cultural blind spots.

Most authors cite few exclusionary criteria but acknowledge that not
all relevant information is psychological in nature. Some may be cultural,
biological, or social. Luborsky and Barrett are representative when they
state that a CCRT formulation "can be applied to people across all levels of
psychiatric severity and ethnic and cultural groups with a nearly unique
pattern for each person" (p. 107). Both Levenson and Strupp as well as
Greenberg and Goldman note selection and exclusionary criteria for the
type of therapy their formulation method is designed for (i.e., time-limited
dynamic therapy and emotion-focused therapy). These criteria are consistent with what is generally understood for brief therapies and include the
absence of psychosis, an ability to interpersonally engage the therapist in a
meaningful way, and the absence of a strong biochemical component to the
disorder treated. As suggested in their chapter titles, the methods presented
by Markowitz and Swartz and by Koerner are best suited for individuals
with either major depressive disorder or borderline personality disorder, respectively. Caspar interestingly notes that with Plan Analysis, "exclusion
criteria are related rather to therapists than to patients," (p. 267) explaining that the method requires therapists to demonstrate a capacity for disciplined reasoning and cognitive complexity.

STEPS IN CASE FORMULATION

Although differing in details, the methods identify the following steps in
constructing a case formulation: (1) observe and describe clinical informa-

tion; (2) infer, interpret, or organize the observed information; and (3) apply the formulation to the case and revise as needed.

Observe and Describe Clinical Information

Most authors endorse the open-ended clinical interview as the most practical and flexible method of data gathering, while also acknowledging the value of other sources of information, including structured interviews, family informants, and psychological testing. Messer and Wolitzky distinguish between content and process aspects of the interview. The first refers to information gathered through the patient's words and cognitive style (e.g., the report of symptoms and problems and personal and family history). The second refers to inferred information based on the manner in which the interviewer and patient relate to each other. From the psychoanalytic perspective, process information leads to inferences about mental status (e.g., mood and affect, thought processes, perceptions, appearance, speech, cognitive functions, and orientation) as well as transference and countertransference themes and associations between topics and heightened affect.

Other authors add to Messer and Wolitzky. Ridley and Kelly, as well as Persons and Tompkins, and others encourage multiple data collection methods, the former emphasizing the gathering of both salient and nonsalient information. Ridley and Kelly advise the use of structured interviews to identify relevant cultural data and avoid stereotyping; Persons and Tompkins put symptom measures in their waiting room to help identify symptom severity at the outset and throughout therapy; Koerner notes the value of structured interview methods to help with diagnosis and the identification of parasuicidal behavior, as well as symptom checklists to help assess quality of life. Markowitz and Swartz use a written interpersonal inventory to gather and organize relationship information as part of an IPT case formulation. The CCRT model focuses on narratives as a way to identify the patient's core conflictual theme. These may be extracted from a clinical interview, obtained from a questionnaire format, or gathered through a "relationships anecdote paradigm" (RAP) structured interview. For most models, the end product of the information gathering stage is a "problem list" (Persons & Tompkins, Chapter 10), set of "phenomena" (Horowitz & Eells, Chapter 5), or "target behaviors" (Koerner, Chapter 11; Nezu, Nezu, & Cos, Chapter 12) that constitute the focus of explanation or organization in the remaining parts of the formulation.

Infer, Interpret, or Organize the Observed Information

Although all authors agree that one must move beyond the collection of descriptive data, the key to what differentiates the methods is how the descriptive information is organized and interpreted. Some models include making a diagnosis as an explicit step in the formulation process. For example, Markowitz and Swartz state the importance of diagnosing depression as a medical illness in order to minimize any stigma attached to this condition. Persons and Tompkins's model involves the selection of an anchoring diagnosis to capitalize on nomothetic data about that diagnosis. A nomothetic formulation provides a template for a hypothesized psychological mechanism that is individualized so that the formulation accounts for idiographic information about the case at hand. Ridley and Kelly criticize DSM-IV for its excessive focus on individual rather than social origins of psychopathology as well as its Eurocentric conceptions of normality but nevertheless see diagnosis as an important aspect of the assessment process.

From description or diagnosis, one then moves to a mechanism that explains the problems. Several models identify information categories to aid in organization and explanation. Messer and Wolitzky distinguish between structural and process categories. The former include autonomous ego functions, such as disruptions in cognition, biological, perceptual, or motor functioning, including reality testing; affects; drives and defenses; object-related functions (i.e., the basic modes of relating to other people); and self-related functions (e.g., a person's stability, coherence, self-valuation, identity, goals, and identifications). Process categories are dynamic features and include a "central conflict," such as between wishes and fears or between basic impulses and the conscience. Other primarily psychodynamic methods employ categories related to those identified by Messer and Wolitzky. Luborsky's categories are wishes of the self, responses from others, and responses back of the self. Horowitz's components include states of mind, role-relationship models, and control processes. The CMP includes acts of the self; expectations of others' reactions; acts of others toward the self; and acts of the self toward the self. Curtis and Silbershatz's (Chapter 7) PFM model identifies the patient's goals for therapy; the obstructions (pathogenic beliefs) that inhibit the patient from pursuing or achieving these goals; the events and experiences (traumas) that lead to the development of the obstructions; the insights that will help the patient achieve therapy goals; and the manner in which the patient will work in therapy to overcome the obstacles and achieve the goals (tests). For some models, the information in these categories and its arrangement into sequences *are* the explanation or the mechanism. Horowitz, for example, arranges his CA components into a wish–fear–compromise format in the form of a role-relationship–model configuration.

The CBT models also include formulation components, such as schemas about the self, others, the world, and the future, in the case of Persons and Tompkins; or ultimate and instrumental outcomes in the case of the problem-solving model of Nezu, Nezu, and Cos. Most CBT models, however, tend to emphasize identifying behavior patterns or processes. All describe the importance of conducting a functional analysis. Nezu, Nezu, and Cos describe functional analysis as "the clinician's assessment-derived integration of the important functional relationships among variables (i.e., the

effects of a given variable on others)" (p. 352). A functional analysis is a
meta-judgment and a synthesis of several judgments about a client's problems and goals, their effects, related causal and mediating variables, and the
functional relationships among such variables. Koerner describes functional analysis as a behavioral theory of change, as where "the rubber
meets the road" and "where general hypotheses regarding problematic behavior guide the analysis of specific antecedents and consequences that
maintain (motivate) current problematic behavior" (p. 323) She uses the
image of links in a chain to describe functional analysis, where the therapist's task is to "pick up the correct length of chain" (p. 338) that leads to
primary treatment targets. It involves clearly identifying problem behavior,
then identifying what left the client vulnerable to the behavior and the specific precipitating events, including thoughts, feelings, and actions that led
the client along the chain to the behavior. Finally, it involves identifying
consequences of the behavior, more adaptive alternative behavior, and what
interfered with the use of more adaptive behavior. Analyses of this type are
at the heart of cognitive-behavioral case formulation.

In contrast to functional analysis, Caspar describes hierarchically organized instrumental relations, which lie at the heart of his Plan Analysis.
This is a purpose-driven, means–ends approach that focuses on a client's
intentions and how he or she goes about attempting to achieve them, consciously or unconsciously. It is similar in some regards to Curtis and
Silberschatz's PFM, which begins with the inference of a client's goal.
Typically, the goal involves an effort to disconfirm a pathogenic belief.

Greenberg's EFT model gives perhaps the least attention to identifying
case formulation components, focusing instead on process and moment-by-
moment emotional experiences. Nevertheless, it does include the identification of a client's emotional processing style, including vocal style and depth
of processing, as well as an assessment of how emotions are regulated and
experienced, and consideration of what constitutes a client's emotional
pain. The technique is aided by identifying and using affective problem
markers and tasks.

Three other areas of overlap among the models may also be identified
in regard to inferential and organizational processes in case formulation:
(1) A developmental focus, (2) provisions to improve clinical judgment, and
(3) the use of graphical representations. Several models explicitly include a
developmental focus to help understand the mechanism, or at minimum, as
an element in information gathering. The PFM model is representative in
its assumption that the identification of traumas can be essential to understanding the meaning of the patient's behaviors. This view is emphasized
most in the psychodynamic models, but it is also a step in Persons and
Tompkins's CBT model, in which the early life origins of mechanisms are
inferred. Functional-analytic models may also draw on developmental
information in order to understand antecedents and consequences or problematic behavior. In all models, the primary emphasis is on the present cir-

cumstances and problems of the client; developmental information is used to provide a sufficiently comprehensive context of understanding. Including developmental information in several models across theoretical frameworks was borne out in empirical analysis of case formulations in which both psychodynamic and cognitive-behavioral therapists valued this information (Eells & Lombart, 2003a), identified it in case formulations, and used it as a basis for inferring mechanisms (Eells, Lombart, Kendjelic, Turner, & Lucas, 2005).

Some methods explicitly include steps to improve quality of one's clinical judgment, or, as Ridley puts it, employing "debiasing strategies." Ridley is particularly concerned about availability, anchoring, and representativeness biases, which in turn, refer to overemphasizing the most salient information a client gives, focusing overly on initial information given and ignoring later information and depending excessively on one's existing cognitive schemas, which can lead to stereotyping and failure to recognize base rates. Ridley identifies several methods for overcoming these biases, including an intentional search for alternative explanations of client behavior (e.g., considering medical causes); conceptualizing alternative interpretations of behavior; reframing apparent weaknesses into strengths; and delaying decision making until one has given sufficient time to hypothesis testing. Given how well documented these judgment biases are, these strategies may be crucial in maximizing the value of a case formulation. As discussed further later on, improved, psychometrically based methods of aggregating and exploiting clinician judgments may be on the horizon (Westen & Weinberger, 2004).

Finally, several of the models include construction of a graphical representation of the formulation in addition to or in place of a narrative. Examples include Nezu, Nezu, and Cos's clinical pathogenesis map (CPM), Caspar's Plan Analysis, and Horowitz's role-relationship–model configuration (RRMC). These pictorial displays may show interrelationships more clearly. They may also serve the practical aim of aiding in framing problems to patients, communicating an understanding of their problems, and ways to address them.

Apply the Formulation to the Case and Revise as Needed

All models incorporate the idea that the formulation is a hypothesis that should be tested with the patient and revised as needed throughout the course of therapy. This step is explicit in MAP, CA, CMP, IPT, CBT, DBT, and EFT. As Koerner notes, the formulation may be refined as more information becomes available and other information is better understood. Alternatively, the formulation may be extensively revised if it does not appear to advance the course of therapy.

With regard to applying the formulation to the case, the CA approach involves planning interventions that address each formulation component individually. For example, one might plan steps to reduce undermodulated states of mind. At the same time, one might also plan how to address a control process involving role reversal and an RRMC involving fear of either being subordinate to others or of dominating others excessively.

APPLICATION TO PSYCHOTHERAPY TECHNIQUE

In this section, authors were asked to discuss how the therapist should use the formulation in therapy—for example, how and whether it is shared directly with the patient. All agree that the primary use of the formulation is to guide and shape the therapist's decision making. Initially, it can be useful to determine suitability of a particularly type of therapy for a patient. It can also help the therapist choose problem areas to focus on, or types of interventions to make. Another point authors made is that the formulation can help alert the therapist to potential problems that may arise in therapy. The DBT model, for example, includes the identification of "therapy-interfering events" as an explicit step in the formulation process. Similarly, Curtis and Silberschatz note that a formulation can help alert the therapist to a patient's pathogenic beliefs that potentially could undermine the therapy. Relatedly, some note that a formulation is particularly helpful when the therapy is not going well because it can provide a framework for understanding and addressing why it is not going better. Persons and Tompkins note that a formulation helps the therapist adapt a nomothetic formulation to the idiographic circumstances of a particular patient. Others have noted that a formulation provides continuity in theme from one session to another and also helps the therapist gain confidence in understanding the patient and being able to choose among a set of interventions. Levenson and Strupp state that the formulation need not be given but that the formulation always guides the therapist to choose facilitative interventions to aid in achieving new insights and new experiences.

Most authors recommend sharing the formulation, but not in a single intervention, which might overwhelm or confuse a patient. Messer and Wolitzky recommend giving an initial tentative, jargon-free formulation to the patient that addresses symptoms and problems. Others have noted that, in a sense, the unfolding of the therapy *is* the presentation of the formulation. This is particularly clear in the EFT model. Greenberg and Goldman note that the therapist "attends, as fully as possible, to the client's momentary experience, and, in response, makes miniformulations of how to facilitate experiential exploration through to resolutions of processing difficulties" (p. 394). The therapist makes judgments as to whether the client is experiencing a primary adaptive emotion or a maladaptive emotional experience and chooses an intervention accordingly.

TRAINING

Authors were asked to address how individuals are best trained to use their case formulation method. Responses included readings on the specifics of a particular method as well as a broad base of knowledge that includes adult and developmental psychopathology, scientific methods, multivariate statistics, clinical judgment, theories of psychotherapy, and assessment methods. Other recommendations included practical skills in therapeutic interviewing and developing skills that illuminate the choice points for intervention as a function of one's theory of psychopathology and of psychotherapy. Some authors recommended self-examination such as personal therapy, efforts to increase one's cognitive complexity and skills in metacognition, and cultural self-awareness. Methods of training ranged from reading, expert and lay consultation, small-group workshops, and use of instructional videotapes. Citing Collins and Messer (1991) and Seitz (1966), Curtis and Silberschatz caution that trainees become well versed in a theoretical position and not underestimate the ease with which differences in operationalizing the approach may arise.

RESEARCH SUPPORT FOR THE APPROACHES

For this section, the authors were asked to summarize evidence of the reliability and validity of their model and any other research using or focused on the model. Although all authors endorse the importance of conducting research on their case formulation method, considerable differences exist in the extent to which such research has occurred as well as on the type of research that is most important to conduct. Several methods have been empirically assessed for their reliability and/or validity, including the CCRT, CA, CMP, PFM, IPT, and CBT models. The most common method to obtain reliability estimates is to ask clinical judges to rate the similarity of two or more independently formulations based on the same clinical material, or more commonly, the similarity of separate components of formulations. These scores are then analyzed, typically using the intraclass correlation coefficient (ICC), a variation of that statistic, or a kappa coefficient. Overall, the results indicate moderate to good reliability among formulations constructed by teams of independent clinicians. Curtis and Silberschatz (Chapter 7, this volume), report coefficient alphas of .90, .84, .85, and .90, respectively, for goals, obstructions, tests, and insights. Similarly, in a review of eight samples examining reliability of the CCRT, Luborsky and Diguer (1998) found that judges agreed on CCRT components in the .64 to .81 range based on a weighted kappa. Eells et al. (1995) reported pooled judge's ICCs of .74 and .89 for ratings of similarity between RRMCs and role relationship models constructed by independent judges. Although most reliability studies have been carried out on the psychodynamic models, Persons and Bertagnolli (1999) replicated an earlier study of cognitive case formulations, finding that therapists on average identified 67% of overt problems in three patients; when reliability ratings were pooled across groups of five judges, interrater agreement was .72 for underlying schemas.

Caution is warranted in applying these reliability estimates to clinical practice, however, because the ratings typically are based on the results of teams of researchers who are well versed in a particular method. When the results are translated to the level of the individual therapist, as would be the case in clinical practice, the reliability estimates plunge. For example, the reliability estimate for identifying underlying schemas in the Persons and Bertagnolli (1999) study drops from .72 for groups of five judges to .37 when an individual judge is the unit of analysis. Horowitz and Eells (1993) found similar results for the RRMC component of CA. One implication of this result is a need for improved methods of formulation in which inferred components can be more reliably identified by individual clinicians. Another implication is that team-based formulation might be relied on more frequently in clinical practice because they are more likely to be reliable. One case formulation method is based on the assumption that consensus among judges provides the most reliable and valid formulation of an individual, including the interpersonal themes most likely to be discussed in therapy (Horowitz & Rosenberg, 1994; Horowitz, Rosenberg, Ureño, Kalehzan, & O'Halloran, 1989). In addition, some formulation components tend to be easier to rate reliably than others—for example, the 68% match on overt problems found by Persons and Bertagnolli (1999) as compared to an interrater reliability of .37 for individual judges found for inferred schemas, a result replicated by Kuyken, Fothergill, Musa, and Chadwick (2005), who used another cognitive formulation method.

Several authors raise concerns about focusing on the reliability of a case formulation model. Messer and Wolitzky cite research by Caston and Martin (1993) showing that even good agreement among judges may lead to a spurious formulation if the areas of agreement are stereotypical in nature and thus not sufficiently individualized to a specific case. Caspar rejects the idea of studying reliability, asserting that "simple coefficients of agreement hide rather than reveal the factors determining the actual accuracy of case conceptualizations" (p. 285). Persons and Tompkins assert that treatment utility, that is, the relationship between a formulation and outcome, is a more important criterion than reliability. They state that if two formulations differ in content but produce equally good outcomes when adhered to by the practitioner, both should be viewed as equally meritorious. Bieling and Kuyken (2003) take a stronger position, however, asserting that an individualized cognitive case formulation is a key tool in evaluating the mechanisms of change proposed for cognitive therapy.

With regard to research on validity of the case formulation models, it is mainly the psychodynamic models that have been studied, and among these, primarily the CCRT. Multiple studies have demonstrated the validity and utility of the CCRT. Interventions based on patients' CCRTs, particularly the combination of wish of self and response from other, correlated significantly and to a moderately strong degree with outcome in a sample of 43 patients undergoing brief psychodynamic therapy (Crits-Christoph, Cooper, & Luborsky, 1988); further, as Luborsky and Barrett summarize, outcome is correlated with changes in CCRT patterns (Crits-Christoph & Luborsky, 1998), reductions in the number of CCRT components that apply across multiple narratives (Cierpka et al., 1998), and mastery of the central relationship patterns (Grenyer & Luborsky, 1996). Luborsky and Barrett cite several other studies that characterize the CCRT, for example, that CCRTs derived from dreams are similar to those derived from waking life (Popp et al., 1996); that narratives told outside a session are similar to those told in sessions (Barber, Luborsky, Crits-Christoph, & Diguer, 1995); and that CCRTs show consistency across different relationships (Fried, Crits-Christoph, & Luborsky, 1992).

Other psychodynamic and interpersonal methods have also been examined for validity. For example, adherence to the PFM has also been shown in multiple small sample studies to predict outcome and depth of experiencing in therapy (e.g., Silberschatz, Curtis, & Nathans, 1989; Silberschatz & Curtis, 1993. In addition, clinically derived formulations based on CA have been shown to converge with quantitatively derived formulations based on ratings or q-sorts by patients (Eells, 1995; Eells, Fridhandler, & Horowitz, 1995).

The foregoing positive findings relating psychodynamic formulations to treatment outcome should be viewed in light of the methodologies used to reach these outcomes. With the exception of the study by Crits-Christoph, Cooper, and Luborsky (1988), all are done on single subjects or small samples that are intensively analyzed at the individual level and then aggregated. These should be contrasted with results of randomized clinical trials cited by Persons and Tompkins in which standardized cognitive-behavioral therapy (CBT) is compared with CBT guided by individualized formulations. These studies show somewhat more equivocal findings, as noted previously. Perhaps the strategy of analyze then aggregate (Thorngate, 1986), as followed by those investigating psychodynamic models, revealed relationships that the studies which followed the aggregate-then-analyze strategy, as is typically seen from the interindividual frame of reference (see Chapter 1), accounts for the difference in outcomes.

Most other authors focus their attention in the research section on efficacy studies of the psychotherapy method in which their case formulation model is embedded. This makes sense considering the pivotal assumed role that case formulation plays in these therapy methods. However, several of these authors also call for more research specifically focused on the case formulation model itself.

THE FUTURE OF PSYCHOTHERAPY CASE FORMULATION IN PSYCHOTHERAPY PRACTICE AND RESEARCH

In this section, I consider where future work on case formulation may go. An assumption underlying these considerations is that the concept of case formulation will likely play an important role as long as the mental health professions continue to employ a nosology that is primarily descriptive rather than explanatory or prescriptive in nature. A descriptive nosology creates a gap between description and treatment that case formulation fills. Even if a more etiological nosology were developed, case formulation would still occupy an important niche in psychotherapy practice because therapists would need to apply a nomothetic etiological explanation to the idiographic context of treating a specific client. It is also likely that considerations about formulation will continue to follow general trends in the psychotherapy literature. For example, authors in this revised edition have made more references to the relationship between case formulation and evidence-based practice (Levant, 2005) as compared to the original volume. In looking ahead, it is helpful to acknowledge the future may already be with us in the form of innovations currently practiced outside of the mainstream. Several case formulation experts have recently addressed where research, clinical, and creative activity related to formulation might be headed (e.g., Bieling & Kuyken, 2003; Tarrier & Calam, 2002; Westmeyer, 2003). Toward this end, I make eight predictions.

First, a case formulation mind-set will become further embedded in psychotherapy treatment. This trend is well developed in the Greenberg and Goldman's emotion-focused approach in which "mini-formulations" of unfolding events in therapy are undertaken. A similar idea is apparent in functional, or chain, analysis by authors such as Koerner; Nezu, Nezu, and Cos; and Persons and Tompkins. These involve close examination of specific events in client's lives or in the client–therapist relationship, rather than of a "case." Persons and Tompkins distinguish three different levels of formulation: symptoms, disorder or problem, and case, each of which focuses the therapist differently. Similarly, Eells and Lombart (2003b) distinguish between a case formulation, a modal formulation for a disorder, and a formulation of situation or episode that arises in or out of therapy. These different foci of formulation are interrelated and mutually inform each other. For example, at the modal case level one might characterize a young man with social phobia as excessively preoccupied by negative self-beliefs and images that lead to heightened self-consciousness and inhibited spontaneity that limits effective social interactions (Clark & Wells, 1995). At the individual case level one might write the following formulation: "This client's social phobia is characterized by a preoccupation with a view of himself as small and vulnerable. When approaching others the client fears that others will see his perceived vulnerability and will laugh at him. Consequently, he withdraws when possible; but when 'trapped' into interacting, he becomes anxious, perspires and shakes; he 'freezes' and 'feels like a fool.' " During a therapy session, the client might describe missing out on going out with a group of others the previous weekend for fear that they would notice his weaknesses and laugh at him. This situational episode could be formulated as demonstrating how his avoidance behavior decreased his enjoyment of life and chances of pleasant interactions with others (see Edwards & Kannan, 2006).

Second, the explanatory mechanism component of case formulations will increasingly be influenced by advances in psychopathology research, including advances in neurobiology, learning theory, and epidemiology. For example, Mineka and Zinbarg (2006) show how contemporary learning theory contributes to understanding the etiologies of anxiety disorders and the course they take, including why some who undergo acute or long-term traumatic experiences develop anxiety disorders whereas others do not. Similarly, Tarrier and Calam (2002) assert that while few would dispute that patients' problems are the product of adverse early life experiences, it is unsatisfactory and potentially tautological to use their retrospective recall as one's sole etiological evidence. One remedy, they claim, is to incorporate epidemiological data on vulnerability factors into historical accounts of the development of a disorder or problem. Incorporating such information sources need not compete with the "evolving narrative structure" that Messer and Wolitzky characterize as part of the course of psychodynamic psychotherapy but can potentially enrich it.

Third, psychotherapy case formulation will increasingly become a focus of research. One can classify research on case formulation into two general categories: Research in which the case formulation is the object of study and research in which case formulation becomes a measurement tool to advance understanding of psychotherapy. In the former category, the following questions are potential objects of research:

- Given that reliability measures of current case formulation models remain based on small samples and are unsatisfyingly low when computations are based on individual clinicians, how can the reliability of case formulation models be improved?
- How do individualized formulations affect psychotherapy outcome?
- To what extent do therapists applying ostensibly standardized treatment protocols tailor those protocols to individual patients, and thus effectively work from individualized case formulations? How

might the process of tailoring standardized protocols best be described?

- What cognitive processes do experts and nonexperts follow when formulating cases?
- How can case formulation skills best be taught to therapists in training?
- What is the relationship between a case formulation and a diagnosis? What similarities can be found for case formulations of individuals who meet criteria for the same diagnosis?
- What criteria should be met for a case formulation to be considered adequate?
- How can well-known biases in clinical judgment be minimized when formulating a case?
- What constitutes an evidence-based formulation?
- What is the effect of communicating case formulation information versus non-case formulation information to patients?

The second set of questions is large because the issue of interest can focus on any substantive question about psychopathology or about psychotherapy. Bieling and Kuyken (2003) term these "top down" questions and focus several in regard to cognitive case formulation. Generalized, they include two kinds of questions:

- Are nomothetic explanatory hypotheses of disorders substantiated at the case formulation level?
- Are the processes proposed to explain the mechanism of action of a model of psychotherapy supported at the individual process and outcome level?

These questions use case formulation as a tool to address the validity of the etiology of a disorder or a proposed mechanism of action in therapy.

Fourth, the future of case formulation will incorporate more quantitative methods that capitalize on skilled clinical observation, resulting in improved clinical judgment and outcomes. Westen and Weinberger (2004) show that clinicians can provide valid and reliability data if we quantify their inferences using psychometric instruments that are designed for experts. Westen and Muderrisoglu (2003) found that clinicians using the SWAP-200 q-sort technique achieved highly reliable classifications of patients into personality disorder categories, as well as evidence of both convergent and discriminant validity. The technique involved quantified judgments of clinically relevant personality characteristics that were then statistically aggregated. It could be possible to develop these methods further to go beyond a DSM-IV diagnosis to a fuller case formulation that includes categories such as self-concept, concepts of others, affect management, defensive and coping behaviors, functional analyses, instrumental and ultimate outcomes, identification of emotion schemas, and identification of instrumental relationships. New case formulation measures could be part of an effort to reduce the arbitrary quality of many metrics measuring psychological constructs, so that it is better known where a given score locates an individual on an underlying psychological dimension (Blanton & Jaccard, 2006).

Fifth, case formulations in the future will incorporate information about the stage of change that best characterizes a client. This prediction is based on work by Prochaska and colleagues (e.g., Prochaska & Norcross, 2001; Prochaska, Velicer, Ross, Redding, & Greene, 2004) demonstrating that psychological interventions are differentially effective depending on where on a continuum of readiness to change an individual lies. Stage-related variables were more powerful than demographics, type and severity of problems, and other client variables in predicting outcome.

Sixth, as the trend toward psychotherapy integration increases, as experts predict it will (Norcross, Hedges, & Prochaska, 2002), so will efforts to develop an integrative model of case formulation. As this review shows, overlap exists among many of the models presented, while each also has its distinctive characteristics. Ideally, an integrative model of case formulation would capture these overlapping concepts in the models presented in this volume while also retaining the distinctive features of each approach. Such an integrative model could be particularly useful in psychotherapy training. Potentially, it could include the following components: current symptoms and problems; consideration of possible nonpsychological explanations; antecedent learning experiences or vulnerabilities; a mechanism explaining the problems (plus an alternative mechanism); adaptive features of the individual; and an application of all components to treatment. The mechanism section might draw from each of the methods presented in this model. Such an integrative model might also be developed for formulating common psychotherapy dilemmas as well. These might include situations such as noncompliance with homework, lateness to sessions, avoidance of central topics, excessive silence, anger at therapist, and placation of the therapist.

Seventh, multicultural competence will increasingly be required of therapists, increasing pressure to incorporate cultural considerations into case formulation. The underlying driver of this prediction is the increasingly diverse demographics in the United States (American Psychological Association, 2003; Committee on Institutional and Policy-Level Strategies for Increasing the Diversity of the U.S. Healthcare Workforce, 2004) as well as evidence, such as that presented by Ridley and Kelly, that failure to account for culture can have deleterious consequences for clients.

Eighth, case formulations in the future will focus more on solutions, strengths, and resilience. This prediction is based on a Delphi poll on the future of psychotherapy (Norcross, Hedges, & Prochaska, 2002), in which experts predicted an increased focus on solution-focused methods, as well as on other psychotherapy methods that focus on case formulation and enhancement of personal resources and strengths (e.g., Benjamin, 2003), the recognition among developmental psychologists of both the ordinariness of resilience in individuals and its protective effects in the face of adverse events (Masten, 2001), and evidence in a mildly depressed population that Internet-based, individualized interventions focused on emphasizing strengths and positive events can reduce self-reported symptoms of depression for up to 6 months (Seligman, Steen, Park, & Peterson, 2005).

In sum, the case formulation models described in this volume share many common features although each is also distinct from the others. Taken together, they provide a complementary set of compasses to orient clinicians trying to understand their patients' problems and to intervene effectively. The contributors to this volume have significantly advanced our understanding of case formulation. It will be exciting to follow advances in coming years.

REFERENCES

American Psychological Association. (2003). Guidelines on multicultural education, training, research, practice, and organizational change for psychologists. *American Psychologist, 58*, 377–402.

APA Presidential Task Force on Evidence-Based Practice (2006). Evidence-based practice in psychology. *American Psychologist, 61*, 271–285.

Barber, J. P., Luborsky, L., Crits-Christoph, P., & Diguer, L. (1995). A comparison of core conflictual relationship themes before psychotherapy and during early sessions. *Journal of Consulting and Clinical Psychology, 63*, 145–148.

Benjamin, L. S. (2003). *Interpersonal reconstructive therapy: Promoting change in nonresponders.* New York: Guilford Press.

Bieling, P. J., & Kuyken, W. (2003). Is cognitive case formulation science or science fiction? *Clinical Psychology: Science and Practice, 10*, 52–69.

Blanton, H., & Jaccard, J. (2006). Arbitrary metrics in psychology. *American Psychologist, 61*, 27–41.

Caston, J., & Martin, E. (1993). Can analysts agree? The problems of consensus and the psychoanalytic mannequin: II. Empirical tests. *Journal of the American Psychoanalytic Association, 41*(2), 513–548.

Cierpka, M., Strack, M., Benninghoven, D., Staats, H., Dahlbender, R., Pokorny, D., et al. (1998). Stereotypical relationship patterns and psychopathology. *Psychotherapy and Psychosomatics, 67*, 241–248.

Clark, D. M., & Wells, A. (1995). A cognitive model of social phobia. In R. G. Heimberg & M. R. Liebowitz (Eds.), *Social phobia: Diagnosis, assessment, and treatment* (pp. 69–93). New York: Guilford Press.

Collins, W. D., & Messer, S. B. (1991). Extending the plan formulation method to an object relations perspective: Reliability, stability, and adaptability. *Psychological Assessment, 3,* 75–81.

Committee on Institutional and Policy-Level Strategies for Increasing the Diversity of the U.S. Healthcare Workforce. (2004). *In the nation's compelling interest: Ensuring diversity in the health case workforce.* Washington, DC: Institute of Medicine.

Crits-Christoph, P., Cooper, A., & Luborsky, L. (1988). The accuracy of therapists' interpretations and the outcome of dynamic psychotherapy. *Journal of Consulting and Clinical Psychology, 56*(4), 490–495.

Crits-Christoph, P., & Luborsky, L. (1998). Changes in CCRT pervasiveness during psychotherapy. In L. Luborsky & P. Crits-Christoph (Eds.), *Understanding transference: The Core Conflictual Relationship Theme method* (2nd ed., pp 151–163). Washington, DC: APA Books.

Edwards, D. J. A., & Kannan, S. (2006). Identifying and targeting idiosyncratic cognitive processes in group therapy for social phobia: The case of Vumile. *Pragmatic Case Studies in Psychotherapy* [Online], 2(1), Article 1. Available: http://hdl.rutgers.edu/1782.1/pcsp2.1.65.

Eells, T. D. (1995). Role reversal: A convergence of clinical and quantitative evidence. *Psychotherapy Research, 5,* 297–312.

Eells, T. D., Fridhandler, B., & Horowitz, M. J. (1995). Self schemas and spousal bereavement: Comparing quantitative and clinical evidence. *Psychotherapy, 32,* 270–282.

Eells, T. D., Horowitz, M. J., Singer, J. L., Salovey, P., Daigle, D., & Turvey, C. (1995). The role-relationship models method: A comparison of independently derived case formulations. *Psychotherapy Research, 5,* 154–168.

Eells, T. D., & Lombart, K. G. (2003a). Case formulation and treatment concepts among novice, experienced, and expert cognitive-behavioral and psychodynamic therapists. *Psychotherapy Research, 13*(2), 187–204.

Eells, T. D., & Lombart, K. G. (2003b). Case formulation: Determining the focus in brief dynamic psychotherapy. In D. P. Charman (Ed.), *Core processes in brief psychodynamic psychotherapy* (pp. 119–144). Mahwah, NJ: Erlbaum.

Eells, T. D., Lombart, K. G., Kendjelic, E. M., Turner, L. C., & Lucas, C. (2005). The quality of psychotherapy case formulations: A comparison of expert, experienced, and novice cognitive-behavioral and psychodynamic therapists. *Journal of Consulting and Clinical Psychology, 73,* 579–589.

Freud, S. (1958a). The dynamics of the transference. In J. Strachey (Ed. and Trans.), *The standard edition of the complete psychological works of Sigmund Freud* (Vol. 12, pp. 99–108). London: Hogarth Press. (Original work published 1912)

Freud, S. (1958b). Recommendations to physicians practicing psycho-analysis. In J. Strachey (Ed. and Trans.), *The standard edition of the complete psychological works of Sigmund Freud* (Vol. 12, pp.111–120). London: Hogarth Press. (Original work published 1912)

Fried, D., Crits-Christoph, P., & Luborsky, L. (1992). The first empirical demonstration of transference in psychotherapy. *Journal of Nervous and Mental Disease, 180,* 326–331.

Grenyer, B. F. S., & Luborsky, L. (1996). Dynamic change in psychotherapy: Mastery of interpersonal conflict. *Journal of Consulting and Clinical Psychology, 64,* 411–416.

Horowitz, M. J., & Eells, T. D. (1993). Case formulations using role-relationship model configurations: A reliability study. *Psychotherapy Research, 3,* 57–68.

Horowitz, L. M., & Rosenberg, S. E. (1994). The Consensual Response Psychodynamic Formulation: Part 1: Method and research results. *Psychotherapy Research, 4,* 222–233.

Horowitz, L. M., Rosenberg, S. E., Ureño, G., Kalehzan, B. M., & O'Halloran, P. (1989). Psychodynamic formulation, consensual response method and interpersonal problems. *Journal of Consulting and Clinical Psychology, 57,* 599–606.

Kuyken, W., Fothergill, C. D., Musa, M., & Chadwick, P. (2005). The reliability and quality of cognitive case formulation. *Behaviour Research and Therapy, 43*(9), 1187–1201.

Luborsky, L., & Diguer, L. (1998). The reliability of the CCRT measure: Results from eight samples. In L. Luborsky & P. Crits-Christoph (Eds.), *Understanding transference: The Core Conflictual Relationship Theme method* (2nd ed., pp. 97–107). Washington, DC: APA Books.

Masten, A. S. (2001). Ordinary magic: Resilience processes in development. *American Psychologist, 56*(3), 227–238.

Mineka, S., & Zinbarg, R. (2006). A contemporary learning theory perspective on the etiology of anxiety disorders: It's not what you thought it was. *American Psychologist, 61*(1), 10–26.

Norcross, J. C., Hedges, M., & Prochaska, J. O. (2002). The face of 2010: A Delphi poll on the future of psychotherapy. *Professional Psychology: Research and Practice, 33,* 316–322.

Persons, J. B., & Bertagnolli, A. (1999). Inter-rater reliability of cognitive-behavioral case formulations of depression: A replication. *Cognitive Therapy and Research, 23*(3), 271–283.

Popp, C., Diguer, L., Luborsky, L., Faude, J., Johnson, S., Morris, M., et al. (1996). Repetitive relationship themes in waking narratives and dreams. *Journal of Consulting and Clinical Psychology, 64,* 1073–1078.

Prochaska, J. O., & Norcross, J. C. (2001). Stages of change. *Psychotherapy: Theory, Research, Practice, Training, 38,* 443–448.

Prochaska, J. O., Velieer, W. F., Rossi, J. S., Redding, C. A, Greene, G. W., Rossi, S. R., et al. (2004). Multiple risk expert systems interventions: Impact of simultaneous stage-matched expert system interventions for smoking, high-fat diet, and sun exposure in a population of parents. *Health Psychology, 23,* 503–516.

Seitz, P. F. (1966). The consensus problem in psychoanalytic research. In L. Gottschalk & L. Auerbach (Eds.), *Methods of research and psychotherapy* (pp. 209–225). New York: Appleton-Century-Crofts.

Seligman, M. E. P., Steen, T. A., Park, N., & Peterson, C. (2005). Positive psychology progress: Empirical validation of interventions. *American Psychologist, 60*(5), 410–421.

Silberschatz, G. (2005). *Transformative relationships: The control-mastery theory of psychotherapy.* New York: Routledge.

Silberschatz, G., & Curtis, J. T. (1993). Measuring the therapist's impact on the patient's therapeutic progress. *Journal of Consulting and Clinical Psychology, 61,* 403–411.

Silberschatz, G., Curtis, J. T., & Nathans, S. (1989). Using the patient's plan to assess progress in psychotherapy. *Psychotherapy, 26,* 40–46.

Tarrier, N., & Calam, R (2002). New developments in cognitive-behavioural case formulation. Epidemiological, systemic and social context: An integrative approach. *Behavioural and Cognitive Psychotherapy, 30*, 311–328.

Thorngate, W. (1986). The production, detection, and explanation of behavioral patterns. In J. Valsiner (Ed.), *The individual subject and scientific psychology* (pp. 71–93). New York: Plenum Press.

Weiss, J. (1993). *How psychotherapy works: Process and technique.* New York: Guilford Press.

Westen, D., & Muderrisoglu, S. (2003). Assessing personality disorders using a systematic clinical interview: Evaluation of an alternate to structured interviews. *Journal of Personality Disorders, 17*(4), 351–369.

Westen, D., & Weinberger, J. (2004). When clinical description becomes statistical prediction. *American Psychologist, 59*, 595–613.

Index